AUTISM and Other
Neurodevelopmental
Disorders

AUTISM and Other **Neurodevelopmental Disorders**

Edited by

Robin L. Hansen, M.D.

Sally J. Rogers, Ph.D.

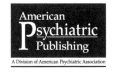

American **Psychiatric** Publishing

A Division of American Psychiatric Association

Washington, DC
London, England

Books published by American Psychiatric Publishing (APP) represent the findings, conclusions, and views of the individual authors and do not necessarily represent the policies and opinions of APP or the American Psychiatric Association.

Quantities of 25–99 copies of this or any other American Psychiatric Publishing title can be purchased at a 20% discount; please contact Customer Service at appi@psych.org or 800-368-5777. If you wish to buy 100 or more copies of the same title, please e-mail us at bulksales@psych.org for a price quote.

Manufactured in the United States of America on acid-free paper
16   15   14   13   12   5   4   3   2   1
First Edition

Typeset in Janson and Futura

American Psychiatric Publishing
A Division of American Psychiatric Association
1000 Wilson Boulevard
Arlington, VA 22209-3901
www.appi.org

Library of Congress Cataloging-in-Publication Data
Autism and other neurodevelopmental disorders / edited by Robin L. Hansen, Sally J. Rogers. — 1st ed.
   p. ; cm.
   Includes bibliographical references and index.
   ISBN 978-1-58562-425-6 (pbk. : alk. paper)
   I. Hansen, Robin L. II. Rogers, Sally J. III. American Psychiatric Publishing.
   [DNLM: 1. Child Development Disorders, Pervasive. 2. Adult. 3. Child.
4. Developmental Disabilities. 5. Nervous System Diseases. WS 350.8.P4]
   616.85'882—dc23

                                                                    2012037982

British Library Cataloguing in Publication Data
A CIP record is available from the British Library.

CONTENTS

CONTRIBUTORS

Kathleen Angkustsiri, M.D.
Assistant Professor, Department of Pediatrics; MIND Institute, University of California Davis School of Medicine, Sacramento, California

Liga Bivina, M.S., C.G.C.
Certified Genetic Counselor, Section of Genetics, Department of Pediatrics, University of California Davis School of Medicine, Sacramento, California

J. Faye Dixon, Ph.D.
Assistant Clinical Professor, Department of Psychiatry and Behavioral Sciences; MIND Institute, University of California School of Medicine, Sacramento, California

Janice L. Enriquez, Ph.D.
Assistant Clinical Professor, Department of Pediatrics, Section of Developmental Behavioral Pediatrics; MIND Institute, University of California Davis School of Medicine, Sacramento, California

Joan R. Gunther, Psy.D.
Clinical Psychologist, MIND Institute, University of California Davis School of Medicine, Sacramento, California

Randi J. Hagerman, M.D.
Professor and Endowed Chair in Fragile X Research, Department of Pediatrics; Medical Director, MIND Institute, University of California Davis School of Medicine, Sacramento, California

Robin L. Hansen, M.D.
Professor, Department of Pediatrics; Director, Center for Excellence in Developmental Disabilities; Director of Clinical Programs, MIND Institute, University of California Davis School of Medicine, Sacramento, California

David Hessl, Ph.D.
Associate Professor, Department of Psychiatry and Behavioral Sciences; MIND Institute, University of California Davis School of Medicine, Sacramento, California

Ingrid N. Leckliter, Ph.D.
Associate Clinical Professor, Department of Pediatrics, Section of Developmental-Behavioral Pediatrics; MIND Institute, University of California Davis School of Medicine, Sacramento, California

Mary Jacena S. Leigh, M.D.
Clinical Fellow, Developmental-Behavioral Pediatrics, Department of Pediatrics; MIND Institute, University of California Davis School of Medicine, Sacramento, California

Ann M. Mastergeorge, Ph.D.
Associate Professor, Department of Family Studies and Human Development, Frances McClelland Institute for Children, Youth, and Families, University of Arizona, Tucson, Arizona

Molly McGinniss, M.S., L.C.G.C.
Certified and Licensed Genetic Counselor, Department of Genetics, The Permanente Medical Group, Sacramento, California

Billur Moghaddam, M.D.
Medical Geneticist, Department of Genetics, The Permanente Medical Group, Sacramento, California

Sally Ozonoff, Ph.D.
Professor, Department of Psychiatry and Behavioral Sciences; MIND Institute, University of California School of Medicine, Sacramento, California

Murat Pakyurek, M.D.
Associate Clinical Professor, Department of Psychiatry and Behavioral Sciences, University of California Davis School of Medicine, Sacramento, California

Sally J. Rogers, Ph.D.
Professor, Department of Psychiatry and Behavioral Sciences; Director of Training and Mentoring, MIND Institute, University of California Davis School of Medicine, Sacramento, California

Julie B. Schweitzer, Ph.D.
Associate Professor, Department of Psychiatry and Behavioral Sciences; MIND Institute, University of California Davis School of Medicine, Sacramento, California

Frank R. Sharp, M.D.
Professor, Department of Neurology; MIND Institute, University of California Davis School of Medicine, Sacramento, California

Tony J. Simon, Ph.D.
Professor, Department of Psychiatry and Behavioral Sciences; MIND Institute, University of California Davis School of Medicine, Sacramento, California

Mary Beth Steinfeld, M.D.
Associate Clinical Professor, Department of Pediatrics, Section of Developmental-Behavioral Pediatrics; MIND Institute, University of California Davis School of Medicine, Sacramento, California

Nicole Tartaglia, M.D.
Assistant Professor, Department of Pediatrics, University of Colorado School of Medicine, Aurora, Colorado

Jeannie Visootsak, M.D.
Associate Professor, Department of Human Genetics, Emory University, Atlanta, Georgia

Terry D. Wardinsky, M.D.
Congenital Defect and Clinical Genetic Consultant, Alta California Regional Center, Sacramento, California

DISCLOSURE OF INTERESTS

Contributors to this book disclosed financial or institutional relationships that could represent or could appear to represent competing interests with their work published in this volume, as follows:

Kathleen Angkustsiri, M.D., has served as investigator or subinvestigator on clinical trials for Curemark, Johnson & Johnson, Novartis, Roche, and Seaside Therapeutics.

Randi J. Hagerman, M.D., receives, has received, or is receiving support from Curemark, Forest Research Institute, Inc., Hoffman-LaRoche, Novartis, and Seaside Therapeutics for clinical trials involving individuals with fragile X syndrome and associated disorders and/or autism. She is on a fragile X advisory committee for Novartis. She also receives support from the Department of Defense, Department of Health and Human Services, Health Resources and Services Administration, National Institute on Aging, National Institute of Child Health and Human Development, National Institute of Dental and Craniofacial Research, National Institute of Mental Health, and National Institutes of Health for studies of patients with fragile X syndrome and associated disorders.

David Hessl, Ph.D., receives, has received, or is receiving support from Hoffman-LaRoche, Novartis, and Seaside Therapeutics for clinical trials involving individuals with fragile X syndrome. He also receives support from the Department of Defense, National Institutes of Health, National Fragile X Foundation, and FRAXA for studies of patients with fragile X syndrome and associated disorders.

The following contributors affirmed that they had no competing interests with regard to their work published in this volume:

Liga Bivina, M.S., C.G.C., J. Faye Dixon, Ph.D., Janice L. Enriquez, Ph.D., Joan R. Gunther, Psy.D., Robin L. Hansen, M.D., Ingrid N. Leckliter, Ph.D., Mary Jacena S. Leigh, M.D., Ann M. Mastergeorge, Ph.D., Billur Moghaddam, M.D., Sally Ozonoff, Ph.D., Murat Pakyurek, M.D., Sally J. Rogers, Ph.D., Julie Schweitzer, Ph.D., Frank R. Sharp, M.D., Tony J. Simon, Ph.D., Mary Beth Steinfeld, M.D., Nicole Tartaglia, M.D., Jeannie Visootsak, M.D.

FOREWORD

This is an exciting but perplexing time for families affected by autism spectrum disorders and other neurodevelopmental disorders, as well as for the professionals who provide care for them. On the one hand, new and promising therapeutics are emerging at a rapid rate, thereby increasing optimism and producing a palpable excitement among families and providers. New pharmacological treatments that target core impairments in autism, fragile X syndrome, Down syndrome, and other neurodevelopmental disorders are being tested in dozens of clinical trials around the globe. Behavioral and educational interventions are continuing to evolve, with many new interventions, including innovative uses of technologies such as video teleconferencing and tablet computing. Alternative and complementary approaches to treatment are also being promoted, such as adding nutritional supplements and using animals to reduce stress and provide comfort. On the other hand, it is difficult for families and professionals alike to evaluate the evidence supporting or refuting these various treatments. Even for treatments that seem to be garnering considerable scientific support, it is often difficult to know when those treatments will be moving from the laboratory to wide public availability. For example, what is a likely timeline for a drug that "rescues" the phenotypes in a mouse model of autism or fragile X syndrome to move to FDA-approved use with humans affected by these disorders? Thus, the optimism and excitement of families and professionals is often combined with confusion and frustration.

The growth in potential therapeutics is occurring at a time when the public's access to information is dramatically increasing as well. For example, a Google search of the term *autism* leads to 76 million hits, and the phrase *autism treatment* results in more than 850,000 hits. Even a search of Amazon.com yields a list of almost 900 books available for purchase. Unfortunately, it is impossible for all of these sources of information to be vetted so that families and professionals can distinguish well-supported, scientifically sound treatments from those that have yet to be evaluated for efficacy or from those that are unsound or even potentially harmful. Making the wrong decision about what treatment to employ or information to believe can be costly in terms of time, money, and effort, and it might actually put a person with a neurodevelopmental disorder at risk for other health problems. Following the wrong path might also mean missed opportunities to provide effective treatments, resulting in days, months, or even years wasted.

The present volume is thus timely and essential reading for professionals charged with caring for individuals with autism or other neurodevelopmental disorders and their families. Dr. Hansen, Dr. Rogers, and their colleagues have created comprehensive and highly readable summaries of more than a dozen common neurodevelopmental disorders. The chapters are similar in format, covering symptom onset and developmental course, epidemiology, etiology, diagnosis, and treatment. Each chapter also includes lists of recommended readings, Web sites, and other sources of information. The authors of each chapter integrate complex and highly nuanced scientific information with keen clinical insight and deliver the information in a manner that will be understood by a diverse audience. They also are careful to present treatment options with appropriate cautions regarding the strength of their evidence base. In short, these authors have sifted and weighed the mass of scientific publications, clinical practice guidelines, and Internet claims to provide families and professionals with a road map for making informed decisions.

I would like to conclude this foreword with a few personal reflections. In 2011, I had the good fortune of becoming the director of the University of California Davis MIND (Medical Investigation of Neurodevelopmental Disorders) Institute. The authors of all the chapters in this volume are either current or former MIND Institute faculty, researchers, clinicians, or trainees. The breadth of this volume is evidence of the impressive range of disciplinary expertise available to families and other professionals who participate in our research, enroll in our educational programs, or receive care in one of our clinical programs. The commitment to this volume by almost two dozen present and former staff is evidence of the spirit of interdisciplinary collaboration that characterizes the MIND Institute. The content of each chapter displays the translational science agenda that has characterized the MIND Institute from its very beginning. This agenda is always focused on finding treatments, cures, and strategies for prevention, but in a way that recognizes that such clinical applications must be based on a firm understanding of the causes, course, and consequences of autism and other neurodevelopmental disorders. It also is noteworthy that the authors of these chapters include some individuals who are likely to self-identify primarily as researchers and others who are likely to view themselves first and foremost as clinicians or educators—again, testimony to the spirit of interdisciplinary collaboration that defines the UC Davis MIND Institute.

And finally, I must comment on the desire to help and support families that is evident in each and every chapter in this volume. The MIND Institute was founded by families who were committed to helping their children and the countless other children affected by a neurodevelopmental disorder. These families recognized that real progress in helping affected individuals and their families required a different approach to thinking about neurodevelopmental disorders, conducting science, and providing care. They invested considerable time, effort, and hope in the MIND Institute. Working on behalf of these founding families and, indeed, all families affected by autism or other neurodevelopmental disorders, is a privilege and a responsibility we take very seriously. I believe the present volume is another important step in fulfilling this responsibility and realizing the vision of our founding families.

Leonard Abbeduto, Ph.D.
Director and Tsakopoulos-Vismara Endowed Chair
UC Davis MIND Institute
Sacramento, California

PREFACE

The field of neurodevelopmental disorders is expanding rapidly, creating a challenge for clinicians who are trying to provide the most up-to-date care for their patients. Clinicians may feel flooded by the many new research findings from multidisciplinary studies covering the range of neurodevelopmental disorders. Daily reports of new genetic findings, new neuroimaging findings, new treatment approaches, and purported successes reach us through the Internet. Patients and families scour online resources for information about their children's conditions, and some may deluge clinicians with questions about the latest treatments, causes, and theories. Here at the MIND Institute, we, too, experience the range of e-mails, information flow, patient questions, and treatment teasers, and we undertook this text to try to help gather and organize the most recent information into a clinically useful volume.

Our focus in this book is on a range of neurodevelopmental disorders commonly seen and managed by both primary and subspecialist health care professionals. For this purpose, we tapped into the multidisciplinary and clinical expertise of our faculty as well as of former trainees who are now leaders in their fields of research and practice. We sought a translational approach and asked each author to cover the newest findings from the biological, behavioral, and clinical sciences in ways that are accessible to clinicians and helpful in meeting family and patient needs.

Each chapter covers presenting signs and symptoms, including onset and developmental course; epidemiology and etiology, including known genetic and environmental contributors; biological mechanisms; and relevant animal models. Diagnostic approaches, differential diagnosis, and evidence-based interventions follow, addressing psychological, behavioral, and medical issues as well as supports and resources for patients, their families, and the community. The authors also provide updates on ongoing research that holds promise for future clinical care.

We begin with autism spectrum disorders (ASDs) (Rogers, Ozonoff, and Hansen, Chapter 1). More words may have been published about ASD in the last few years than about any other neurodevelopmental disorder (NDD), with the possible exception of attention-deficit/hyperactivity disorder (ADHD). The amount of information available on the Internet about ASD has expanded exponentially. Among recent developments that affect clinical practice in ASD are these:

- The emphasis on empirically supported practice in education, medical care, and all types of treatment
- The changes in diagnostic criteria that will come with DSM-5
- The latest in psychopharmacology
- The recent and unexpected findings coming from studies of infants in terms of onset patterns, early signs, and sometimes dramatic response to early intervention
- Continuing worldwide increases in prevalence according to the latest studies

In Chapter 2, Schweitzer, Pakyurek, and Dixon address recent findings in ADHD. ADHD co-occurs frequently in most other NDDs, as well as in many other diagnostic conditions, and is managed by both primary and subspecialty clinicians. ADHD dramatically affects long-term outcomes and quality of life for patients and families. The interdisciplinary team of authors addresses the challenges of diagnosis as well as approaches to treatment that include both behavioral and psychopharmacological practice. They highlight developmental aspects of ADHD across the life span; brain changes that are being recognized as important to understanding the disorder; comorbid learning disorders; and targeted treatments.

Fragile X syndrome, the most common inherited cause of intellectual disability and a major risk for ASD, is just one of a multigenerational group of disorders resulting from instability of the trinucleotide promotor region of the fragile X mental retardation-1 gene (*FMR1*) on the X chromosome. Authors Leigh, Hagerman, and Hessl are actively involved as both clinicians and pioneering researchers in developing diagnostic as well as targeted treatments. In Chapter 3, they point out the importance of recognizing the early signs of these associated disorders in family members of probands with fragile X syndrome, establishing accurate diagnosis, and addressing the intervention needs of all individuals affected by this family of disorders. The authors also highlight new research in targeted treatments, based on our understanding of the role of fragile X mental retardation protein (FMRP), that holds promise for many other neurodevelopmental disorders beyond fragile X syndrome.

In Chapter 4, Angkustsiri and Simon provide updates on chromosome 22q11.2 deletion syndrome (22q11.2DS), the most common microdeletion syndrome, including an extensive overview of the myriad medical and mental health issues as well as cognitive and behavioral difficulties that need to be addressed across the life span. Their research has highlighted high rates of unrecognized anxiety and the possible association with high rates of psychosis in 22q11.2DS, and they present ongoing research that suggests possibilities for treatment that may reduce or prolong the onset of psychosis.

In Chapter 5, Gunther and Sharp address tic disorders, including Tourette syndrome, with a unique focus on the emergence and differentiation of tics. They examine, too, the associated comorbidities that occur over the developmental course (such as ADHD, obsessive-compulsive disorder, anxiety, and depression) and significantly affect intervention needs and outcomes. Highlighted as well are new research findings in genetics, epigenetics, and biology that provide exciting opportunities to improve diagnosis, specify the impact of comorbid disorders, and design more effective interventions.

Down syndrome is one of the first and most readily recognized genetic syndromes resulting in neurodevelopmental disability. In Chapter 6, Bivina, Moghaddam, and Wardinsky provide a fascinating history of the syndrome itself and note the important historical role that individuals and their families have played in expanding hopes for community inclusion and self-determination for all individuals with neurodevelopmental disabilities. In addition to providing comprehensive guidelines important for prevention and intervention across the life span for medical and mental health care, the authors also describe new advances in understanding the developmental onset of and recommended treatments for dementia.

In Chapter 7, McGinniss and Moghaddam provide an important update on Prader-Willi syndrome and Angelman syndrome that highlights our expanding knowledge about the mechanisms of imprinting and new approaches to genetic diagnosis and mechanisms of gene expression or silencing. They also provide key resources for professionals to share with families.

The neurocognitive discrepancies and behavioral challenges of the socially outgoing, effusive, and empathetic individuals with Williams syndrome have fascinated neuroscientists and clinicians since the syndrome was first described by a group of cardiologists almost 50 years ago. In Chapter 8, Steinfeld and Hansen review key clinical information important across the life span, describe the variability within the phenotype, and provide an update on research that has helped us understand gene-brain-behavior links underlying the unique cognitive-behavioral phenotype in Williams syndrome.

In Chapter 9, on sex chromosome aneuploidy, Visootsak and Tartaglia describe a group of chromosomal disorders, common but largely unrecognized, that are very important for clinicians to diagnose as early as possible so that the physical, cognitive, and behavioral concerns can be addressed appropriately. The authors have done an excellent job of describing the clinical aspects of several of the most common disorders, the importance of increased professional and public awareness, and new research on medical and mental health interventions.

In Chapter 10, on learning disorders and disabilities (LDs), Leckliter and Enriquez cover the four main types of LDs that commonly occur: dyslexia, dyscalculia, dysgraphia, and nonverbal learning disorders. The authors provide a life span description of the course of these disorders, summarized in very helpful tables that lay out the developmental trajectories of each. They also address current draft DSM-5 diagnoses as well as those included in DSM-IV-TR. Considerable emphasis is placed on the importance of ongoing surveillance, both to recognize LD risk and to provide preventive interventions in the preschool and early elementary school years. The new information on neuroimaging studies of the parietotemporal system and its role in mapping print to language provides a way of characterizing brain-behavior relations in dyslexia. Information about current case law concerning educational rights of students with LD will help clinicians who are providing recommendations to parents. Finally, the authors describe new findings from treatment studies involving effective interventions using computerized instruction.

Every neurodevelopmental disorder described in this text affects language and social communication in some way. In Chapter 11, on language development and disability, Mastergeorge describes the various patterns and types of language disorders that arise in childhood. Enlarging clinical concepts of language disorders, she describes specific deficits in the pragmatics of social communication—the ways in which we use both language and nonverbal communication skills to influence others. The author makes clear the relationship between language disorders and literacy skills, and in so doing, underlines the importance of recognizing and intervening early in the course of language disorders. She encourages clinicians who are assessing the presence of other neurodevelopmental and psychiatric disorders to assess co-occurring problems with language development as well. New biological findings expand our information about gene-environment interactions in language disorders, and the emerging use of animal models helps us to understand neurogenetic mechanisms underlying language development and disorders. In addition, the author describes in detail the language phenotypes associated with many of the neurodevelopmental disorders covered in this book.

ACKNOWLEDGMENTS

We thank Dr. Robert Hales for making this book possible and for his persistent encouragement and gentle prodding. We also thank Tina Coltri-Marshall for supportively keeping us on track despite many obstacles.

We owe a huge debt of gratitude to our colleagues at the MIND Institute for providing a rich, exciting, and collaborative environment for translational research and clinical practice, and particularly to our colleagues who agreed to contribute their time and expertise to this project. It is rare to have such a wealth of talent in one institution, and it attests to the commitment to excellence and support provided by the University of California Davis School of Medicine and Health System.

We thank our executive director, Dr. Len Abbeduto, for affirming the importance of providing comprehensive, family-centered clinical care that is embedded in cutting-edge science.

We acknowledge and thank our patients and their families as well, both for teaching us about the day-to-day challenges of living rich, satisfying, included lives in their communities and for their willingness to participate in research that advances our knowledge and helps us provide better care for other families in the future. We are thankful on a daily basis for their generosity of spirit.

Diane Larzelere, Catherine Martin, and Patricia Johnson-Haynes provided outstanding administrative support to us and the other chapter authors, for which we are eternally grateful. Thank you from all of us.

We thank William Frankenburg, who brought us together at the JFK Child Development Center in Denver several decades ago and impressed us with the importance of uniting research and clinical care in interdisciplinary training centers such as the UC Davis Center for Excellence in Developmental Disabilities. He provided us with the lifelong opportunity to work, learn, teach, and play together.

And to our own families—our parents, siblings, daughters, and life partners—thank you for your patience, your support, and your affirmation of how we share our lives with you and our work.

CHAPTER 1

AUTISM SPECTRUM DISORDERS

Sally J. Rogers, Ph.D.
Sally Ozonoff, Ph.D.
Robin L. Hansen, M.D.

In the space of 50 years, infantile autism has evolved from a rather obscure and very rare disorder involving children with remarkably aberrant behavior, seldom seen by child clinicians in a professional lifetime, to what is now recognized as a spectrum disorder, autism spectrum disorder (ASD), occurring in more than 1 out of every 100 children and adults (Centers for Disease Control and Prevention 2012). ASD is now known widely, both by name and through personal experience, by the lay public and the clinical community. It encompasses children and adults with severe and classic symptoms as well as those whose symptoms are mild enough that the disorder may remain unidentified for many years. The combination of increasing prevalence, unusual onset patterns, varying symptoms within and across ages, and at times remarkable response to treatment has stimulated scientists and clinicians to conduct an exponentially greater amount of research decade by decade, although the underlying etiologies for most people with ASD remain elusive.

Findings from the past 5–10 years concerning etiology, symptomatology, course, and treatment response require adjustments in clinical practice, new ways of thinking about ASD, and a change in dialogues between practitioners and parents. In this chapter, we review these findings and their implications for clinicians.

Signs and Symptoms

ASDs have three core symptom domains: impaired social relatedness, communication deficits, and repetitive/restricted behaviors and interests. In the social domain, symptoms include impaired use of nonverbal behaviors (such as eye contact, facial expression, gestures) to regulate social interaction, failure to develop age-appropriate relationships with peers and others, decreased seeking to share enjoyment and interests with other people, and limited social-emotional reciprocity. Communication deficits include delay in or absence of spoken language, difficulty initiating or sustaining conversation, idiosyncratic or repetitive language, and deficits of imitation and pretend play. Behavioral features include unusual interests, inflexible adherence to nonfunctional routines, stereotyped body movements, and preoccupation with details or sensory qualities of objects (American Psychiatric Association 2000).

Onset

The onset of ASD always occurs before age 3 years, at two peak periods. The majority of children (approximately two-thirds) display developmental abnormalities within the first 2 years of life. A smaller group of children with autism display a period of normal or mostly normal development, followed by a loss of communication and social skills and onset of autism (Lord et al. 2004). Frequently, onset, parental recognition, and clinical diagnosis do not coincide. Parents often begin to be concerned when a child's language fails to develop as expected (De Giacomo and Fombonne 1998). However, several other behavioral differences may predate the language delays that parents report at the time of recognition: less looking at faces, infrequent responding to name, less pointing, and a lack of sharing of enjoyment and interests with others (Lord 1995; Nadig et al. 2007; Osterling and Dawson 1994; Wetherby et al. 2004; Zwaigenbaum et al. 2005).

In the regressive pattern of onset, there is a period of mostly typical development, followed by a loss of some previously acquired social and communicative behaviors and onset of autistic symptoms. The average age at onset of regression across studies is between 14 and 24 months (Fombonne and Chakrabarti 2001). Regression typically progresses gradually, although onset can be sudden in a minority of cases. Loss of language is the most commonly described and perhaps most salient manifestation of regression (Goldberg et al. 2003; Siperstein and Volkmar 2004). Virtually all children who lose language also lose social behaviors, such as eye contact, social interest, and engagement with others (Hansen et al. 2008; Lord et al. 2004; Ozonoff et al. 2005). It may be difficult to distinguish regression from a different onset pattern, developmental plateau (Jones and Campbell 2010; Kalb et al. 2010), in which children fail to progress as expected and do not gain new skills but experience no loss of previously acquired skills.

Developmental Course

ASDs are considered lifelong conditions, but usually symptoms improve with age and development, and often periods of waxing or waning of particular symptoms occur. Existing literature suggests that once diagnosed with ASD, the vast majority of children will retain this diagnosis into adulthood (Howlin et al. 2004; Piven et al. 1996); however, this situation may change in another generation, given advances in intervention science and practice. Some children appear to recover from an ASD diagnosis (Lovaas 1987; Perry et al. 1995), although some of these individuals continue to have difficulties in other areas (Fein et al. 2005).

Over the long term, functional and adaptive outcome is highly related to overall cognitive ability. To date, the most powerful predictors of outcome continue to be IQ scores and verbal ability at age 5 (Lotter 1974; Rutter 1984). Most individuals with ASD studied longitudinally present with functional impairment throughout life (Billstedt et al. 2005; Howlin 2003; Howlin et al. 2004; Seltzer et al. 2003). Educational, vocational, economic, community, and family supports appear to play an important role in promoting positive adaptation and may be important factors in explaining variability in outcome. In addition, the availability of high-quality intensive early intervention for an increasing number of young children may change the frequency of what are considered to be "best outcomes" for ASD.

Epidemiology

Autism as first described by Kanner (1943) was considered a rare disorder. In the mid-1970s, prevalence in the United Kingdom, Denmark, and the United States was estimated at 5 in 10,000 (Wing et al. 1976). Reported prevalence has been increasing rapidly since then (Fombonne 2002; Wing and Potter 2002), and the most recent estimated prevalence of ASD in the United States is 11.3 per 1,000 or 1 in 88 (Centers for Disease Control and Prevention 2012). Clearly, some of the increase is attributable to better detection, increased awareness, and use of broader diagnostic criteria, although some studies suggest that environmental factors must be considered, because other factors do not fully explain the dramatic rise in ASD (Hertz-Picciotto and Delwiche 2009). ASDs affect individuals of all social strata and ethnicities, with a 4:1 male-to-female ratio. Elsabbagh et al. (2012) provide a systematic review of epidemiological surveys of ASD worldwide. Rates vary widely, from a high of 189 per 10,000 in South Korea (Kim et al. 2011) to lower rates in low- and middle-income countries (e.g., 14 in 10,000 in Mexico).

Etiology

ASDs are biologically based conditions that are thought to involve complex interactions between multiple genetic and environmental factors. ASDs are highly heritable, with a recurrence rate of 18.7% (Ozonoff et al. 2011), based on a large, multisite longitudinal study of infant siblings with an older sibling with ASD. The concordance rates for ASDs are 60%–92% in monozygotic twins compared with 0%–10% in dizygotic twins, supporting a strong genetic component (Bailey et al. 1995). Although genetic causes, such as chromosomal abnormalities and de novo copy number variations, are implicated in 10%–20% of cases of ASD, no single genetic etiology accounts for more than 1%–2% of cases (Abrahams and Geschwind 2008). ASD-associated syndromes (e.g., fragile X syndrome, tuberous sclerosis, chromosome 15q duplication syndrome) contribute to autism risk through common neural pathways related to early brain development (Spence 2001). Current theories propose that genetic susceptibility modulated by environmental factors is involved in the etiology of ASDs (Hertz-Picciotto et al. 2006; Schmidt et al. 2011).

Environmental influences that have been implicated include prenatal exposure to rubella, thalidomide, and valproic acid. Other potential risk factors include prematurity, low birth weight (Reichenberg et al. 2006), and advanced parental age (Croen et al. 2007). Although some individuals with ASD have dysfunctional immune responses (Braunschweig et al. 2008, 2011; Enstrom et al. 2009; Heuer et al. 2008), epidemiological studies have not supported a causal link between immunization and the development of ASD (Fombonne et al. 2006; Offit and Coffin 2003; Parker et al. 2004). Carnitine deficiency and mitochondrial dysfunction may also be related to autism risk in some individuals (Filipek et al. 2004; Giulivi et al. 2010).

Diagnostic Criteria

Five pervasive developmental disorders (PDDs) are defined in DSM-IV-TR (American Psychiatric Association 2000): autistic disorder, Asperger disorder, Rett disorder, childhood disintegrative disorder, and PDD not otherwise specified. However, DSM-5 will use one diagnostic label, autism spectrum disorder, to refer to the entire group and will provide severity indices rather than different diagnoses to reflect severity of core symptoms. The scientific rationales for using one diagnostic label rather than many in

DSM-5 were as follows: 1) the failure of studies to find meaningful distinctions among the various DSM-IV-TR PDD conditions; 2) the demonstration that the various DSM-IV-TR PDD conditions are genetically similar (identical twins can have different PDD subtypes); and 3) the movement from one category to another over time (e.g., a child who has more symptoms early in life, suggestive of autistic disorder, but improves greatly over time and presents in adolescence as a highly verbal and engaging, but odd, child having symptoms more like those of Asperger disorder).

At the time of this writing, the DSM-5 criteria have not been finalized, so we cannot provide the final criteria in this text. The reader is referred to DSM-5 for revised diagnostic criteria. The new diagnosis provides two main symptom categories: social communication and repetitive, restricted behaviors and interests. An ASD diagnosis requires multiple symptoms in both areas.

Asperger disorder was a diagnostic label used in DSM-IV (American Psychiatric Association 1994) to describe persons who did not meet criteria for autistic disorder but who had some of the social, pragmatic, and restricted, repetitive behavior symptoms seen in autism, along with intact intellectual, adaptive, and language functioning. Asperger disorder was first described almost 60 years ago by Austrian pediatrician Hans Asperger (1944). Studies comparing Asperger disorder and high-functioning autism, however, have provided mixed evidence of their external validity. Although differences between the disorders were evident during children's early years, follow-up studies demonstrated similar adaptive and functional outcomes (Ozonoff and Griffith 2000; Szatmari et al. 2000).

Assessment

Specific practice parameters for the assessment of ASD have been published by the American Academy of Neurology (Filipek et al. 2000), the American Academy of Pediatrics (Johnson et al. 2007), and the American Academy of Child and Adolescent Psychiatry (Volkmar et al. 1999). These practice parameters describe two levels of screening/evaluation. Level 1 screening involves routine developmental surveillance by primary care physicians for young children. Level 2 evaluation involves a diagnostic assessment by experienced clinicians for children who fail the initial screening.

A diagnostic assessment has three essential parts: 1) developmental history and review of presenting problems with parents, 2) review of available records (e.g., medical, school, previous testing, intervention reports), and 3) direct observation of and interaction with the child. Assessment of intellectual, language, and adaptive functioning usually rounds out the core assessment. Additional domains evaluated in more comprehensive assessments include neuropsychological functioning (e.g., attention, memory, executive function), academic abilities, motor function, and psychiatric and behavioral comorbidities.

Multiple measures are available for collecting information from parents and for direct assessment of children suspected of having ASD; each measure has strengths and weaknesses (see Ozonoff et al. 2005 for a more complete discussion). The current gold-standard diagnostic tool for an observational and direct assessment of symptoms is the Autism Diagnostic Observation Schedule (Lord et al. 2001), which involves a 40-minute semistructured interview specifically formatted in various modules so that it is developmentally appropriate for persons from infancy through adulthood and across the range of functioning levels. The current gold-standard diagnostic tool for gathering information concerning symptoms observed in other settings, as well as the evolution of symptoms, is the Autism Diagnostic Interview—Revised (ADI-R; Rutter et al. 2003b), a detailed, semistructured interview format for caregivers. The authors of the ADI-R have also developed a briefer version, the Social Communication Questionnaire (SCQ; Rutter et al. 2003a), from the key ADI-R items. The SCQ consists of 40 questions and is built as a 10- to 15-minute parent questionnaire, which gives information about both current and lifetime symptoms and has good discriminative validity for differentiating ASD from non-ASD (Berument et al. 1999).

Medical assessment needs to occur when ASD is suspected or diagnosed to identify potential etiological factors, address prognosis, guide treatment decisions, and determine the need for additional family assessment. A careful medical history, including prenatal, perinatal, postnatal, and early childhood history, is important to assess risk factors associated with ASD, such as maternal illness or exposure to teratogens during pregnancy, prematurity, low birth weight, newborn encephalopathy, congenital anomalies, and serious illnesses. Sleep disturbances, dietary restrictions by either the child or the family, and gastrointestinal symptoms are common and important to elicit as well. Family and social histories help identify other family members with developmental, educational, and social difficulties, as well as psychiatric disorders. Family history of autoimmune disorders has been elevated in some studies (Croen et al. 2005; Zimmerman et al. 2007). Physical and neurological examination is critical to identify recognizable genetic syndromes highly associated with ASD, such as fragile X syndrome, tuberous sclerosis, Timothy syndrome, and 15q duplication, as well as to recognize abnormal neurological findings suggestive of overt central nervous system insult or sensory impairment, such as hearing loss or visual abnormalities. Growth parameters, including head circumference, should be carefully assessed. Macrocephaly that develops during the first 1–2 years due to accelerated head growth has been reported in a subset of children with ASD (Courchesne et al. 2003; Nordahl et al. 2011).

Referral for hearing and/or vision assessment is important if any concerns are raised by history or examination. Lead or other testing is appropriate if environmental risk factors exist, particularly if children persist in mouthing objects. Chromosomal microarray is recommended for all individuals diagnosed with ASD, because chromosomal abnormalities and de novo copy number variants are implicated in 10%–20% of ASD cases (Manning and Hudgins 2010; Miller et al. 2010; Shen et al. 2010). Targeted genetic testing, such as fragile X DNA or methyl-CpG-binding protein 2 gene (*MECP2*) mutations in females with clinical presentation consistent with Rett disorder (acquired microcephaly, regression, stereotypical hand movements), is recommended. Metabolic studies should be considered when indicated by the history or examination (cyclic vomiting or lethargy associated with mild illness, unusual odors, poor growth). Routine magnetic resonance imaging and electroencephalography are not recommended unless a person has clinically relevant symptoms, such as focal neurological signs or signs of increased intracranial pressure, examination findings suggesting tuberous sclerosis, or history suggestive of seizures (Johnson et al. 2007; Myers et al. 2007). Seizures have been reported in 25%–30% of individuals with ASD, with a bimodal distribution of onset in early childhood and adolescence. Abnormal electroencephalograms often occur in the absence of clinical seizures, although the treatment of these abnormalities in the absence of clinical symptoms has little evidence base (Spence and Schneider 2009).

Differential Diagnosis and Comorbidities

ASDs can co-occur with a variety of additional disorders (Deprey and Ozonoff 2009) and associated symptoms. The most common comorbid conditions in the ASD population are intellectual disability, seizure disorders, hyperactivity, anxiety disorders, and depressed mood (Kim et al. 2000; Leyfer et al. 2006; Myers et al. 2007). Despite general agreement that rates of affective disorders are higher in the ASD population than in the general population, few epidemiological studies of comorbidity prevalence have been done. Another common comorbidity is disturbance in attention and activity levels (Goldstein and Schwebach 2004). DSM-IV-TR did not permit the diagnosis of attention-deficit/hyperactivity disorder in individuals with ASD, but this exclusion will be dropped in DSM-5 (Frazier et al. 2001). Other common comorbidities include seizures, gastrointestinal symptoms, tics, aggression, and problems with sleep and appetite (Buie et al. 2010; Deprey and Ozonoff 2009; Tuchman and Rapin 2002). A critical part of the process of case formulation is differential diagnosis, with the goal of determining whether presenting symptoms are due to ASD, a different condition, or the presence of two comorbid disorders. For example, poor eye contact and low social initiative may be indicative of ASD or of depression. Examining the developmental history for the consistency of symptoms over time and their pervasiveness across situations will help the clinician immensely in the process of differential diagnosis. The package of social and communication limitations, combined with odd or repetitive behaviors, expressed consistently throughout the lifetime, should alert the clinician that ASD must be part of the differential diagnosis. Comorbidity should be considered if additional problems not encompassed by the ASD criteria are present, or if there are changes from baseline indicating onset of new difficulties, or if the individual is not responding as expected to treatment (Lainhart 1999).

Early Detection

Over the last two decades, the age at first diagnosis of ASD has remained steady at 4–5 years (Centers for Disease Control and Prevention 2009; Shattuck et al. 2009), despite parents' first concerns about development occurring at a mean age of 14 months (Chawarska et al. 2007). Early intensive treatment has been shown to be highly promising for young children with ASD (Dawson et al. 2010; Rogers and Vismara 2008), but such interventions are typically reserved for children with a formal diagnosis, making early accurate identification imperative. The American Academy of Pediatrics recommends screening all children for ASD during regular checkups at ages 18 and 24 months (Johnson et al. 2007). Although brief screening measures appropriate for the second year of life have been developed and used in the general population (e.g., Pierce et al. 2011; Robins et al. 2001; Wetherby et al. 2004), the sensitivity and long-term predictive value of each are difficult to ascertain until the initially screened population has been followed to school age. Initially promising instruments turned out to have high false-negative rates when screened toddlers were reassessed at age 7 years (Baird et al. 2000). For this and other reasons, some researchers have suggested that routine universal screening for ASD is premature (Al-Qabandi et al. 2011).

One of the primary methods used to learn about the earliest signs of ASD is the prospective infant sibling design. A key finding from these studies—the lack of behavioral differences before the first birthday in children who are later diagnosed with autism (Landa and Garrett-Mayer 2006; Zwaigenbaum et al. 2005)—suggests that autism signs are not present early in infancy in most of these children, as once suggested by Kanner (1943), but rather emerge over time through a process of diminishment of key social and communication behaviors. This finding also suggests that early social regression, subtle and difficult for parents to detect, may be a more common feature of autism onset than previously realized.

Interventions

Medical Interventions

Medical treatments at this point are largely effective in treating associated or comorbid symptoms of ASD rather than core symptoms (Anagnostou and Hansen 2011; McPheeters et al. 2011). Medical interventions to treat associated symptoms of aggression, irritability, and repetitive behaviors with risperidone and aripiprazole have evidence to support their benefit, although significant adverse effects, including somnolence and weight gain, also occur. The Research Units on Pediatric Psychopharmacology Autism Network (2005) completed a randomized, placebo-controlled crossover trial of methylphenidate versus placebo in children and adolescents with ASD and found that each of three dosing levels performed better than placebo on hyperactivity, although parents reported higher withdrawal and lethargy at the highest dose. In a small randomized trial of atomoxetine in children ages 5–15 with ASD, the drug produced significant improvement in hyperactivity and was well tolerated, suggesting the need for further trials (Arnold et al. 2006).

The use of serotonin reuptake inhibitors or stimulant medications lacks sufficient strength of evidence to evaluate benefit/risk profiles (McPheeters et al. 2011), although the medications are used clinically for repetitive behaviors and anxiety.

Behavioral Interventions

Behavioral interventions are the most successful approaches for treating core symptoms and improving outcomes in people with ASDs. Initial diagnosis needs to be followed by validated behavioral treatments as soon as possible. All states offer publicly funded services for children younger than 3 years with autism spectrum disorders as well as many other developmental difficulties. These intervention services, often referred to as "Birth to Three" services, do not require specific medical diagnoses and can be located via city and county systems. Fortunately for practitioners and parents, a number of systematic reviews of effective interventions and educational strategies have been published in the last few years (National Autism Center 2012; Odom et al. 2010; Reichow and Wolery 2009; Virues-Ortega 2010; Vismara and Rogers 2010). The references for these reviews can be provided to parents to help them make choices about services for their children with ASD. The majority of the reviewed studies involve interventions for preschoolers and school-age children, but older children and adolescents are also included in many. Interventions tend to be clustered by age group and by the focus of the intervention (e.g., social, language, behavior).

Few types of early intervention approaches have been evaluated with rigorous research designs. Two approaches stand out from the rest based on the quality of research and outcomes (see Odom et al. 2010 for a review of comprehensive interventions): Lovaas's Early Intensive Behavioral Intervention (EIBI; Lovaas 1987) and the Early Start Denver Model (ESDM; Rogers and Dawson 2010). Both the EIBI and the ESDM have well-defined curricula, clearly defined teaching approaches with fidelity measurement tools that define the method, embedded data systems that record daily progress, and specific methods for dealing with child error or failure to progress.

Lovaas's Model

Lovaas's EIBI (McEachin et al. 1993) is the best-studied approach, with two well-controlled studies (one a randomized controlled design) and one long-term outcome study. Two different meta-analyses (Reichow and Wolery 2009; Virues-Ortega 2010) have demonstrated medium to large effect sizes. This approach involves several years of 35–40 hours per week of one-to-one intervention carried out in the home (and in community settings as children progress) by trained paraprofessionals closely supervised by a senior therapist certified in the model. Outcome studies demonstrate large and significant gains in IQ and language in children participating in the EIBI compared with control subjects, and gains that continue throughout childhood and into adolescence were documented from one study.

Early Start Denver Model

The ESDM is a recent treatment, with a manual (Rogers and Dawson 2010), curriculum, and outcomes paper (Dawson et al. 2010) from a randomized controlled study. The ESDM was designed for toddlers and has been tested on children ranging in age from 18 to 30 months. The curriculum follows typical sequences in early childhood developmental areas and is based on developmental science. The teaching approach focuses on dyadic, responsive, developmentally specified joint play and activity routines between adult and child, in which individualized and specified teaching opportunities are embedded in the play. The adult's ability to stimulate and support the targeted skills in the child and reward the child within the play, using the intrinsic reward value of the activity itself, follows the principles of applied behavior analysis. The approach can be delivered, after specific training, by many different persons: speech pathologists, early childhood professionals, occupational therapists, psychologists, parents, and paraprofessionals when under the supervision of a trained professional interventionist. In a randomized controlled trial, children who received up to 20 hours of the ESDM per week of one-to-one instruction in their homes from a trained person as well as 5 or more hours per week of instruction from their parents (who also received training) showed large and significant gains in IQ, language, and adaptive behavior compared with the contrast group, who received their intervention in the community.

Other Intervention Practices

A number of other comprehensive interventions that have specific curricula, specific sets of teaching practices, and specified measurement systems for child progress have gained much publicity and large followings but lack rigorous outcome data that provide empirical support. However, a large number of individual teaching practices are backed by solid empirical support. These practices, when combined with a specific curriculum, also allow early educators and interventionists to use empirically supported practices, assembled individually, to deliver a rigorous, individualized intervention to a specific child. Well over 25 individual teaching practices have solid empirical support, but they need to be used to teach skills that are identified for the individual with ASD from appropriate assessment practices and task analyses. Several groups have conducted systematic reviews of the treatment literature to identify these successful practices. Boyd et al. (2010) provide a list of effective preschool practices. The National Autism Center's (2009) National Standards Report represents a multiyear national effort to review the research on effective interventions for ASD. Finally, the National Professional Development Center on Autism Spectrum Disorders, a project located at the Frank Porter Graham Child Development Institute, has developed a comprehensive list of effective practices and related teaching materials (available at http://autismpdc.fpg .unc.edu).

Many of the treatment referrals most commonly made for persons with ASD have surprisingly little scientific evidence behind them. Occupational therapy and one of its derivative treatments, sensory integration therapy, are excellent examples. Randomized trials of these treatments are just beginning (Pfeiffer et al. 2011).

Speech therapy presents a more complex picture. Speech and language development is directly affected by autism, and needs habilitation. However, speech and language therapy alone for 1–2 hours per week is unlikely to result in substantial effect. Positive gain is much more likely when speech and language therapists are part of a more comprehensive approach and when they include parents in the sessions and help them develop skills in sensitivity and responsivity to children's cues, thereby supporting their children's communicative development step by step; there is evidence of positive effects on outcomes with this approach (Siller and Sigman 2002, 2008).

Medical and Alternative Biomedical Treatments

Efficacy has not been established for some popular and widespread practices, particularly interventions classified as complementary and alternative medicine (CAM; Akins et al. 2010). Although they are used clinically, serotonin reuptake inhibitors and stimulant medications, as mentioned earlier, lack sufficient strength of evidence to evaluate benefit/risk profiles (McPheeters et al. 2011). Melatonin is the only biologically based CAM intervention that has shown efficacy in controlled trials for sleep onset difficulties in people with autism, and the long-acting form may be helpful in maintaining sleep, although this is still under investigation (Akins et al. 2010). Physicians can help families by steering them toward interventions based on peer-reviewed literature, explaining the reasons for prioritizing evidence-based behavioral interventions over medications, openly discussing CAM therapies that parents may be interested in trying relative to any unknown benefits and known or potential risks (Akins et al. 2010), and helping them locate services or advocates to assist them in requesting that educators and therapists specify the evidence-based practices to be used in Individualized Education Programs (IEPs) and Individualized Family Service Plans (IFSPs).

Equally important, physicians should take care not to write prescriptions that unnecessarily tie the hands of service deliverers. Specifying in a clinical report that a child needs "3 hours per week of speech therapy" or "40 hours per week of early intervention" does not reflect best practice, and such specification may set up antagonistic relations between families and service providers. It is more useful to recommend that children with ASD receive "empirically supported early intervention practices" or "empirically supported teaching practices for communication, social, and academic skill development." This practice focuses both family and service providers on the empirical evidence of child intervention.

Family Issues

The impact of a diagnosis of a child's major health disorder causes repercussions throughout the family system. (Because of major differences across cultures in beliefs about autism, cultural family values, and availability of services, we focus on current knowledge about the impact of ASD on American families.) Whereas earlier literature assumed the five-stage grief response first described by Kübler-Ross (1969), it is now clear that many different types of reactions occur in individual family responses to diagnosis. Cultural differences in the meaning of a disability to a family and the types of coping strategies that families use add to the variability of family responses seen in ASD (Smith and Elder 2010). Professionals need to listen carefully to each family's experience rather than assume an expected pattern or response based on the family's having a child with ASD.

When a child is first diagnosed with a major health disorder, families often respond initially with denial, emotional devastation, and distancing from others (Altiere and von Kluge 2009). As a long-term predictor of adjustment, the type of reaction may be less important than the "resolution of diagnosis" (Pianta and Marvin 1993)—the ability to adjust over time to the diagnosis and the changes it brings to life while also resisting self-blame and other distressing chronic emotions and cognitions (Wachtel and Carter 2008). Mothers' emotional resolution of diagnosis has significant effects on the quality of the emotional and cognitive support they provide to their young children with autism (Koren-Karie et al. 2009; Wachtel and Carter 2008), independent of child characteristics (fathers have not been reported on yet). Maternal resolution of diagnosis and sensitivity to children's experiences are also related to children's attachment security (Oppenheim et al. 2009). Parents' cognitive appraisals of their situation also appear to have significant effects on their coping (McCubbin and McCubbin 1987). Families who find some benefits in their situation are likely to be happier and better adjusted (Suedfeld 1997).

Family social supports affect family functioning and happiness over time as well. Families typically turn to formal supports—professionals, teachers, and other helpers—early on after diagnosis, but over the years, families develop more informal supports (friends, other families whose children have similar disorders) (Sharpley et al. 1997). These informal supports from partners, friends, and family members contribute to parental sense of well-being, life satisfaction, and positive affect, although each source operates in somewhat different ways (Ekas et al. 2010). Unfortunately, for many families, extended family members may not be a support initially, because they are also reacting to the diagnosis (Altiere and von Kluge 2009).

One significant effect of autism diagnosis is maternal depression. In a large study of highly educated mothers, Carter et al. (2009) reported elevated and long-lasting (over 2 years) depressive symptoms in 28%–42% of the mothers of toddlers with ASD. Surprisingly, child characteristics did not affect maternal symptoms over time. Professionals working with families of children with ASD need to be aware of potential depression, anxiety, and other mental health symptoms in parents so that needed interventions are put in place for parents as well as children.

Another important factor in family life related to autism is increased parental stress. A number of comparative studies have demonstrated that parents of children with autism experience more stress than parents of children with any other type of developmental disorder (Estes et al. 2009). Financial pressures mount for families of children with ASD, and many families experience a significant reduction of income, due to both the need for a parent to be at home and the need to pay for expensive services (Montes and Halterman 2008). The combination of problem behaviors, impaired social communication, and need for ongoing assistance and close supervision seen in children with ASD places many additional daily demands on their parents. Of these, problem behaviors have the clearest ties to parental stress (Estes et al. 2009). Problem behaviors have a much greater direct relationship with parental stress and distress than does severity of the core ASD symptoms, although severity is also a contributor (Ekas and Whitman 2010). Some evidence suggests that in families of children with ASD, mothers report higher levels of stress than do fathers, a finding that does not necessarily occur in families of children with other disorders (Dabrowski and Pisula 2010). Fatigue, anxiety, depression, and stress (Giallo et al. 2011) affect parental sense of self-efficacy and, likely, parenting skills. Children's sleep disorders and behavior problems, as well as familial isolation from social support systems, contribute to parental symptoms and indicate important areas for specific assessments and interventions in families of children with ASD (Giallo et al. 2011).

Parental stress takes its toll on marriages and families. In a large and carefully done recent study, the divorce rate in families of children with ASD was significantly higher (24%) than in economically and ethnically matched families of typically developing children (14%). Unlike these comparison families, for whom the divorce rate is high during the school years and then drops significantly, divorce rates among families of children with ASD continue to be high until children are well into adulthood (Hartley et al. 2010). Quality of the marital relationship is related to quality of parenting experiences, and it has direct links with the closeness of the father-child relationship, regardless of whether the child has ASD or is developing typically (Hartley et al. 2011). Parenting stress negatively affects the amount of progress children with ASD make in intervention (Osborne et al. 2008), and it likely affects the quality of interactions with the other children in the family as well.

New questions have arisen in recent literature about the contribution of the broader autism phenotype as it occurs in parents to effects seen in families. Pollman et al. (2010) report that in fathers, more symptoms of ASD are related to less emotional intimacy and satisfaction with the marital relationship, but this was not true for their wives, whose marital and emotional satisfaction were unrelated to the degree of their husbands' symptoms. Interestingly, wives' autism symptoms did not demonstrate any relationships with partners' marital satisfaction, and no relationships were found between the number of symptoms in wives and the number of symptoms in their husbands, a finding that does not support the hypothesis about assortative mating in the broader autism phenotype (Baron-Cohen 2006).

Perhaps surprising to some, parents also report some positive results of their altered life experiences. Personal benefits that some family members report are a new level of gratitude for the "smaller" things in life, new levels of acceptance of persons with disabilities, new levels of care and empathy for their partners, spiritual growth, and changes for the better in personal value systems ("what is really important in life"). They also report positive emotional experiences as they come to know and love their child with autism as a whole person, with unique and lovable characteristics. Some families grow closer together, spend more time with their children, and feel stronger as a family unit (Altiere and von Kluge 2009). Family optimism also affects the family's social support network directly, enhancing contacts and ties, and these in turn provide further well-being (Ekas et al. 2010). This ability of families to reflect on their life-changing experience and to value some of the changes likely reflects a deep process of resolution and cognitive as well as emotional acceptance of their new status and situation.

In the home, siblings of a child with ASD experience the increased parental stress, fatigue, and depression, and they live daily with their sibling's behavior problems, communication challenges, problems with social reciprocity, and increased need for caregiving and supervision. Although the large majority of siblings show typical adjustment patterns (Pilowsky et al. 2004; see Smith and Elder 2010 for a review), these stressors take their toll on siblings, as they do on their parents.

Professional Support

How can professionals add to families' needed supports? Several recommendations can be gleaned from the preceding discussion:

1. Professional supports: At the time of diagnosis, professionals need to help parents understand the importance of high-quality intervention for their child's current and future functioning, and to provide parents with specific referrals to intervention sources. Written information, including names and phone numbers, should supplement verbal recommendations.

2. Emotional supports: Professionals need to consider parental emotional responses and consider the number and severity of stressors affecting the parents, including symptoms of significant depression, anxiety, marital or family discord, and isolation. Referrals for needed supports or treatment for parent difficulties should be provided, and follow-up should occur.

3. Social supports: Professionals can enhance parental social supports through specific referrals to parent support groups and through provision of opportunities for extended family members and other family supports to join the parents in a feedback session with the professional.

4. Support of child's strengths: Professionals need to provide reports that detail a child's strengths as well as needs, point out the positive supports already in place, detail the family strengths, and paint a picture of potential for improvement as well as needs. Such reporting can help foster parental optimism in the face of diagnosis.

5. Support of advocacy: By providing written information that details a child's rights to intervention and education, professionals can support parents' sense of advocacy and empowerment as they move forward to find the best services for their child. Providing written documentation of Web sites that provide balanced, empirically based information in family-friendly language helps families evaluate the quality of Web-based information they come across. The Autism Speaks Web site has a 100 Day Kit, which is an especially useful tool for families with a new diagnosis (www.autismspeaks.org/family-services/tool-kits/100-day-kit).

6. Support for siblings: Professional sensitivity can support sibling needs as well. Professionals should screen for possible sibling risk for ASD or related conditions as part of the child's diagnosis and treatment. Newly developing behavior difficulties in siblings may indicate the need for direct supports through referral to sibling groups. Interventionists working with the child with ASD should be alert to parent comments about sibling difficulties and be ready to listen and provide support and referrals as needed for siblings. Family therapy sessions may be useful for siblings and parents who are having difficulties adjusting to the new demands that the needs of a child with ASD places on family structure.

New Research Directions

Etiology

ASDs are known to be highly heritable, with a concordance rate as high as 92% in monozygotic twins and 10% in dizygotic twins (Bailey et al. 1995). Single-gene disorders, such as fragile X syndrome, that are highly associated with ASD account for a small percentage of children diagnosed, and it is believed that a "second hit" or multiple additional contributing factors are necessary in these disorders for ASD symptomatology to develop (Christian et al. 2008). Emerging technologies for looking at genetic variability in structure and function, such as expanded comparative genomic hybridization microarray testing and genome-wide sequencing, will likely increase the percentage of individuals with identified genetic causes for ASD above the current 10%–20% range (Miller et al. 2010). Complex genetic susceptibility profiles from multiple contributing genes and epigenetic alterations interacting with environmental factors are beginning to be implicated in explaining the heterogeneity of ASD (Schmidt et al. 2011). Studies implicating immune dysfunction in a subset of both mothers (Braunschweig et al. 2008) and children with ASD (Ashwood et al. 2006) may prove important for early diagnosis as well as treatment. Many different gene-environment interactions are hypothesized to lead to similar alterations in common neural pathways during early brain development.

Behavioral Interventions

Unfortunately, the progress made in scientific studies in early intervention has not been matched by similar bodies of work focused on older persons with ASD. Although the literature includes a plethora of well-designed single-subject studies in older persons that describe successful interventions targeted at increasing behaviors involving social and communicative skills, decreasing unwanted behaviors, and improving academic, recreational, or vocational skills, group designs and randomized studies are almost absent from the literature on older persons with ASD. Controlled or randomized group designs to identify intervention efficacy are necessary in studies of older children, youth, and adults with ASD to be able to generalize from more data than studies involving 1–3 subjects. Treatment studies of older children and adults will benefit from multisite network studies that can examine the response of persons with relatively similar learning abilities and communication skills to various intervention approaches for a specific set of skills (e.g., social recreational skills, job training involving independence, personal independence related to the first year in college, management of personal time after work for those living in apartments).

Another area of need for intervention science in ASD involves development of more advanced linguistic functions for people using augmentative communication devices. With increasing technological developments, an abundance of personal devices are becoming available for communicative use. However, people often use augmentative devices only for simple requesting. Concerted effort by linguists and communication scientists is needed to develop interventions that will promote elaborated spontaneous language using augmentative devices across a wide range of pragmatic functions. Studies are also needed that are aimed at understanding whether the group of people with ASD without useful verbal skills can acquire complex language using augmentative devices, or whether their verbal language output reflects a deep linguistic impairment rather than a modality impairment.

Behavioral intervention studies should lead to studies that examine the relation of brain changes to behavioral changes. Demonstrating the biological concomitants of intervention should assist with gains in understanding the brain bases of ASD, as well as provide a mechanism for explaining the power of early intervention. In fact, biological changes likely underlie all successful interventions, because adults as well as children show brain-based differences after specific task learning. It is quite possible that connectivity differences in ASD, for instance, may diminish in children with positive responses to early intervention. Demonstrating this effect would show that core biological deficits in ASD may in fact be reversible, which would change the whole understanding of ASD as a chronic, lifelong disability. This finding would also lead people away from the tendency to attribute positive change to "compensatory mechanisms" rather than deep, biological growth and development.

Medical Interventions

As the fields of genomics and molecular neuroscience advance, researchers are better positioned to identify molecular targets for treating core ASD symptoms. A series of independent but related studies have documented abnormalities in candidate genes (e.g., *SHANK3*, neuroligins) (Pinto et al. 2010), peripheral markers (Aldred et al. 2003; Shinohe et al. 2006), animal models (e.g., fragile X) (Kelleher and Bear 2008), and neuropathology (Fatemi et al. 2002; Purcell et al. 2001) that implicate the glutamate and γ-aminobutyric acid (GABA) neurotransmitter systems in the pathophysiology of ASD. Medications affecting the N-methyl-D-aspartate (NMDA) receptor, such as amantadine (King et al. 2001), dextromethorphan (Woodard et al. 2005, 2007), and memantine (Chez et al. 2007; Erickson et al. 2007; Niederhofer 2007; Owley et al. 2006), have preliminary evidence to support further studies in the treatment of ASD. Metabotropic glutamate receptor 5 (mGlur5) inhibitors are in Phase II and early Phase III trials (Silverman et al. 2010).

Oxytocin has been linked to modulation of social cognition and function in multiple animal models and in humans, although the data for oxytocin involvement in the pathophysiology of ASD remain limited. However, both genomic and peripheral biomarker data suggest that at least in a subgroup of individuals with ASD, this system may be implicated in the neurobiology of the disorder (Green et al. 2001; Jacob et al. 2007; Modahl et al. 1998; Wu et al. 2005), and preliminary studies have provided proof of concept for the potential therapeutic role of oxytocin in facilitating social cognition in ASD (Hollander et al. 2007).

Finally, ongoing neuroinflammatory processes in the cortex, white matter, and cerebellum have been reported in postmortem brain tissue (Vargas et al. 2005), as well as increases in cerebrospinal fluid proinflammatory factors (Pardo et al. 2005; Zimmerman et al. 2005, 2006), and dysregulation of both cellular and innate immune response has been found (Ashwood et al. 2006; Braunschweig et al. 2008) in a subset of individuals with ASD. Multiple agents are available that may modulate the immune system in children with ASD; however, the evidence for any of these is currently lacking, and well-controlled randomized trials are urgently needed.

Key Points

- The findings summarized in this chapter require differences in clinical practice and different dialogues between practitioners and parents from those of 10 years ago.

- DSM-5 will provide one diagnosis, autism spectrum disorder (ASD), for all patients on this spectrum. Severity will be described by function rather than by diagnosis. Comorbid psychiatric disorders and medical disorders will be recognized, diagnosed, and treated as separate conditions.

- Onset of autism has a variety of patterns, rather than the previously used dichotomous early-onset and regressive categories. Clinicians need to listen for and report the pattern of symptom emergence that each parent describes, without trying to impose a particular pattern.

- A thorough medical examination should occur at initial diagnosis to aid in etiological evaluation and treatment of comorbid associated disorders or symptoms, such as seizure disorders, gastrointestinal disorders, feeding problems and nutritional deficiencies, sleep disorders, and aggressive or self-injurious behaviors.

- Many behavioral symptoms that used to be attributed to ASD but are not part of the definition should be evaluated both medically and functionally, diagnosed, and treated with empirically supported approaches. The most common are attention-deficit/hyperactivity disorder, depression, anxiety, sleep disorders, aggression, and self-injury. Behavior therapy approaches rather than medications should be considered as the first line of treatment for sleep disorders, aggression, and self-injury if no underlying medical conditions are identified, because of the efficacy of behavioral treatments for these conditions.

- Clinicians should refer children for empirically based behavioral intervention services at the first signs of ASD, rather than waiting until the diagnosis is established with certainty. For infants and toddlers, taking a wait-and-see approach precludes the earliest treatment and may forfeit the child's best opportunity for significant improvement.

- The message to parents that ASD is a severe and lifelong disorder is no longer accurate. ASD has a very wide range of outcomes, and persons with ASD of all ages and all levels of functioning are responsive to well-delivered, empirically supported treatment and education. It is not possible to predict a young child's eventual outcome from data gathered at first assessment, or even from repeated assessments over childhood. For families of young children, it is accurate to predict that their child, as an adult, could live separately from the parents, work, and have a fulfilling life, often with some level of support. It is possible that a young child with autism will grow up to go to a university, marry and have children, and be independent. A family's ability to locate and provide the best quality of care and treatment available in their community throughout their child's developmental years will lead to the best outcome possible for that particular child. However, outcomes are quite variable even among children receiving the best interventions possible. Parents need to learn as much as they can about ASD in general, their own child's strengths and needs, and the range of services available to them, and they need to work closely with providers to ensure best quality of care and education throughout childhood and adolescence.

Recommended Readings

Autism Speaks (Web site). 100-Day Kit. Available at: http://www.autismspeaks.org/family-services/tool-kits/100-day-kit. Accessed August 16, 2012.

Lord C, Jones RM: Annual research review: re-thinking the classification of autism spectrum disorders. J Child Psychol Psychiatry 53:490–509, 2012

Odom SL, Boyd BA, Hall LJ, et al: Evaluation of comprehensive treatment models for individuals with autism spectrum disorders. J Autism Dev Disord 40:425–436, 2010

Yirmiya N, Charman T: The prodrome of autism: early behavioral and biological signs, regression, peri- and post-natal development and genetics. J Child Psychol Psychiatry 51:432–458, 2010

References

Abrahams BS, Geschwind DH: Advances in autism genetics: on the threshold of a new neurobiology. Nat Rev Genet 9:341–355, 2008 [erratum in: Nat Rev Genet 9:493, 2008]

Akins RS, Angkustsiri K, Hansen R: Complementary and alternative medicine in autism: an evidence-based approach to negotiating safe and efficacious interventions with families. Neurotherapeutics 7:307–319, 2010

Aldred S, Moore KM, Fitzgerald M, et al: Plasma amino acid levels in children with autism and their families. J Autism Dev Disord 33:93–97, 2003

Al-Qabandi M, Gorter JW, Rosenbaum P: Early autism detection: are we ready for routine screening? Pediatrics 128:e211–e117, 2011

Altiere MJ, von Kluge S: Family functioning and coping behaviors in parents of children with autism. J Child Fam Stud 18:83–92, 2009

American Psychiatric Association: Diagnostic and Statistical Manual of Mental Disorders, 4th Edition. Washington, DC, American Psychiatric Association, 1994

American Psychiatric Association: Diagnostic and Statistical Manual of Mental Disorders, 4th Edition, Text Revision. Washington, DC, American Psychiatric Association, 2000

Anagnostou E, Hansen R: Medical treatment overview: traditional and novel psycho-pharmacological and complementary and alternative medications. Curr Opin Pediatr 23:621–627, 2011

Arnold LE, Aman MG, Cook AM, et al: Atomoxetine for hyperactivity in autism spectrum disorders: placebo-controlled crossover pilot trial. J Am Acad Child Adolesc Psychiatry 45:1196–1205, 2006

Ashwood P, Wills S, Van de Water J: The immune response in autism: a new frontier for autism research. J Leukoc Biol 80:1–15, 2006

Asperger H: Die Autistischen Psychopathen im Kindesalter. Arch Psychiatr Nervenkr 177:76–136, 1944

Bailey A, Le Couteur A, Gottesman I, et al: Autism as a strongly genetic disorder: evidence from a British twin study. Psychol Med 25:63–77, 1995

Baird G, Charman T, Baron-Cohen S, et al: A screening instrument for autism at 18 months of age: a 6-year follow-up study. J Am Acad Child Adolesc Psychiatry 39:694–702, 2000

Baron-Cohen S: The hyper-systemizing, assortative mating theory of autism. Prog Neuropsychopharmacol Biol Psychiatry 30:865–872, 2006

Berument SK, Rutter M, Lord C, et al: Autism Screening Questionnaire: diagnostic validity. Br J Psychiatry 175:444–451, 1999

Billstedt E, Gillberg IC, Gillberg C: Autism after adolescence: population-based 13- to 22-year follow-up study of 120 individuals with autism diagnosed in childhood. J Autism Dev Disord 35:351–360, 2005

Boyd BA, Odom SL, Humphreys BP, et al: Infants and toddlers with autism spectrum disorder: early identification and early intervention. J Early Interv 32:75–98, 2010

Braunschweig D, Ashwood P, Krakowiak P, et al: Autism: maternally derived antibodies specific for fetal brain proteins. Neurotoxicology 29:226–231, 2008

Braunschweig D, Duncanson P, Boyce R, et al: Behavioral correlates of maternal antibody status among children with autism. J Autism Dev Disord Oct 20, 2011 [Epub ahead of print]

Buie T, Campbell DB, Fuchs GJ, et al: Evaluation, diagnosis, and treatment of gastrointestinal disorders in individuals with ASDs: a consensus report. Pediatrics 125 (suppl 1):S1–S18, 2010

Carter AS, Martínez-Pedraza Fde L, Gray SA: Stability and individual change in depressive symptoms among mothers raising young children with ASD: maternal and child correlates. J Clin Psychol 65:1270–1280, 2009

Centers for Disease Control and Prevention: Prevalence of autism spectrum disorders—Autism and Developmental Disabilities Monitoring Network, United States, 2008. MMWR Surveill Summ 61:1–24, 2012

Chawarska K, Paul R, Klin A, et al: Parental recognition of developmental problems in toddlers with autism spectrum disorders. J Autism Dev Disord 37:62–72, 2007

Chez MB, Burton Q, Dowling T, et al: Memantine as adjunctive therapy in children diagnosed with autistic spectrum disorders: an observation of initial clinical response and maintenance tolerability. J Child Neurol 22:574–579, 2007

Christian SL, Brune CW, Sudi J, et al: Novel submicroscope chromosomal abnormalities detected in autism spectrum disorder. Biol Psychiatry 63:1111–1117, 2008

Courchesne E, Carper R, Akshoomoff N: Evidence of brain overgrowth in the first year of life in autism. JAMA 290:337–344, 2003

Croen LA, Grether JK, Yoshida CK, et al: Maternal autoimmune diseases, asthma and allergies, and childhood autism spectrum disorders. Arch Pediatr Adolesc Med 159:151–157, 2005

Croen LA, Najjar DV, Fireman B, et al: Maternal and paternal age and risk of autism spectrum disorders. Arch Pediatr Adolesc Med 161:334–340, 2007

Dabrowski A, Pisula E: Parenting stress and coping styles in mothers and fathers of pre-school children with autism and Down syndrome. J Intellect Disabil Res 53:266–280, 2010

Dawson G, Rogers S, Munson J, et al: Randomized, controlled trial for toddlers with autism: the Early Start Denver Model. Pediatrics 125:e17–e23, 2010

De Giacomo A, Fombonne E: Parental recognition of developmental abnormalities in autism. Eur Child Adolesc Psychiatry 7:131–136, 1998

Deprey L, Ozonoff S: Assessment of psychiatric conditions in autism spectrum disorders, in Assessment of Autism Spectrum Disorders. Edited by Goldstein S, Naglieri J, Ozonoff S. New York, Guilford, 2009, pp 290–317

Ekas N, Whitman TL: Autism symptom topography and maternal socioemotional functioning. Am J Intellect Dev Disabil 115:234–249, 2010

Ekas NV, Lickenbrock DM, Whitman TL: Optimism, social support, and well-being in mothers of children with autism spectrum disorder. J Autism Dev Disord 40:1274–1284, 2010

Elsabbagh M, Divan G, Koh, YJ, et al: Global prevalence of autism and other PDDs. Autism Res 5:160–179, 2012

Enstrom AM, Van de Water JA, Ashwood P: Autoimmunity in autism. Curr Opin Investig Drugs 10:463–475, 2009

Erickson CA, Posey DJ, Stigler KA, et al: A retrospective study of memantine in children and adolescents with pervasive developmental disorders. Psychopharmacology (Berl) 191:141–147, 2007

Estes A, Munson J, Dawson G, et al: Parenting stress and psychological functioning among mothers of preschool children with autism and developmental disorders. Autism 13:375–387, 2009

Fatemi SH, Halt AR, Stary JM, et al: Glutamic acid decarboxylase 65 and 67 kDa proteins are reduced in autistic parietal and cerebellar cortices. Biol Psychiatry 52:805–810, 2002

Fein D, Dixon P, Paul J, et al: Brief report: pervasive developmental disorder can evolve into ADHD: case illustrations. J Autism Dev Disord 35:525–534, 2005

Filipek PA, Accardo PJ, Ashwal S, et al: Practice parameter: screening and diagnosis of autism. Report of the Quality Standards Subcommittee of the American Academy of Neurology and the Child Neurology Society. Neurology 55:468–479, 2000

Filipek PA, Juranek J, Nguyen MT, et al: Relative carnitine deficiency in autism. J Autism Dev Disord 34:615–623, 2004

Fombonne E: Epidemiological trends in autism. Mol Psychiatry 7 (suppl 2):S4–S6, 2002

Fombonne E, Chakrabarti S: No evidence for a new variant of measles-mumps-rubella–induced autism. Pediatrics 108:e58, 2001

Fombonne E, Zakarian R, Bennett A, et al: Pervasive developmental disorders in Montreal, Quebec, Canada: prevalence and links with immunizations. Pediatrics 118:e139–e150, 2006

Frazier JA, Biederman J, Bellorde CA, et al: Should the diagnosis of attention-deficit/hyperactivity disorder be considered in children with pervasive developmental disorder? J Atten Disord 4:203–211, 2001

Giallo R, Wood CE, Jellett R, et al: Fatigue, wellbeing and parental self-efficacy in mothers of children with an autism spectrum disorder. Autism July 25, 2011 [Epub ahead of print]

Giulivi C, Zhang YF, Omanska-Klusek A, et al: Mitochondrial dysfunction in autism. JAMA 304:2389–2396, 2010

Goldberg WA, Osann K, Filipek PA, et al: Language and other regression: assessment and timing. J Autism Dev Disord 33:607–616, 2003

Goldstein S, Schwebach AJ: The comorbidity of pervasive developmental disorder and attention deficit hyperactivity disorder: results of a retrospective chart review. J Autism Dev Disord 34:329–339, 2004

Green LA, Fein D, Modahl C, et al: Oxytocin and autistic disorder: alterations in peptide forms. Biol Psychiatry 50:609–613, 2001

Hansen RL, Ozonoff S, Krakowiak P, et al: Regression in autism: prevalence and associated factors in the CHARGE study. Ambul Pediatr 8:25–31, 2008

Hartley SL, Barker ET, Seltzer MM, et al: The relative risk and timing of divorce in families of children with an autism spectrum disorder. J Fam Psychol 24:449–457, 2010

Hartley SL, Barker ET, Seltzer MM, et al: Marital satisfaction and parenting experiences of mothers and fathers of adolescents and adults with autism. Am J Intellect Dev Disabil 116:81–95, 2011

Hertz-Picciotto I, Delwiche L: The rise in autism and the role of age at diagnosis. Epidemiology 20:84–90, 2009

Hertz-Picciotto I, Croen LA, Hansen R, et al: The CHARGE study: an epidemiologic investigation of genetic and environmental factors contributing to autism. Environ Health Perspect 114:1119–1125, 2006

Heuer L, Ashwood P, Van de Water J: The immune system in autism: is there a connection? Autism 4:271–288, 2008

Hollander E, Bartz J, Chaplin W, et al: Oxytocin increases retention of social cognition in autism. Biol Psychiatry 61:498–503, 2007

Howlin P: Outcome in high-functioning adults with autism with and without early language delays: implications for the differentiation between autism and Asperger syndrome. J Autism Dev Disord 33:3–13, 2003

Howlin P, Goode S, Hutton J, et al: Adult outcome for children with autism. J Child Psychol Psychiatry 45:212–229, 2004

Jacob S, Brune CW, Carter CS, et al: Association of the oxytocin receptor gene (OXTR) in Caucasian children and adolescents with autism. Neurosci Lett 417:6–9, 2007

Johnson CP, Myers SM; American Academy of Pediatrics Council on Children With Disabilities: Identification and evaluation of children with autism spectrum disorders. Pediatrics 120:1183–1215, 2007

Jones LA, Campbell JM: Clinical characteristics associated with language regression for children with autism spectrum disorders. J Autism Dev Disord 40:54–62, 2010

Kalb LG, Law JK, Landa R, et al: Onset patterns prior to 36 months in autism spectrum disorders. J Autism Dev Disord 40:1389–1402, 2010

Kanner L: Autistic disturbances of affective contact. Nerv Child 2:217–250, 1943

Kawamura Y, Takahashi O, Ishii T: Reevaluating the incidence of pervasive developmental disorders: impact of elevated rates of detection through implementation of an integrated system of screening in Toyota, Japan. Psychiatry Clin Neurosci 62:152–159, 2008

Kelleher RJ, Bear MF: The autistic neuron: troubled translation. Cell 135:401–406, 2008

Kim JA, Szatmari P, Bryson SE, et al: The prevalence of anxiety and mood problems among children with autism and Asperger syndrome. Autism 4:117–132, 2000

Kim YS, Leventhal BL, Koh YJ, et al: Prevalence of ASDs in a total population sample. Am J Psychiatry 168:904–912, 2011

King BH, Wright DM, Handen BL, et al: Double-blind, placebo-controlled study of amantadine hydrochloride in the treatment of children with autistic disorder. J Am Acad Child Adolesc Psychiatry 40:658–665, 2001

Koren-Karie N, Oppenheim D, Dolev S, et al: Mothers of securely attached children with autism spectrum disorder are more sensitive than mothers of insecurely attached children. J Child Psychol Psychiatry 50:643–650, 2009

Kübler-Ross E: On Death and Dying. New York, Macmillan, 1969

Lainhart JE: Psychiatric problems in individuals with autism, their parents, and siblings. Int J Psychiatry 11:278–298, 1999

Landa R, Garrett-Mayer E: Development in infants with autism spectrum disorders: a prospective study. J Child Psychol Psychiatry 47:629–638, 2006

Leyfer OT, Folstein SE, Bacalman S, et al: Comorbid psychiatric disorders in children with autism: interview development and rates of disorders. J Autism Dev Disord 36:849–861, 2006

Lord C: Follow-up of two-year-olds referred for possible autism. J Child Psychol Psychiatry 36:1365–1382, 1995

Lord C, Rutter M, DiLavore P, et al: Autism Diagnostic Observation Schedule (ADOS) Manual. Los Angeles, CA, Western Psychological Services, 2001

Lord C, Shulman C, DiLavore P: Regression and word loss in autistic spectrum disorders. J Child Psychol Psychiatry 45:936–955, 2004

Lotter V: Factors related to outcome in autistic children. J Autism Dev Disord 4:263–277, 1974

Lovaas OI: Behavioral treatment and normal educational and intellectual functioning in young autistic children. J Consult Clin Psychol 55:3–9, 1987

Manning M, Hudgins L: Array-based technology and recommendations for utilization in medical genetics practice for detection of chromosomal abnormalities. Genet Med 12:742–745, 2010

McCubbin HI, McCubbin MA: Family stress theory and assessment: the T-double ABCX model of family adjustment and adaptation, in Family Assessment Inventories for Research and Practice. Edited by McCubbin HI, Thompson AI. Madison, University of Wisconsin–Madison, 1987, pp 203–216

McEachin JJ, Smith T, Lovaas OI: Long-term outcome for children with autism who received early intensive behavioral treatment. Am J Ment Retard 97:359–372, 1993

McPheeters ML, Warren Z, Sathe N, et al: A systematic review of treatments for children with autism spectrum disorders. Pediatrics 127:e1312–e1321, 2011

Miller DT, Adam MP, Aradhya S, et al: Consensus statement: chromosomal microarray is a first-tier clinical diagnostic test for individuals with developmental disabilities or congenital anomalies. Am J Hum Genet 86:749–764, 2010

Modahl C, Green LA, Fein D, et al: Oxytocin in autism. Biol Psychiatry 43:270–277, 1998

Montes G, Halterman JS: Association of childhood autism spectrum disorders and loss of family income. Pediatrics 121:e821–e826, 2008

Myers SM, Johnson CP; American Academy of Pediatrics Council on Children with Disabilities: Management of children with autism spectrum disorders. Pediatrics 120:1162–1182, 2007

Nadig A, Ozonoff S, Young GS, et al: A prospective study of response to name in infants at risk for autism. Arch Pediatr Adolesc Med 161:378–383, 2007

National Autism Center: National standards report. 2009. Available at: http://www.nationalautismcenter.org/pdf/NAC%20Standards%20Report.pdf. Accessed April 18, 2012.

National Autism Center: Resource guides. 2012. Available at: http://www.nationalautismcenter.org/learning/guides.php. Accessed April 4, 2012.

Niederhofer H: Glutamate antagonists seem to be slightly effective in psychopharmacologic treatment of autism. J Clin Psychopharmacol 27:317–318, 2007

Nordahl CW, Lange N, Li DD, et al: Brain enlargement is associated with regression in preschool-age boys with autism spectrum disorders. Proc Natl Acad Sci USA 108:20195–20200, 2011

Odom SL, Collet-Klingenberg L, Rogers SJ, et al: Evidence-based practices in interventions for children and youth with autism spectrum disorders. Preventing School Failure 54:275–282, 2010

Offit PA, Coffin SE: Communicating science to the public: MMR vaccine and autism. Vaccine 22:1–6, 2003

Oppenheim D, Koren-Karie N, Dolev S, et al: Maternal insightfulness and resolution of the diagnosis are associated with secure attachment in preschoolers with autism spectrum disorders. Child Dev 80:519–527, 2009

Osborne LA, McHugh L, Saunders J, et al: Parenting stress reduces the effectiveness of early teaching interventions for autistic spectrum disorders. J Autism Dev Disord 38:1092–1103, 2008

Osterling J, Dawson G: Early recognition of children with autism: a study of first birthday home videotapes. J Autism Dev Disord 24:247–257, 1994

Owley T, Salt J, Guter S, et al: A prospective, open-label trial of memantine in the treatment of cognitive, behavioral, and memory dysfunction in pervasive developmental disorders. J Child Adolesc Psychopharmacol 16:517–524, 2006

Ozonoff S, Griffith EM: Neuropsychological function and the external validity of Asperger syndrome, in Asperger Syndrome. Edited by Klin A, Volkmar FR, Sparrow SS. New York, Guilford, 2000, pp 72–96

Ozonoff S, Williams BJ, Landa R: Parental report of the early development of children with regression autism: the delays-plus-regression phenotype. Autism 9:461–486, 2005

Ozonoff S, Young GS, Carter A, et al: Recurrence risk for autism spectrum disorders: a Baby Siblings Research Consortium study. Pediatrics 128:e488–e495, 2011

Pardo CA, Vargas DL, Zimmerman AW: Immunity, neuroglia and neuroinflammation in autism. Int Rev Psychiatry 17:485–495, 2005

Parker SK, Schwartz B, Todd J, et al: Thimerosal-containing vaccines and autistic spectrum disorder: a critical review of published original data. Pediatrics 114:793–804, 2004

Perry R, Cohen I, DeCarlo R: Case study: deterioration, autism, and recovery in two siblings. J Am Acad Child Adolesc Psychiatry 34:232–237, 1995

Pfeiffer BA, Koenig K, Kinnealey M, et al: Effectiveness of sensory integration interventions in children with autism spectrum disorders: a pilot study. Am J Occup Ther 65:76–85, 2011

Pianta RC, Marvin RS: Patterns of parents' reactions to their child's diagnosis: relations with parent-child interaction. Paper presented at the biennial meeting of the Society for Research in Child Development, New Orleans, LA, 1993

Pierce K, Carter C, Weinfeld M, et al: Detecting, studying, and treating autism early: the one-year well-baby check-up approach. J Pediatr 159:458–465, 2011

Pilowsky T, Yirmiya N, Doppelt O, et al: Social and emotional adjustment of siblings of children with autism. J Child Psychol Psychiatry 45:855–865, 2004

Pinto D, Pagnamenta AT, Klei L, et al: Functional impact of global rare copy number variation in autism spectrum disorders. Nature 466:368–372, 2010

Piven J, Harper J, Palmer P, et al: Course of behavioral change in autism: a retrospective study of high-IQ adolescents and adults. J Am Acad Child Adolesc Psychiatry 35:523–529, 1996

Pollman MM, Finkenauer C, Begeer S: Mediators of the link between autistic traits and relationship satisfaction in a non-clinical sample. J Autism Dev Disord 40:470–478, 2010

Purcell AE, Jeon OH, Zimmerman AW, et al: Postmortem brain abnormalities of the glutamate neurotransmitter system in autism. Neurology 57:1618–1628, 2001

Reichenberg A, Gross R, Weiser M, et al: Advancing paternal age and autism. Arch Gen Psychiatry 63:1026–1032, 2006

Reichow B, Wolery M: Comprehensive synthesis of early intensive behavioral interventions for young children with autism based on the UCLA Young Autism Project Model. J Autism Dev Disord 39:23–41, 2009

Research Units on Pediatric Psychopharmacology Autism Network: Randomized, controlled, crossover trial of methylphenidate in pervasive developmental disorders with hyperactivity. Arch Gen Psychiatry 62:1266–1274, 2005

Robins DL, Fein D, Barton ML, et al: The Modified Checklist for Autism in Toddlers: an initial study investigating the early detection of autism and pervasive developmental disorders. J Autism Dev Disord 31:131–144, 2001

Rogers SJ, Dawson G: Early Start Denver Model for Young Children With Autism: Promoting Language, Learning, and Engagement. New York, Guilford, 2010

Rogers SJ, Vismara L: Evidence-based comprehensive treatments for early autism. J Clin Child Adolesc Psychol 37:8–38, 2008

Rutter M: Autistic children growing up. Dev Med Child Neurol 26:122–129, 1984

Rutter M, Bailey A, Lord C: Social Communication Questionnaire. Los Angeles, CA, Western Psychological Services, 2003a

Rutter M, Le Couteur A, Lord C: ADI-R: Autism Diagnostic Interview—Revised. Los Angeles, CA, Western Psychological Services, 2003b

Schmidt RJ, Hansen RL, Hartiala J, et al: Prenatal vitamins, one-carbon metabolism gene variants, and risk for autism. Epidemiology 22:476–485, 2011

Seltzer MM, Krauss MW, Shattuck PT, et al: The symptoms of autism spectrum disorders in adolescence and adulthood. J Autism Dev Disord 33:565–581, 2003

Sharpley CF, Bitsika V, Efremidis B: Influence of gender, parental health, and perceived expertise of assistance upon stress, anxiety, and depression among parents of children with autism. J Intellect Dev Disabil 22:19–28, 1997

Shattuck PT, Durkin M, Maenner M, et al: Timing of identification among children with an autism spectrum disorder: findings from a population-based surveillance study. J Am Acad Child Adolesc Psychiatry 48:474–483, 2009

Shen Y, Dies KA, Holm IA, et al: Clinical genetic testing for patients with autism spectrum disorders. Pediatrics 125:e727–e735, 2010

Shinohe A, Hashimoto K, Nakamura K, et al: Increased serum levels of glutamate in adult patients with autism. Prog Neuropsychopharmacol Biol Psychiatry 30:1472–1477, 2006

Siller M, Sigman M: The behaviors of parents of children with autism predict the subsequent development of their children's communication. J Autism Dev Disord 32:77–89, 2002

Siller M, Sigman M: Modeling longitudinal change in the language abilities of children with autism: parent behaviors and child characteristics as predictors of change. Dev Psychol 44:1691–1704, 2008

Silverman JL, Tolu SS, Barkan CL, et al: Repetitive self-grooming behavior in the BTBR mouse model of autism is blocked by the mGluR5 antagonist MPEP. Neuropsychopharmacology 35:976–989, 2010

Siperstein R, Volkmar F: Brief report: parental reporting of regression in children with pervasive developmental disorders. J Autism Dev Disord 34:731–734, 2004

Smith LO, Elder JH: Siblings and family environments of persons with autism spectrum disorder: a review of the literature. J Child Adolesc Psychiatr Nurs 23:189–195, 2010

Spence MA: The genetics of autism. Curr Opin Pediatr 13:561–565, 2001

Spence SJ, Schneider MT: The role of epilepsy and epileptiform EEGs in autism spectrum disorders. Pediatr Res 65:599–606, 2009

Suedfeld P: Reactions to societal trauma: distress and/or eustress. Polit Psychol 18:849–861, 1997

Szatmari P, Bryson SE, Streiner DL, et al: Two-year outcome of preschool children with autism or Asperger's syndrome. Am J Psychiatry 157:1980–1987, 2000

Tuchman R, Rapin I: Epilepsy in autism. Lancet Neurol 1:352–358, 2002

Tuman JP, Roth-Johnson D, Baker DL, et al: Autism and special education policy in Mexico. Global Health Governance 2, 2008. Available at: http://ssrn.com/abstract=1578963. Accessed April 6, 2012.

Vargas DL, Nascimbene C, Krishnan C, et al: Neuroglial activation and neuroinflammation in the brain of patients with autism. Ann Neurol 57:67–81, 2005

Virues-Ortega J: Applied behavior analytic intervention for autism in early childhood: meta-analysis, meta-regression and dose-response meta-analysis of multiple outcomes. Clin Psychol Rev 30:387–399, 2010

Vismara LA, Rogers SJ: Behavioral treatments in autism spectrum disorder: what do we know? Annu Rev Clin Psychol 6:447–468, 2010

Volkmar F, Cook EH, Pomeroy J, et al: Practice parameters for the assessment and treatment of children, adolescents and adults with autism and other pervasive developmental disorders. J Am Acad Child Adolesc Psychiatry 38(suppl):32S–54S, 1999

Wachtel K, Carter AS: Reaction to diagnosis and parenting styles among mothers of young children with ASDs. Autism 12:575–594, 2008

Wetherby AM, Woods J, Allen L, et al: Early indicators of autism spectrum disorders in the second year of life. J Autism Dev Disord 34:473–493, 2004

Wing L, Potter D: The epidemiology of autistic spectrum disorders: is the prevalence rising? Ment Retard Dev Disabil Res Rev 8:151–161, 2002

Wing L, Yeates SR, Brierley LM, et al: The prevalence of early childhood autism: comparison of administrative and epidemiological studies. Psychol Med 6:89–100, 1976

Woodard C, Groden J, Goodwin M, et al: The treatment of the behavioral sequelae of autism with dextromethorphan: a case report. J Autism Dev Disord 35:515–518, 2005

Woodard C, Groden J, Goodwin M, et al: A placebo double-blind pilot study of dextromethorphan for problematic behaviors in children with autism. Autism 11:29–41, 2007

Wu S, Jia M, Ruan Y, et al: Positive association of the oxytocin receptor gene (OXTR) with autism in the Chinese Han population. Biol Psychiatry 58:74–77, 2005

Zimmerman AW, Jyonouchi H, Comi AM, et al: Cerebrospinal fluid and serum markers of inflammation in autism. Pediatr Neurol 33:195–201, 2005

Zimmerman AW, Connors SL, Pardo CA: Neuroimmunology and neurotransmitters in autism, in Autism: A Neurological Disorder of Early Brain Development. Edited by Tuchman R, Rapin I. London, MacKeith Press, 2006, pp 141–159

Zimmerman AW, Connors SL, Matteson KJ, et al: Maternal antibrain antibodies in autism. Brain Behav Immun 21:351–357, 2007

Zwaigenbaum L, Bryson S, Rogers T, et al: Behavioral manifestations of autism in the first year of life. Int J Dev Neurosci 23:143–152, 2005

CHAPTER 2

ATTENTION-DEFICIT/HYPERACTIVITY DISORDER

Julie B. Schweitzer, Ph.D.
Murat Pakyurek, M.D.
J. Faye Dixon, Ph.D.

Signs, Symptoms, and Developmental Course

Attention-deficit/hyperactivity disorder (ADHD) is characterized by age-inappropriate, significant, and chronic inattention and/or excessive motor restlessness and impulsivity. To qualify for a diagnosis of ADHD, these symptoms must occur across settings, including home and school for children or home and work for adults. Common inattentive symptoms may include difficulty maintaining attention, poor organizational skills, careless mistakes, forgetfulness, trouble listening, and distractibility. Hyperactive/impulsive symptoms include restlessness, excessive talking, poor self-control, and interrupting.

In recent years, the field has invoked cognitive neuroscience terminology to describe and tease apart more finely the symptoms associated with the disorder. Many of the common symptoms of ADHD are now subsumed under umbrella terms such as executive dysfunction, cognitive control (i.e., flexible responding to meet current demands by focusing on task-relevant over irrel-

Support provided to J.B. Schweitzer by the UC Davis Center for Excellence in Developmental Disabilities and by Department of Health and Human Services Administration for Children and Families Grant 90DD0596/01.

evant stimuli), response inhibition, and motivational impairments. *Executive functioning* is a broad term that encompasses many of the processes that seem to be impaired in ADHD. These processes include but are not limited to working memory, response inhibition, attention, planning, monitoring, and behavior adjustment according to task demands. Working memory deficits, which include difficulty in the ongoing maintenance and manipulation of information to be used in the future, may be subsumed under executive and cognitive control dysfunction, and they present the most robust evidence of cognitive deficits in ADHD (Willcutt et al. 2005).

ADHD is also typically characterized by high degrees of intraindividual variability in reaction time (e.g., Castellanos et al. 2005). Intraindividual variability has emerged as an important endophenotype for the disorder. Increased reaction time variability has been associated with fluctuations in attention or arousal (Bellgrove et al. 2004; Cao et al. 2008; Stuss et al. 2003), with response to medication, and with the DAT-1 dopamine transporter genotype. On a clinical level, these intraindividual fluctuations seem to correspond with the characterization of children with ADHD as showing great variability from day to day and even hour to hour in their performance at home or school. Parents and teachers are often perplexed by the variability they see in school and home settings day to day within a child. This variability can be frustrating for caregivers and the children with ADHD because they may not understand why attention and performance may be far superior at some times than others. These studies on intraindividual variability and reaction time suggest that this variability is a common and core problem associated with ADHD.

The core symptoms of ADHD can change dramatically with development (Biederman et al. 2000). The cognitive symptoms of ADHD, including inattention and distractibility, are most likely to continue through adolescence and adulthood for about two-thirds of individuals with ADHD (Turgay et al. 2012). Problems with impulsivity may decrease for some adolescents, and the form of impulsivity may decrease from overt physical acts to other more subtle yet significant high-risk behaviors. These behaviors may include greater substance abuse, traffic accidents, and earlier initiation of sexual activity and intercourse. Hyperactivity is the behavior that declines the greatest with development. Rather than demonstrating the excessive running and climbing associated with childhood, adolescents and adults with ADHD may appear more fidgety and report a cognitive "restlessness." Other related problems associated with ADHD, including poor peer relationships, may remain throughout development.

DSM-IV-TR lists three ADHD subtypes: predominantly inattentive, predominantly hyperactive-impulsive, and combined. Individuals diagnosed with the combined subtype exhibit both inattentive and hyperactive-impulsive symptoms to a significant degree. Individuals identified with the inattentive or hyperactive-impulsive subtype present with predominantly inattention or with predominantly hyperactive-impulsive symptoms, respectively. Developmental changes also appear to affect subtype classification. The hyperactive-impulsive subtype is most common among young children, who may be better characterized as having the combined type as the individuals mature and the inattentive symptoms become more observable. Many individuals with the combined subtype during the primary grades are more likely to meet criteria only for the inattentive subtype during adolescence and young adulthood, when they no longer exhibit the same degree of hyperactive or impulsive symptoms. A substantial portion of the adolescents and young adults may exhibit a more subtle motor restlessness or impulsivity as they mature and may be better characterized as having a subthreshold combined subtype. Another type of ADHD under discussion in the field is sluggish cognitive tempo ADHD, which is not a DSM category (Baumeister et al. 2012; Jacobson et al. 2012; McBurnett et al. 2001). Sluggish cognitive tempo ADHD is most closely associated with an inattentive type of ADHD and is characterized by *hypo*activity, apparent daydreaming, sluggishness, and inconsistent alertness. The sluggish cognitive tempo type may be distinct from the other types of ADHD.

A better understanding of subtypes or subgroups within the broad category of ADHD is likely to lead to improved diagnosis and personalized treatments. Increasing evidence suggests that genetic profile, treatment response, and brain activity differ across subtypes; however, consistent, robust differences on a neuropsychological level are difficult to identify across ADHD subtypes. Most neuropsychological research studies suggest that the inattentive subtype is on a continuum with the combined subtype. New research using more sensitive measures of brain functioning, such as functional magnetic resonance imaging (fMRI) and event-related potentials, is beginning to show that there are distinct differences in brain functioning across subtypes that may not be apparent via neuropsychological measures. A great deal of current research and interest is focused on possible associations between brain development changes during adolescence and young adulthood and changes in the symptom presentation in ADHD. This work includes trying to predict who may outgrow ADHD symptoms and "remit" with maturity. DSM-5 is likely to include some changes in regard to how subtypes are addressed; however, the issue is still under debate.

Epidemiology

ADHD is considered the most common childhood behavioral disorder. Prevalence rates of ADHD in the childhood population vary. DSM-IV-TR

(American Psychiatric Association 2000) reports 3%–7% among school-age children (American Psychiatric Association 2000), whereas other studies cite estimates of 5%–10% (Scahill and Schwab-Stone 2000). Preschool rates of prevalence are less known; however, reported rates vary from 2% to 11.4%, depending on the instruments and informants used to assess the disorder (Lavigne et al. 2009). ADHD continues to be a common disorder among adults as well. Approximately two-thirds of children and adolescents with the disorder continue to exhibit significant symptoms as adults. Prevalence rates in adults are estimated to be about 4.4%, based on estimates from the National Comorbidity Survey Replication (Kessler et al. 2006). The worldwide estimate of ADHD prevalence is 5.29%, with considerable variability across countries. Prevalence estimates in North America and those in Africa and the Middle East vary significantly; however, there are no significant differences in prevalence rates between North America and Europe, South America, Asia, or Oceania (Polanczyk et al. 2007). Methodological differences in how the children were diagnosed (i.e., criteria for diagnosis, source of information on functioning, whether or not criteria needed to be met across situations) were primarily responsible for the great heterogeneity found in prevalence estimates.

Males are more likely than females to be referred for evaluation and diagnosed with ADHD; however, the ratio of boys to girls is greater in clinical samples (approximately 9:1) than in epidemiological samples (3:1). In adult clinical samples, the ratio is closer to 1:1 males to females.

Etiology

Genetic Risk Factors

Strong evidence indicates that ADHD is a genetically predisposed disorder. Estimated heritability for ADHD, based on various twin studies, is around 76% (Faraone et al. 2005). In addition to twin studies, adoption and family studies on ADHD also support the heritable nature of the disorder. Several genomewide linkage studies (Fisher et al. 2002; Smalley et al. 2002) as well as candidate gene studies (Pliszka et al. 1996) assist further understanding of the genetics of ADHD. Possible linkage with moderate effect was found for chromosome bands 5q12, 10q26, 12q23, and 16p13. Examples of the candidate genes for ADHD are dopamine transporter gene *DAT*, D_2 dopamine receptor gene *DRD2*, and D_5 dopamine receptor gene *DRD5*. Other examples are serotonin transporter gene *DRD3* and dopamine beta-hydroxylase gene *DBH*. It is very clear that although ADHD is a genetically predisposed disorder, it does not follow Mendelian patterns of inheritance.

Developmental and Environmental Risk Factors

Prematurity, including moderately preterm (33–36 weeks) delivery, is associated with ADHD, with degree of immaturity significantly increasing risk (Lindstrom et al. 2011). Additional factors thought to contribute to ADHD include environmental toxins, such as prenatal exposure to maternal smoking and alcohol consumption and postnatal exposure to lead. Recently, increased rates of ADHD have been associated with early exposure to even low levels of organophosphates or organochlorine compounds. These compounds are commonly used as pesticides and may be found in fruits and vegetables. The organophosphates may increase the risk of ADHD by interfering with the development of neurotransmitters associated with ADHD.

Associated Neural Alterations in Functioning

ADHD is most commonly associated with impairments in the dopaminergic and noradrenergic neurotransmitter systems. Dopamine is thought to be dysregulated in frontal, striatal, and limbic regions. In a study in adults with ADHD, Volkow et al. (2009) identified decreased dopamine D_2/D_3 receptor and dopamine transporter availability in both the nucleus accumbens and the midbrain. This decreased level of dopamine is theorized to drive individuals with ADHD to "feed" the dopamine system by engaging in high-risk behaviors that may raise the level of dopamine in their system. This area of research also provides an understanding of how a deficiency in the dopamine system, which regulates reward and motivation, has functional outcomes for an individual with ADHD. This research provides clues as to how to design behavioral therapy programs that emphasize the use of rewards (e.g., highly salient, novel, and more immediately delivered rewards) that may be more likely to increase dopamine levels, a topic that is addressed later in this chapter (see "Behavioral and Educational Interventions"). Stimulant medication, such as methylphenidate or dextroamphetamine, is known to alter the dopamine system by blocking the dopamine transporters and increasing the amount of dopamine in the basal ganglia. The medications most commonly prescribed to treat ADHD also affect the noradrenergic system. The noradrenergic system, in concert with the dopaminergic system, regulates attention and arousal.

Several studies have shown decreased frontal cortical brain volume and global brain volume in individuals with ADHD. A longitudinal study (Shaw et al. 2007) measuring cortical thickness suggested that ADHD is a developmental disorder of brain maturation; compared with a typically developing comparison group, the group with ADHD experienced a 3-year delay in attaining peak thickness throughout the cerebrum. Delays in development ranged from 2 to 5 years for peak thickness of the prefrontal regions in the ADHD group. Notably, compared to the control group, the ADHD group had slightly (about 4 months) earlier peak thickness in the primary motor cortex.

Functional neuroimaging research repeatedly finds significant differences between those with ADHD and typically developing groups in brain activity in frontal, anterior cingulate, basal ganglia, and cerebellar function. Most but not all functional imaging studies find decreased brain activation in parts of the frontal cortex and anterior cingulate cortex in ADHD. However, a number of studies have also shown relatively increased brain activation in ADHD (see Fassbender and Schweitzer 2006). Abnormalities in basal ganglia activation are implicated in ADHD, with mixed evidence on whether the alteration in basal ganglia activity is increased or decreased (see Fassbender and Schweitzer 2006). Other subcortical brain regions, including the cerebellum and posterior brain regions, such as the posterior parietal lobe, are also implicated in ADHD and show either significantly increased or decreased brain activity during task and resting-state conditions. Measures of brain connectivity are becoming more frequent in ADHD research and suggest altered connectivity between prefrontal and posterior brain regions during task-related fMRI and resting-state fMRI studies (Konrad and Eickhoff 2010). Decreased connectivity between prefrontal and posterior brain regions would likely lead to less coordinated and efficient processing of information during tasks requiring active attention and working memory.

Differential relationships between altered functional neuroanatomy and the inattentive versus impulsive symptoms in ADHD are captured in the dual- or multiple-pathway model of ADHD (Castellanos et al. 2006; Sonuga-Barke 2003, 2005). This model attempts to characterize the contributions of executive functioning deficits of ADHD ("cool processes") associated with cognitive processes such as inattention versus those of reward responsivity/motivational impairments ("hot processes") associated with impulsivity and responding to affective, salient stimuli. The model addresses the individual variation found in ADHD (Castellanos et al. 2006; Sonuga-Barke 2003). Some children may experience greater impairment in one pathway, whereas other children may experience impairment along both or multiple pathways. The framework suggests that ADHD symptoms arise from 1) a deficit in executive functioning related to improper functioning of the dorsolateral prefrontal cortex and/or 2) an overdependence on immediate rewards and mesolimbic dopamine dysfunction. Furthermore, there is an imbalance and a failure of the executive function–prefrontal cortical regions to modulate hyperactive reward–striatal regions in ADHD. Those individuals who are experiencing greater impairments in the executive system display greater problems with attention, whereas individuals with greater impairments in the reward–dopamine system are likely to display more impulsive behavior. Persons with ADHD who experience impairments in both systems will be less likely to engage the executive system to modulate their behavior and are more likely to display impulsivity, hyperactivity, and inattention. Sonuga-Barke (2005) has proposed an updated version of this model, suggesting that temporal processing deficits should be considered in future models. The overall idea of trying to develop a model to account for the heterogeneity of ADHD is an advance and will continue to be influential in the field and will likely stimulate future research in identifying subgroups under the umbrella diagnosis of ADHD.

Animal Models

Animal models permit the study of specific neurotransmitters on a much finer-grained level than can be done in humans. This research can further the understanding of a disorder and lead to better genetic models. These models can also be useful for testing novel behavioral and pharmacological treatments in developing organisms that could not be tested in humans. The most commonly studied animal model of ADHD is the spontaneously hypertensive rat (SHR; Sagvolden et al. 2005). The SHR has good face validity for ADHD in that, similar to children with ADHD, the rat has decreased response inhibition, high rates of hyperactivity and impulsivity that increase as novelty decreases, heightened sensitivity to delays in delayed reward paradigms, and poor sustained attention. Similar to persons with ADHD, the rat also has impaired dopaminergic and noradrenergic systems. Unlike children with ADHD, however, the rat also is hypertensive. More recently, a variant of the SHR was developed by crossbreeding the SHR with the Wistar-Kyoto rat to produce the Wistar-Kyoto "hyperactive" (WKHA) rat. This model may be superior to the SHR model because the WKHA rat does not have hypertension.

Another recent development in animal models for ADHD is the development of mouse models (Fan et al. 2012). The availability of mouse models greatly facilitates the use of genetic studies in ADHD because mouse models of gene-behavior interactions are more established. Mouse models include a dopamine transporter knockout mouse model and the coloboma mutant mouse (Cm/+) that displays hyperactivity associated with the SNAP-25 mutant allele. These mouse models, however, have fewer of the behavioral characteristics of ADHD than are found in the SHR or WKHA rat models.

Other investigators are studying the potential of a domestic dog genetic and behavioral model of ADHD. The dog has more complex social behavior than rodent models and is genetically closer to humans than humans are to rodents. Use of an ADHD rating scale developed for children has been shown to result in owner-rated dog scores that are reliable on "inattention" and "hyperactivity-impulsivity" axes (Lit et al. 2010). The domestic dog model requires further validation to assess its full potential as an ADHD model.

ADHD and Comorbid Disorders

ADHD increases a person's risk of experiencing additional cognitive, emotional, or behavior disorders across the life span (Brown 2009). Consideration of comorbidity is crucial, because it may affect the presentation of both ADHD and the comorbid disorder. The exact prevalence of comorbidity appears to vary based on what methodological procedures are used and whether a study uses a cross-sectional or longitudinal design. A consistent conclusion, however, is that comorbid psychiatric conditions are common with ADHD. It appears that comorbidity is influenced by genetics, because persons with ADHD may be more vulnerable to particular comorbidities depending on heredity. Relatives of children with ADHD not only have increased rates of ADHD but also have higher than expected rates of antisocial personality, alcoholism, and substance abuse (Angold et al. 1999).

According to Wilens et al. (2002), 74% of preschoolers with ADHD had at least one other comorbid diagnosis. In the Preschool ADHD Treatment Study, Posner et al. (2007) reported that 52% of participants met criteria for oppositional defiant disorder, 24.7% for communication disorders, and 14% for anxiety disorders. Comorbidity also contributed to a lower clinician rating of functioning compared with ratings for preschoolers with ADHD alone. In school-age children with ADHD, approximately 30% met criteria for a learning disability (DuPaul and Stoner 2003). (See Chapter 10 for further discussion of the evaluation and treatment of learning disorders.) According to Barkley (2006), children with ADHD are at higher risk for developing behavior problems such as aggression and noncompliance at home and school. Children with a tic or Tourette's disorder should also be assessed for ADHD because these disorders are highly comorbid with ADHD. During adolescence, there may be greater concern regarding substance use disorders and conduct disorders in individuals with ADHD. Adolescents with ADHD also have high rates of comorbid oppositional defiant disorder (59%–65%) and major depressive disorder (29%). In addition, 11% of adolescents with ADHD manifest bipolar disorder (Robin 1998). Adults with ADHD have an increased risk for academic impairment, occupational problems (including underemployment and lower pay), and relationship difficulties (higher rates of separation and divorce). Psychiatric comorbidities in adults with ADHD include major depressive disorder, 20%; anxiety disorders, 25%; bipolar disorder, 10%; and antisocial personality disorder, 10% and higher (based on various research studies).

ADHD and high-functioning autism have a high rate of overlapping deficits (e.g., executive dysfunction), yet DSM-IV-TR does not permit a diagnosis of autism comorbid with ADHD; that fact is expected to change with DSM-5. Differentiating between high-functioning autism and ADHD can be a diagnostic challenge but is important, particularly for those children with autism who respond well to early intervention. Children with both ADHD and autism have higher rates of poor attention and organizational skills, problems following rules, and difficulty in social relationships. Persons with either ADHD or autism should be evaluated for these common symptoms. The type of intervention, its effectiveness, and side effects may differ depending on whether an individual's primary symptoms are those of ADHD or autism. For instance, stimulant medications tend to be effective in treating ADHD symptoms in autism but may have greater side effects in autism than in ADHD. Many ongoing studies are exploring the relationship between symptoms in these two neurodevelopmental disorders, which should aid in the assessment and treatment of both in the future.

The presence of a comorbid disorder may also affect the treatment plan for ADHD and the comorbid disorder. Previous studies (MTA Cooperative Group 1999) found that when a child had comorbid anxiety or oppositional defiant disorder, the choice of combined parent education with medication was more beneficial than medication alone. Treating patients with comorbid substance use disorder and ADHD may be particularly challenging, because these patients may be less likely to be prescribed a stimulant medication due to concerns about its abuse. There are also alternative delivery forms of stimulant medication with less potential for abuse, such as the transdermal patch delivery of methylphenidate. The decision regarding how to treat a patient with ADHD and a comorbid substance use disorder should be made on an individual basis.

Occasionally, a patient with ADHD may have a concomitant medical condition that may influence treatment decisions. For example, comorbid ADHD and a medical condition, such as asthma or a seizure disorder, may occur and will require appropriate consultation and ongoing communication between care providers to better prioritize presenting difficulties and minimize any potential problems, such as lower seizure threshold due to use of stimulant medications.

In conclusion, psychiatric comorbidity with ADHD is common. It is, therefore, very important for the clinician to properly assess patients and diagnose not only ADHD but also any comorbid conditions. Careful diagnosis will help determine the treatment strategy and most effective services within the framework of a multimodal approach.

Behavioral and Psychological Evaluation

DSM-IV-TR lists nine possible inattentive and nine hyperactive-impulsive symptoms of ADHD. A child or adolescent must have six or more symptoms for at least 6 months to meet criteria for either symptom category. These symptoms must cause functional impairment in two or more settings, and the onset of symptoms must generally occur prior to age 7 years. Diagnostic subtypes include predominantly inattentive, predominantly hyperactive-impulsive, and both symptom categories, also known as combined type. Some of these criteria, such as age at onset, are likely to change with the publication of DSM-5.

The American Academy of Child and Adolescent Psychiatry practice guidelines for assessment of youth with ADHD (Pliszka 2007) recommend a comprehensive evaluation including a clinical interview of the child and parent, collection of a teacher or day care provider report of child functioning, and evaluation for ADHD psychiatric comorbidities. Typically, assessment also involves a complete medical and family history, physical examination, and behavior rating scales completed by parents and teachers. Neuroimaging (single-photon emission computed tomography, MRI, fMRI) or electroencephalography (EEG) is not necessary or recommended for diagnosing ADHD. MRI or EEG may be indicated if a person has other neurological symptoms (e.g., seizures, changes in behavior after a head injury) that need to be ruled out. Psychological assessment in the form of cognitive and academic testing can be included, but this is done primarily to address comorbid learning issues and is not required to make an accurate diagnosis of ADHD.

Parent and teacher interviews and rating scales are recommended for both the evaluation of ADHD and the monitoring of treatment response. DSM-IV rating scales assess symptoms specific to ADHD and include measures such as the SNAP-IV Teacher and Parent Rating Scale (Swanson 1992), the Vanderbilt AD/HD Diagnostic Teacher Rating Scale (Wolraich et al. 1998), and the Child Symptom Inventory—4 (Gadow and Sprafkin 2002). Broadband measures such as the Child Behavior Checklist (Achenbach 1991), the Behavior Assessment System for Children, 2nd Edition (Reynolds and Kamphaus 2004), and Conners' Rating Scales, 3rd Edition (Conners 2008), not only include ADHD symptoms but are helpful in rating other possible comorbidities, such as aggression, conduct disorder, oppositional behavior, learning problems, and family relations. Structured and semistructured interviews such as the Diagnostic Interview for Children and Adolescents (Reich 2000) and the Schedule for Affective Disorders and Schizophrenia for School-Age Children (Kaufman et al. 1996) provide further utility by encompassing both the rating of symptoms and in-depth clinician interviews to also assess disorders such as depression, anxiety, or other disruptive behavior conditions.

Supplementation by other rating scales that specifically target the evaluation of comorbid disorders highly associated with ADHD can be helpful. These scales include the Revised Children's Manifest Anxiety Scale, 2nd Edition (Reynolds and Richmond 2000) and the Multidimensional Anxiety Scale for Children (March 1997). Measures of depression, including the Children's Depression Inventory—2 (Kovacs 1992), Children's Depression Rating Scale, Revised (Poznanski and Mokros 1996), and Beck Depression Inventory for Youth, 2nd Edition (Beck et al. 1996), may also be indicated. The Children's Yale-Brown Obsessive Compulsive Scale (Scahill et al. 1997) can be used to diagnose the severity of obsessive and compulsive behavior. The Child Mania Rating Scale for Parents (Pavuluri et al. 2006) can help distinguish between mania and ADHD, whereas the Overt Aggression Scale (Coccaro et al. 1991) can be used to assess aggressive behaviors. As mentioned earlier, the presence of a tic or Tourette's disorder should be assessed because such a disorder is commonly comorbid with ADHD and, if present, may influence treatment decisions.

Environmental factors and the psychological health and stress levels of family members should be ascertained during the evaluation. Understanding the context of the child will be important and may influence treatment decision making. Moderators such as parental depression have been shown to influence the efficacy of various treatments for children with ADHD (Hinshaw 2007). Therefore, researchers are now recommending that parents of children with ADHD who are experiencing depression should have the depression addressed.

Academic Impact of ADHD With or Without Learning Disabilities

ADHD is a chronic, persistent disorder with substantial impact on school, peer, and home functioning extending beyond childhood and into adulthood for at least 50%–70% of individuals with the disorder. School performance is often significantly affected in children with ADHD and is often typified by less work completion, more inaccuracy, and more off-task and disruptive classroom behavior. Academic underachievement is estimated to occur in 18%–53% of children with ADHD (Anastopoulos and Shelton 2001). Untreated or undertreated ADHD is associated with higher school failure, suspension, and dropout rates, and also leads to increased rates of unemployment or underemployment, more relationship problems, and increased alcohol and substance use (Barkley 2006; Breslau et al. 2011;

Hinshaw et al. 2002). Consequently, special education services are often needed to facilitate academic success. Research by Breslau et al. (2009) revealed that attentional functioning at age 6 is one of the strongest predictors of academic achievement at age 17. Those data suggest that failure to address attentional problems in young children has long-term significant negative ramifications for children with ADHD.

For many children, the behavioral and attentional challenges inherent in ADHD interfere with satisfactory academic progress. However, a significant number of children exhibit both ADHD and distinct learning disabilities that further complicate academic achievement. Diagnostic assessment by a psychologist, neuropsychologist, or speech pathologist may be necessary for ascertaining the presence of other developmental disorders, such as learning disabilities or language disorders, in children with ADHD. ADHD most frequently co-occurs with reading challenges (dyslexia), and there is an overlap of 25%–45% between these diagnoses, especially for the inattentive subtype of ADHD (Willcutt et al. 2005). Differentiating between learning disabilities and ADHD can sometimes be a challenge, because both can affect attention and persistence of effort during academic performance. Children with dyslexia, however, experience difficulty with phonological awareness, fluency, and automaticity, whereas youths with ADHD manifest problems with behavioral regulation and attention. Deficits in working memory and processing speed common to both ADHD and learning disabilities appear to account for the strong link between the two (Willcutt et al. 2010). For the student who meets criteria for both ADHD and a learning disability, the intervention strategies must include both behavioral and educational interventions and medication, when indicated.

Educational and behavioral interventions for children with ADHD may be provided under Section 504 of the Rehabilitation Act of 1973, a civil rights law, or the Individuals With Disabilities Education Act Amendments of 1997 (IDEA), a special education law. Both laws guarantee eligible students a free and appropriate public education. Psychologists and educational professionals can assist families in determining which law is most appropriate for their child's specific educational and behavioral needs.

Interventions

Psychopharmacological Treatment

Stimulant Medications

Psychopharmacological treatment should be part of a multimodal treatment approach for the best possible results. Although there are various options, stimulant medications are the recommended initial line of treatment for ADHD. The two broad categories of stimulant medications are methylphenidate and amphetamine-based drugs (e.g., dextroamphetamine, mixed amphetamine salts) (Table 2–1).

Table 2–1. Stimulants for treating attention-deficit/hyperactivity disorder

Methylphenidate

Short acting: Ritalin, Focalin

Long acting: Concerta, Metadate ER, Methylin ER, Ritalin LA, Ritalin SR, Focalin XR

Transdermal: Daytrana patch

Dextroamphetamine

Short acting: Dexedrine

Long acting: Dexedrine Spansule, Vyvanse[a]

Mixed amphetamine salts

Short acting: Adderall

Long acting: Adderall XR

[a]Vyvanse is an amphetamine prodrug.

These categories appear to be equivalent in efficacy and overall side-effect profile; however, individuals may respond differently to them based on genetic factors or the presence of comorbid psychiatric conditions. Generally, a patient should be switched from one to the other stimulant class if, during treatment, a stimulant medication remains limited in its efficacy despite adequate dosing. Similarly, if one stimulant cannot be tolerated due to an adverse effect, a trial with a stimulant from the other class may be considered.

In recent years, new and innovative stimulant delivery systems have emerged, such as OROS (osmotic-controlled release oral delivery system) and transdermal delivery systems, that result in improved tolerability and better treatment compliance. Patients now have more consistent symptom control throughout the day. An advantage of stimulant medications is that their clinical effect is evident within the first few days. Although these medications can be stopped abruptly, so-called drug holidays are no longer recommended, at least for the majority of patients with ADHD.

Nonstimulant Medications

Nonstimulant medications are usually considered for individuals who have failed at least two stimulant trials, those who have a history of severe adverse effects with stimulant medications, and individuals with significant potential for abuse. In some cases, parental or patient preference may be the main reason for a nonstimulant medication trial. Atomoxetine, a nonstimulant medication, is a selective norepinephrine reuptake inhibitor that has received U.S. Food and Drug Administration (FDA) approval for individuals age 6 and older with ADHD. Atomoxetine is a useful option, especially for youth with ADHD and comorbid anxiety. In addition, atomoxetine may be preferred by some families because it is not a controlled substance. Certain side effects, including appetite suppression, may be less of a problem than with stimulant medications. Atomoxetine is a slow-acting medication, and several weeks may be necessary to achieve the full effect (Hammerness et al. 2009). A potential concern is the 2005 FDA boxed warning that resulted from a reported increase in suicidal thinking. The suicidal thinking in placebo-controlled trials was four cases per 1,000 patients in atomoxetine treatment versus no such events in placebo-treated patients (www.fda.gov/Drugs/DrugSafety).

The α_2-adrenergic agonists clonidine and guanfacine are commonly used for ADHD symptom control, usually in cases with poor or limited response to FDA-approved treatments. They are essentially antihypertensive medications with potential for abrupt increase in blood pressure when stopped suddenly by the patient. Therefore, patient and family education at the outset is of paramount importance. Available newer delivery systems for these medications, such as OROS and beaded delivery systems, are likely to help with compliance and tolerability.

Tricyclic antidepressants (TCAs) are also off label for ADHD treatment. Due to their cardiac effects, they require baseline and follow-up electrocardiographic (ECG) monitoring. They may cause a prolonged QT interval, which can be life threatening (Sicouri and Antzelevitch 2008). In case of overdose, TCAs have high risk of fatality.

Bupropion is an antidepressant with a recent FDA boxed warning for suicidal thinking, depressed mood, hostility, and change in behaviors (www.fda.gov/Drugs/DrugSafety). The medication has short and extended forms. Its use for ADHD treatment remains off label.

Side Effects and Treatment Monitoring

Stimulant medications may lead to decreased appetite, sleep difficulties, irritability, transient tics, an increase in pulse and blood pressure, and sudden death. Appetite suppression is a particular concern in younger children and needs to be monitored closely with regular vital signs and basal metabolic index calculation. Pediatric consultation should be used when necessary, as in the case of children with abnormal laboratory results (hyperthyroidism), with questionable facial dysmorphisms, or with a significant personal or family history of cardiac problems. To address insomnia, strategies include earlier administration of the medication, dose reduction, efforts to improve general sleep behaviors, and switching to a shorter-acting form of the medication (Kratochvil et al. 2005). Although stimulant medications can be used in individuals with tic disorders, careful and close monitoring are necessary (Shprecher and Kurlan 2009). Currently, ECG screening is used for those with identified cardiovascular risk factors. Sudden death is rare, but it is a genuine side effect of stimulant medications in children (Gould et al. 2009).

The prescribing of medication for a chronic disorder such as ADHD requires close monitoring to track the behavioral and functional benefits. The functioning of a child with ADHD can be altered by changes in the child's environment, structure, and development. Thus, it is important to assess whether the prescribed medication is still efficacious and has limited side effects. This can be achieved by implementing checklists in addition to obtaining a history from the child's parents and, if possible, teachers. A careful review of side effects at regular periods is also necessary.

Behavioral and Educational Interventions

Behavioral Interventions

Findings from the Multimodal Treatment Study of ADHD (MTA Cooperative Group 1999) suggest that medication, behavioral parent training/education, and classroom behavior contingency management all represent effective treatment modalities. Maximum treatment effects are reported for treatments that include medication and behavioral interventions (Conners et al. 2001). Although studies examining parental preference for treatment modalities show that most parents prefer behavioral intervention, with fewer parents expressing a preference for medication combined with behavioral treatments (Johnston et al. 2008), continued findings from the MTA group indicate that medication therapy alone consistently provides significant symptom reduction in core deficits such as inattention and hyperactivity. The MTA group also found that the combination of medication therapy and behavioral interventions provided better social and family functioning as well. Behavioral interventions are less likely than medication to address the core symptoms of ADHD, but their positive effect on social and family functioning is valuable. Behavioral interventions can also help address common comorbid symptoms, such as anxiety and oppositionality.

Behavioral parent education and training have been shown to consistently improve child functioning in the home and facilitate better parent-child relationships (Pelham and Fabiano 1998). Behavioral parent education typically constitutes a group format that varies in length from 6 to 24 weeks. Content focuses on use of positive attention, reinforcement contingencies, and behavioral structure in the home. Similarly, school-based interventions, such as classroom-wide behavioral programs that include daily report cards, clear behavioral expectations, and reinforcement plans, also result in improved school behavior (Pelham and Fabiano 2008). The daily report card programs provide consistency of treatment approaches between home and school settings because they are a mechanism for parents to deliver positive consequences at home based on behavior exhibited at school (Chronis et al. 2006). Clinical and school psychologists typically provide guidance to teachers and parents about implementation of these strategies. As in pharmacological interventions, development and changes in the environment can affect targets for treatment, the modality of its delivery (e.g., parent vs. child/adolescent/adult, individual vs. group), and its effectiveness. Thus, ongoing treatment monitoring is important. Major milestones, such as entering middle school, high school, or college, where the responsibility on the patient becomes greater, can add stress and responsibilities that require good preventive planning to minimize potential problems. Checking in with the family around the time of added responsibilities or stressors is recommended.

Educational and Cognitive Training Interventions

Successful educational interventions include a combination of academic and behavioral interventions. Work by Raggi and Chronis (2006) and Langberg et al. (2008) supports the use of organizational skill training, peer tutoring, task/instructional modifications, computer-assisted instruction (e.g., reading and math software), and homework-focused interventions for improving the academic outcomes of students with ADHD. For children with comorbid learning disabilities, these interventions will also include specialized direct instruction and intervention in reading, writing, and mathematics.

Computerized cognitive training programs that target working memory and attention have shown some effectiveness in changing ADHD symptoms as rated by parents but not by teachers. These clinical trials have been conducted with different experimental designs, including some with randomized trials with a waitlist control group and others with double-blind placebo control groups. Working memory training appears to enhance performance on nontrained visuospatial and verbal working memory tasks, with improvements persisting at 3- and 6-month intervals after the training period ceases (Holmes et al. 2009, 2010; Klingberg et al. 2005).

Working memory training also generalized to more global functioning on parent (but not teacher) ADHD rating scales, including measures of executive functioning and measures of complex reasoning (e.g., Klingberg et al. 2005) and on-task behavior during a simulated academic task (Green et al. 2012). The mechanisms underlying the generalization are not clear, but active development and neural plasticity in the frontotemporoparietal executive networks between ages 8 and 18 may make that a critical period to facilitate generalization. We recognize that cognitive training programs for ADHD (Beck et al. 2010; Klingberg 2010; Klingberg et al. 2002, 2005; Olesen et al. 2004) are becoming increasingly popular in research and the commercial sector; however, the evidence base for these programs is still emerging, with few randomized, placebo-controlled studies involving well-characterized samples (see the review by Klingberg 2010; Rutledge et al. 2012).

Studies of the neural mechanism of action underlying cognitive training in ADHD have been promising, but these studies are few and of limited scope (see McNab et al. 2009). Results from modestly sized fMRI studies in healthy adults ($N=3$ and $N=8$ in Westerberg and Klingberg 2007 and Olesen et al. 2004, respectively) and in a group of children with ADHD (Hoekzema et al. 2010) suggest that working memory training increases brain activity in the prefrontal and parietal cortices (Hoekzema et al. 2010), regions frequently associated with working memory processing and executive functioning in general. In a positron emission tomography study of 13 healthy adults, McNab et al. (2009) investigated the neurochemical underpinnings of cognitive training. The study showed increased density of cortical dopamine D_1 receptor binding in the prefrontal cortex and parietal cortex. Thus, cognitive training may improve behavioral and cognitive impairments of ADHD related to disturbances of the dopamine system (Volkow et al. 2007, 2009). These training benefits may extend beyond the active training period, giving cognitive training a distinct advantage over medication and most behavioral training. To our knowledge, the effect of working memory training on neural functioning in ADHD in isolation from broader cognitive training has not been studied.

Family Issues

The presence of parenting stress associated with caregiving for children with ADHD is well established in the research literature (Anastopoulos et al. 1992; Podolski and Nigg 2001). Parenting demands are frequently increased in families with ADHD; parents of children with ADHD report less compliance and higher levels of negative interactions and conflicts.

The most significant predictor of parenting stress is the severity of ADHD symptoms, combined with the presence of oppositional and aggressive behaviors. Additionally, maternal negativity about the child's behavior predicts greater child noncompliance (Hinshaw et al. 2000). A modest relationship between factual knowledge about ADHD and parental stress has been established in at least one study (Harrison and Sofronoff 2002); however, it remains unclear how this relationship is mediated by severity of symptoms and parental attributions and beliefs about the causes of ADHD. Ongoing updates from the MTA group (Molina et al. 2009) support the use of behaviorally focused parent education and training groups to improve family functioning. A recent study by Pfiffner et al. (2011) found improved school and home functioning with use of skill-focused groups for parents, teachers, and children that targeted problem behaviors, social skills, and organizational skills.

Outcomes

ADHD is associated with negative outcomes throughout the life span. In the primary school years, ADHD symptoms are associated with increased odds of injury in fifth graders (Schwebel et al. 2011). Academic achievement is one area that is most readily recognized as being affected by ADHD, and concerns about academic functioning frequently serve as a catalyst for parents to pursue evaluation and treatment. Not only is academic achievement in children with ADHD decreased, but rates of on-time high school graduation also are affected: one-third of children with ADHD do not graduate from high school on time. As noted in the earlier section "ADHD and Comorbid Disorders," rates of substance use disorders are higher in individuals with ADHD, and teenagers with ADHD start smoking cigarettes 1 year earlier than their peers without ADHD (Milberger et al. 1997). In adults, ADHD is associated with poor work performance, greater underemployment and unemployment, higher divorce rates, and greater engagement in criminal behavior (Barkley 2006). Treatment for ADHD does not appear to alter these negative outcomes substantially. Most likely the treatment will be more efficacious over time if it is closely monitored and continued for as long as the child is symptomatic.

New Research Directions

Significant improvements have been made in the conceptualization of ADHD, including advances in understanding the basic neural correlates of the disorder. The majority of the neuroimaging and genetic studies, however, include relatively small sample sizes. International groups of researchers studying ADHD are now working together to try to accelerate understanding of the disorder, including the identification of subgroups; to better characterize the disorder using more objective and perhaps biological methods, in conjunction with interviews and ratings; and to develop more effective treatments. The recognition that approximately one-third of patients with ADHD will no longer be symptomatic in adulthood has invigorated efforts to try to understand and predict for whom the symptoms may remit and to determine whether there are methods to promote the remittance of the symptoms.

Prevention of ADHD is rarely discussed, but there is new interest in thinking about how to prevent or reduce the severity of symptoms in ADHD at all ages. Prevention involves identifying environmental (pre- and postnatal) and genetic factors or early intervention that is timed optimally to reduce the severity of the disorder (e.g., Halperin and Healey 2011).

One of the greatest barriers in the field has been the continued use of diagnostic procedures that rely heavily on parent and teacher reports, which may be fairly subjective. Rating scales are crucial to assist in the evaluation of ADHD, but they cannot assess whether other underlying reasons might explain the behavioral manifestation of symptoms. In-depth interviewing and observations can assist but are not always sufficient. Neuropsychological testing is no longer considered to be required or to be as illuminating for evaluating ADHD as testing in a clinician's office and may not necessarily be reflective of how persons with ADHD behave in the home or school setting. Reliability of neuropsychological methods in ADHD is particularly concerning when one considers that intraindividual variability is a hallmark of ADHD. Measures to quantify inattention versus hyperactivity and impulsivity are particularly challenging to develop, because these symptoms may be difficult to observe and measure easily in a clinical setting.

Another difficulty for persons with ADHD remains the lack of tools to predict treatment response. Children may need to try a few medications before finding a satisfactory balance of symptom relief and side effects. The need to try several different formulations of medications is a frequent complaint of children with ADHD and their parents. Pharmacogenomics and other biomedical technology advances may help better predict medication response and potential side effects in both children and adults with ADHD, as well as help minimize problems with compliance.

In many communities, families have limited access to proper evaluation of ADHD and its common comorbid conditions and to treatment. Creative strategies are needed to improve access for these families. Recent advances in technology make new strategies such as telepsychiatry possible for increased access to specialist assessments and treatment recommendations for ADHD. Telepsychiatry may have a significant advantage over existing and more conventional methods of diagnosing and treating patients with ADHD in parts of the world with difficult access to specialty care. Recent work by Pfiffner et al. (2011) also supports the idea of exporting clinic-based behavioral interventions into an educational setting by partnering with school-based mental health professionals to develop more comprehensive social and behavioral interventions for better coordination between home and school.

Treatment options for ADHD need to be increased for children and adults with the disorder. The number of new agents in the pharmacological pipeline to address ADHD needs to be increased. Despite significant progress in treatment strategies for ADHD over the past several decades, new medications with fewer side effects are needed to address symptoms. There is a need to develop new nonpharmacological treatments (e.g., cognitive training) that can be used alone or in combination with pharmacotherapy across the life span for persons with ADHD. Furthermore, treatments need to be developed that are more effective in working with subgroups within ADHD. Such treatments will enhance the ability to personalize and predict treatment response.

Involving the whole family in addressing ADHD-related difficulties in children is also likely to lead to significantly better treatment compliance. Finally, an important goal is to incorporate a culturally aware approach to educating and supporting families of children with ADHD.

Summary

ADHD is a highly prevalent disorder in children and adults. It is highly heterogeneous in presentation, with the degree and co-occurrence of the symptoms of inattention, hyperactivity, and impulsivity varying in intensity and frequency from one individual to the next. The presentation of these symptoms may change dramatically with development, particularly during adolescence and young adulthood. The changes in symptom presentation are thought to reflect changes in brain development, including maturation in the frontal and parietal lobes, cerebellum, and connectivity between brain regions. ADHD commonly is accompanied by comorbid learning and emotional disorders. These common comorbid disorders need to be considered and addressed as well for optimal quality of life.

Pharmacological intervention frequently works to reduce the core symptoms of ADHD, but it does not cure the disorder and it needs to be continued if the child continues to exhibit symptoms. A variety of novel delivery systems and stimulant and nonstimulant medications for ADHD are available. We recommend that children receive pharmacological treatment and that parents receive education and skill building to improve child functioning and parent-child relationships. Working with parents to assist them in working with their child's school is an important part of the parent education and therapy. Similarly, it is important to work with the child's school to implement behavioral and educational procedures that will maximize the child's success. Most importantly, there needs to be good consistency and communication between the home and school regarding expectations, goals and rewards, and response-cost measures for responding to positive and negative behavior. The outcomes for children and adolescents with ADHD remain a concern, although more treatments than ever before are available for children with this disorder. The majority of children with ADHD who receive high-quality pharmacological and behavioral treatment at some point in their childhood still perform worse on 91% of outcome measures in comparison to their peers without ADHD when assessed several years after the treatment was administered (Molina et al. 2009). Thus, although the previous decade has seen important advancements in the field, a great deal of work still needs to be accomplished to improve the quality of life for children with ADHD and their families.

Key Points

- Attention-deficit/hyperactivity disorder (ADHD) symptoms include inattention, hyperactivity, and impulsivity; however, recent conceptualizations recognize heightened intraindividual variability and include impairments in executive functioning, cognitive control, and reward/motivation.

- Brain imaging studies repeatedly demonstrate differences in groups with ADHD versus healthy control groups; however, brain imaging studies have insufficient support to be used for diagnostic purposes.

- The expression and degree of ADHD symptoms can change with maturity from childhood to adolescence.

- Multi-informant (parent and teacher) rating scales should be used to assess core ADHD symptoms, common comorbid conditions, or conditions mimicking ADHD.

- The gold-standard treatment for ADHD includes a combination of stimulant medication and behavioral therapy approaches to address core symptoms and comorbid conditions.

- Novel pharmacological and nonpharmacological treatments may also provide symptom relief.

Recommended Readings

Barkley RA: Attention-Deficit Hyperactivity Disorder: A Handbook for Diagnosis and Treatment, 3rd Edition. New York, Guilford, 2006

Brown TE (ed): ADHD Comorbidities: Handbook of ADHD Complications in Children and Adults. Washington, DC, American Psychiatric Publishing, 2009

Hinshaw SP: Moderators and mediators of treatment outcome for youth with ADHD: understanding for whom and how interventions work. J Pediatr Psychol 32:664-675, 2007

Minzenberg M: Pharmacotherapy for attention-deficit/hyperactivity disorder: from cells to circuits. Neurotherapeutics, 2012. doi: 10.1007/s13311-012-0128-7

Pelham WE Jr, Fabiano GA: Evidence-based psychosocial treatments for attention-deficit/hyperactivity disorder. J Clin Child Adolesc Psychol 37:184-214, 2008

Pfiffner L: All About ADHD: The Complete Practical Guide for Classroom Teachers, 2nd Edition. New York, Scholastic Professional Books, 2011

Pliszka S: Practice parameter for the assessment and treatment of children and adolescents with attention-deficit/hyperactivity disorder. J Am Acad Child Adolesc Psychiatry 46:894-921, 2007

References

Achenbach TM: Child Behavior Checklist—Cross-Informant Version. Burlington, University of Vermont, Department of Psychology, 1991

American Psychiatric Association: Diagnostic and Statistical Manual of Mental Disorders, 4th Edition, Text Revision. Washington, DC, American Psychiatric Association, 2000

Anastopoulos A, Shelton T: Assessing Attention-Deficit/Hyperactivity Disorder. New York, Kluwer Academic/Plenum Publishers, 2001

Anastopoulos AD, Guevremont D, Shelton T, et al: Parenting stress among families of children with attention deficit hyperactivity disorder. J Abnorm Child Psychol 20:503–520, 1992

Angold A, Costello EJ, Erkanli A: Comorbidity. J Child Psychol Psychiatry 40:57–87, 1999

Barkley RA: Attention-Deficit Hyperactivity Disorder: A Handbook for Diagnosis and Treatment, 3rd Edition. New York, Guilford, 2006

Bauermeister JJ, Barkley RA, Bauermeister JA, et al: Validity of the sluggish cognitive tempo, inattention, and hyperactivity symptom dimensions: neuropsychological and psychosocial correlates. J Abnorm Child Psychol 40:683–697, 2012

Beck JS, Beck AT, Jolly JB: Beck Youth Inventory, 2nd Edition. San Antonio, TX, Pearson, 2005

Beck SJ, Hanson CA, Puffenberger SS, et al: A controlled trial of working memory training for children and adolescents with ADHD. J Clin Child Adolesc Psychol 39:825–836, 2010

Bellgrove MA, Hester R, Garavan H: The functional neuroanatomical correlates of response variability: evidence from a response inhibition task. Neuropsychologia 42:1910–1916, 2004

Biederman J, Mick E, Faraone SV: Age-dependent decline of symptoms of attention deficit hyperactivity disorder: impact of remission definition and symptom type. Am J Psychiatry 157:816–818, 2000

Breslau J, Miller E, Breslau N, et al: The impact of early behavior disturbances on academic achievement in high school. Pediatrics 123:1472–1476, 2009

Breslau J, Miller E, Joanie Chung WJ, et al: Childhood and adolescent onset psychiatric disorders, substance use, and failure to graduate high school on time. J Psychiatr Res 45:295–301, 2011

Brown TE (ed): ADHD Comorbidities: Handbook of ADHD Complications in Children and Adults. Washington, DC, American Psychiatric Publishing, 2009

Cao Q, Zang Y, Zhu C, et al: Alerting deficits in children with attention deficit/hyperactivity disorder: event-related fMRI evidence. Brain Res 1219:159–168, 2008

Castellanos FX, Sonuga-Barke EJ, Scheres A, et al: Varieties of attention-deficit/hyperactivity disorder-related intra-individual variability. Biol Psychiatry 57:1416–1423, 2005

Castellanos FX, Sonuga-Barke EJ, Milham MP, et al: Characterizing cognition in ADHD: beyond executive dysfunction. Trends Cogn Sci 10:117–123, 2006

Chronis AM, Jones HA, Raggi VL: Evidence-based psychosocial treatments for children and adolescents with attention-deficit/hyperactivity disorder. Clin Psychol Rev 26:486–502, 2006

Coccaro EF, Harvey PO, Kupsaw-Lawrence E, et al: Development of neuropharmacologically based behavioral assessments of impulsive aggressive behavior. J Neuropsychiatry Clin Neurosci 3:S44–S51, 1991

Conners CK: Conners' 3rd Edition Manual. Toronto, ON, Canada, Multi-Health Systems, 2008

Conners CK, Epstein JN, March JS, et al: Multimodal treatment of ADHD in the MTA: an alternative outcome analysis. J Am Acad Child Adolesc Psychiatry 40:159–167, 2001

DuPaul GJ, Stoner G: ADHD in the Schools: Assessment and Intervention Strategies, 2nd Edition. New York, Guilford, 2003

Fan X, Bruno KJ. Hess EJ: Rodent models of ADHD. Behavioral Neuroscience of Attention Deficit Hyperactivity Disorder and Its Treatment. Curr Top Behav Neurosci, 9:273-300, 2012. doi: 10.1007/7854_2011_121

Faraone SV, Perlis RH, Doyle AE, et al: Molecular genetics of attention-deficit/hyperactivity disorder. Biol Psychiatry 57:1313–1323, 2005

Fassbender C, Schweitzer JB: Is there evidence for neural compensation in attention deficit hyperactivity disorder? A review of the functional neuroimaging literature. Clin Psychol Rev 26:445–465, 2006

Fisher SE, Francks C, McCracken JT, et al: A genomewide scan for loci involved in attention-deficit/hyperactivity disorder. Am J Hum Genet 70:1183–1196, 2002

Gadow KD, Sprafkin J: Child Symptom Inventory–4: Screening and Norms Manual. Stony Brook, NY, Checkmate Plus, 2002

Gould MS, Walsh BT, Munfakh JL, et al: Sudden death and use of stimulant medications in youths. Am J Psychiatry 166:992–1001, 2009

Green CT, Long DL, Green D, et al: Will working memory training generalize to improve off-task behavior in children with attention-deficit/hyperactivity disorder? Neurotherapeutics, 2012. doi: 10.1007/s13311-012-0124-y

Halperin JM, Healey DM: The influences of environmental enrichment, cognitive enhancement, and physical exercise on brain development: can we alter the developmental trajectory of ADHD? Neurosci Biobehav Rev 35:621–634, 2011

Hammerness P, McCarthy K, Mancuso E, et al: Atomoxetine for the treatment of attention-deficit/hyperactivity disorder in children and adolescents: a review. Neuropsychiatr Dis Treat 5:215–226, 2009

Harrison C, Sofronoff K: ADHD and parental psychological distress: role of demographics, child behavioral characteristics, and parental cognitions. J Am Acad Child Adolesc Psychiatry 41:703–711, 2002

Hinshaw SP: Moderators and mediators of treatment outcome for youth with ADHD: understanding for whom and how interventions work. J Pediatr Psychol 32:664–675, 2007

Hinshaw SP, Owens EB, Wells KC, et al: Family processes and treatment outcome in the MTA: negative/ineffective parenting practices in relation to multimodal treatment. J Abnorm Child Psychol 28:555–568, 2000

Hinshaw SP, Klein RG, Abikoff H: Childhood attention deficit hyperactivity disorder: nonpharmacological and combination treatments, in A Guide to Treatments That Work. Edited by Nathan PE, Gorman JM. New York, Oxford University Press, 2002, pp 3–23

Hoekzema E, Carmona S, Tremols V, et al: Enhanced neural activity in frontal and cerebellar circuits after cognitive training in children with attention-deficit/hyperactivity disorder. Hum Brain Mapp 31:1942–1950, 2010

Holmes J, Gathercole SE, Dunning DL: Adaptive training leads to sustained enhancement of poor working memory in children. Dev Sci 12:F9–F15, 2009

Holmes J, Gathercole SE, Place M, et al: Working memory deficits can be overcome: impacts of training and medication on working memory in children with ADHD. Appl Cogn Psychol 24:827–836, 2010

Jacobson LA, Murphy-Bowman SC, Pritchard AE, et al: Structure of a sluggish cognitive tempo scale in clinically-referred children. J Abnorm Child Psychol May 8, 2012 [Epub ahead of print]

Johnston C, Hommersen P, Seip C: Acceptability of behavioral and pharmacological treatment for attention-deficit/hyperactivity disorder: relations to child and parent characteristics. Behav Ther 39:22–32, 2008

Kaufman J, Birmaher B, Rao U, et al: The Schedule for Affective Disorders and Schizophrenia for School-Age Children. Pittsburgh, PA, University of Pittsburgh Medical Center, 1996

Kessler RC, Adler L, Barkley R, et al: The prevalence and correlates of adult ADHD in the United States: results from the National Comorbidity Survey Replication. Am J Psychiatry 163:716–723, 2006

Klingberg T: Training and plasticity of working memory. Trends Cogn Sci 14:317–324, 2010

Klingberg T, Forssberg H, Westerberg H: Training of working memory in children with ADHD. J Clin Exp Neuropsychol 24:781–791, 2002

Klingberg T, Fernell E, Olesen PJ, et al: Computerized training of working memory in children with ADHD: a randomized, controlled trial. J Am Acad Child Adolesc Psychiatry 44:177–186, 2005

Konrad K, Eickhoff SB: Is the ADHD brain wired differently? A review on structural and functional connectivity in attention deficit hyperactivity disorder. Hum Brain Mapp 31:904–916, 2010

Kovacs M: The Children's Depression Inventory Manual—2. Toronto, ON, Canada, Multi-Health Systems, 2010

Kratochvil CJ, Lake M, Pliszka SR, et al: Pharmacological management of treatment-induced insomnia in ADHD. J Am Acad Child Adolesc Psychiatry 44:499–501, 2005

Langberg JM, Epstein JN, Graham AJ: Organizational-skills interventions in the treatment of ADHD. Expert Rev Neurother 8:1549–1561, 2008

Lavigne JV, Lebailly SA, Hopkins J, et al: The prevalence of ADHD, ODD, depression, and anxiety in a community sample of 4-year-olds. J Clin Child Adolesc Psychol 38:315–328, 2009

Lindstrom K, Lindblad F, Hjern A: Preterm birth and attention-deficit/hyperactivity disorder in schoolchildren. Pediatrics 127:858–865, 2011

Lit L, Schweitzer JB, Iosif AM, et al: Owner reports of attention, activity, and impulsivity in dogs: a replication study. Behav Brain Funct 6:1, 2010

March JS: Manual for the Multidimensional Anxiety Scale for Children. Toronto, ON, Canada, Multi-Health Systems, 1997

McBurnett K, Pfiffner LJ, Frick PJ: Symptom properties as a function of ADHD type: an argument for continued study of sluggish cognitive tempo. J Abnorm Child Psychol 29:207–213, 2001

McNab F, Varrone A, Farde L, et al: Changes in cortical dopamine D1 receptor binding associated with cognitive training. Science 323:800–802, 2009

Milberger S, Biederman J, Faraone SV, et al: ADHD is associated with early initiation of cigarette smoking in children and adolescents. J Am Acad Child Adolesc Psychiatry 36:37–44, 1997

Molina BS, Hinshaw SP, Swanson JM, et al: The MTA at 8 years: prospective follow-up of children treated for combined-type ADHD in a multisite study. J Am Acad Child Adolesc Psychiatry 48:484–500, 2009

MTA Cooperative Group: A 14-month randomized clinical trial of treatment strategies for attention-deficit/hyperactivity disorder. Arch Gen Psychiatry 56:1073–1086, 1999

Olesen PJ, Westerberg H, Klingberg T: Increased prefrontal and parietal activity after training of working memory. Nat Neurosci 7:75–79, 2004

Pavuluri MN, Henry DB, Devineni B, et al: Child Mania Rating Scale: development, reliability and validity. J Am Acad Child Adolesc Psychiatry 45:550–560, 2006

Pelham WE Jr, Fabiano GA: Evidence-based psychosocial treatments for attention-deficit/hyperactivity disorder. J Clin Child Adolesc Psychol 37:184–214, 2008

Pfiffner LJ, Kaiser NM, Burner C, et al: From clinic to school: translating a collaborative school-home behavioral intervention for ADHD. School Ment Health 3:127–142, 2011

Pliszka S: Practice parameter for the assessment and treatment of children and adolescents with attention-deficit/hyperactivity disorder. J Am Acad Child Adolesc Psychiatry 46:894–921, 2007

Pliszka SR, McCracken JT, Maas JW: Catecholamines in attention-deficit hyperactivity disorder: current perspectives. J Am Acad Child Adolesc Psychiatry 35:264–272, 1996

Podolski CL, Nigg JT: Parent stress and coping in relation to child ADHD severity and associated child disruptive behavior problems. J Clin Child Psychol 30:503–513, 2001

Polanczyk G, de Lima MS, Horta BL, et al: The worldwide prevalence of ADHD: a systematic review and metaregression analysis. Am J Psychiatry 164:942–948, 2007

Posner K, Melvin GA, Murray DW, et al: Clinical presentation of attention-deficit/hyperactivity disorder in preschool children: the Preschoolers with Attention-Deficit/Hyperactivity Disorder Treatment Study (PATS). J Child Adolesc Psychopharmacol 17:547–562, 2007

Poznanski EO, Mokros HB: Children's Depression Rating Scale, Revised. Los Angeles, CA, Western Psychological Services, 1996

Raggi VL, Chronis AM: Interventions to address the academic impairment of children and adolescents with ADHD. Clin Child Fam Psychol Rev 9:85–111, 2006

Reich W: Diagnostic Interview for Children and Adolescents (DICA). J Am Acad Child Adolesc Psychiatry 39:59–66, 2000

Reynolds CR, Kamphaus RW: BASC-2: Behavior Assessment System for Children, 2nd Edition. Circle Pines, MN, American Guidance Service, 2004

Reynolds CR, Richmond BO: Revised Children's Manifest Anxiety Scale, 2nd Edition. Los Angeles, CA, Western Psychological Services, 2000

Robin AL: ADHD in Adolescents: Diagnosis and Treatment. New York, Guilford, 1998

Rutledge KJ, van den Bos W, McClure SM, et al: Training cognition in ADHD: current findings, borrowed concepts and future directions. Neurotherapeutics, 2012. doi: 10.1007/s13311-012-0134-9

Sagvolden T, Russell VA, Aase H, et al: Rodent models of attention-deficit/hyperactivity disorder. Biol Psychiatry 57:1239-1247, 2005

Scahill L, Schwab-Stone M: Epidemiology of ADHD in school-age children. Child Adolesc Psychiatr Clin N Am 9:541–555, vii, 2000

Scahill L, Riddle MA, McSwiggin-Hardin M, et al: Children's Yale-Brown Obsessive Compulsive Scale: reliability and validity. J Am Acad Child Adolesc Psychiatry 36:844–852, 1997

Schwebel DC, Roth DL, Elliott MN, et al: Association of externalizing behavior disorder symptoms and injury among fifth graders. Acad Pediatr 11:427–431, 2011

Shaw P, Eckstrand K, Sharp W, et al: Attention-deficit/hyperactivity disorder is characterized by a delay in cortical maturation. Proc Natl Acad Sci U S A 104:19649–19654, 2007

Shprecher D, Kurlan R: The management of tics. Mov Disord 24:15–24, 2009

Sicouri S, Antzelevitch C: Sudden cardiac death secondary to antidepressant and antipsychotic drugs. Expert Opin Drug Saf 7:181–194, 2008

Smalley SL, Kustanovich V, Minassian SL, et al: Genetic linkage of attention-deficit/hyperactivity disorder on chromosome 16p13, in a region implicated in autism. Am J Hum Genet 71:959–963, 2002

Sonuga-Barke EJ: The dual pathway model of AD/HD: an elaboration of neurodevelopmental characteristics. Neurosci Biobehav Rev 27:593–604, 2003

Sonuga-Barke EJ: Causal models of attention-deficit/hyperactivity disorder: from common simple deficits to multiple developmental pathways. Biol Psychiatry 57:1231–1238, 2005

Steer RA, Kumar G, Beck JS, et al: Evidence for the construct validities of the Beck Youth Inventories with child psychiatric outpatients. Psychol Rep 89:559–565, 2001

Stuss DT, Murphy KJ, Binns MA, et al: Staying on the job: the frontal lobes control individual performance variability. Brain 126:2363–2380, 2003

Swanson JM: The SNAP-IV Teacher and Parent Rating Scale. Irvine, University of California, Irvine, 1992

Turgay A, Goodman DW, Asherson P, et al; ADHD Transition Phase Model Working Group: Lifespan persistence of ADHD: the life transition model and its application. J Clin Psychiatry 73:192–201, 2012

Volkow ND, Wang GJ, Newcorn J, et al: Depressed dopamine activity in caudate and preliminary evidence of limbic involvement in adults with attention-deficit/hyperactivity disorder. Arch Gen Psychiatry 64:932–940, 2007

Volkow ND, Wang GJ, Kollins SH, et al: Evaluating dopamine reward pathway in ADHD: clinical implications. JAMA 302:1084–1091, 2009

Westerberg H, Klingberg T: Changes in cortical activity after training of working memory—a single-subject analysis. Physiol Behav 92:186–192, 2007

Wilens TE, Biederman J, Brown S, et al: Psychiatric comorbidity and functioning in clinically referred preschool children and school-age youths with ADHD. J Am Acad Child Adolesc Psychiatry 41:262–268, 2002

Willcutt EG, Doyle AE, Nigg JT, et al: Validity of the executive function theory of attention-deficit/hyperactivity disorder: a meta-analytic review. Biol Psychiatry 57:1336–1346, 2005

Willcutt EG, Betjemann RS, McGrath LM, et al: Etiology and neuropsychology of comorbidity between RD and ADHD: the case for multiple-deficit models. Cortex 46:1345–1361, 2010

Wolraich ML, Feurer ID, Hannah JN, et al: Obtaining systematic teacher reports of disruptive behavior disorders utilizing DSM-IV. J Abnorm Child Psychol 26:141–152, 1998

CHAPTER 3

FRAGILE X SYNDROME

Mary Jacena S. Leigh, M.D.
Randi J. Hagerman, M.D.
David Hessl, Ph.D.

A 3-year-old boy is seen in your office with his mother and maternal grand-parents for evaluation of developmental delays and frequent tantrums. He had trouble gaining weight as a baby, and when his parents picked him up, they felt that he was going to "slip through our arms." He currently is non-verbal and has been diagnosed with autism. His mother is anxious and un-derwent menopause at age 35 years. You notice the boy's grandfather has difficulty walking and has a tremor. The child sometimes bites his fingers and his collar. On physical examination, he has a round face, prominent ears, flexible fingers, and the smoothest skin you have ever felt. DNA test-ing for the fragile X mental retardation-1 gene *FMR1* reveals 600 fully methylated CGG repeats.

The preceding case illustrates some of the physical and behavior symptoms that may be present when individuals with fragile X syndrome (FXS) are young. Disorders associated with the fragile X premutation are also present in the child's mother (fragile X premature ovarian insufficiency [FXPOI]) and maternal grandfather (fragile X–associated tremor-ataxia syndrome [FXTAS]). This case highlights the multigenerational effects of fragile X that make knowledge about the characteristics, etiology, and recommended interventions for the fragile X family of disorders essential across a multitude of disciplines.

This work was supported by National Institutes of Health Grants HD036071, HD02274, DE019583, DA024854, AG032119, AG032115, MH77554, and MH078041; National Center for Resources Grant UL1RR024146; and Health and Human Services Administration of Developmental Disabilities Grant 90DD05969.

Signs and Symptoms

First described in the 1940s, FXS is the most common inherited cause of intellectual disability. Signs and symptoms of the fragile X family of disorders, which includes the full mutation causing FXS and the premutation causing several additional disorders, can be seen from birth and can emerge throughout the lifetime. Some of these features may be nonspecific, and the phenotypes can be quite broad.

Full Mutation

At the time of birth, infants with FXS may be hypotonic and may have oral-motor dyspraxia, as manifested by a poor suck. Individuals with FXS can often have problems with gastrointestinal reflux and commonly spit up. Failure to thrive can also occur. Congenital abnormalities such as clubfoot, cleft palate, and hip dislocation are sometimes observed. Individuals with FXS can have connective tissue abnormalities, such as hyperextensibility of joints, soft velvety skin, and flat feet (Table 3–1). Hyperextensibility can be assessed by examining metacarpal-phalangeal joint extension; extension greater than or equal to 90 degrees is considered hyperextension. In the standing position, hyperextensibility can be seen in individuals with FXS, as demonstrated by flat feet that are often pronated. Mitral valve prolapse, a high arched palate, and pectus excavatum (hollowed chest) can be manifestations of connective tissue abnormalities as well.

Table 3–1. Physical features of fragile X syndrome

System	Common features
Constitutional	Macrocephaly
Head	Long face, large and prominent ears with cupping, ptosis, prominent jaw
Eyes	Strabismus
Ears	Frequent otitis media
Throat	Abnormal palate, may be high arched
Cardiovascular	Mitral valve prolapse
Genitourinary	Macro-orchidism
Musculoskeletal	Joint laxity, flat or pronated feet, congenital malformations such as clubfoot or hip dislocation
Skin	Single or bridged palmar crease, soft skin
Neurological	Seizures, spike wave discharges on electroencephalogram

Male individuals with FXS often have distinctive facial features, such as large or prominent ears (Figure 3–1). There may be "cupping" of the outer helix, which occurs due to loss of the antihelical fold (Figure 3–2). Other facial features may include a long or narrow face and prominent jaw, which usually develop only after puberty. Females with FXS can also have some of the physical features, including mildly prominent ears and hyperextensibility.

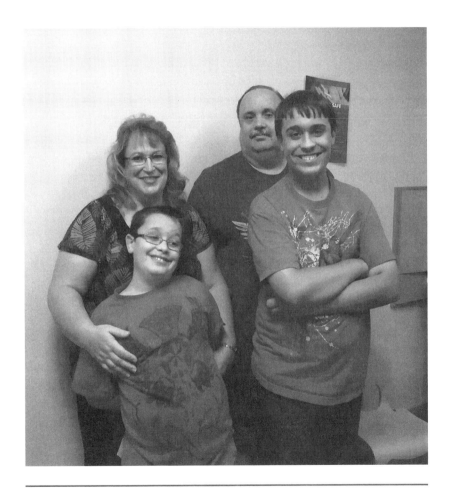

FIGURE 3–1. Mother with the premutation, father who is unaffected, and their two sons with FXS, one (at left) with mildly prominent ears and the other without typical FXS facial features.

Source. Image used with parental permission.

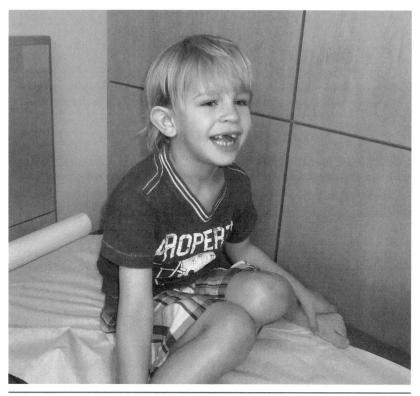

FIGURE 3–2. A young boy with fragile X syndrome who has prominent ears with cupping.

Source. Image used with parental permission.

Growth patterns in FXS can be abnormal. Macrocephaly is commonly seen in individuals with FXS. Short stature has also been noted in both males and females with FXS as adults; however, increased height for age may be present during childhood. Macro-orchidism is a very common feature in males with FXS. This does not typically emerge before age 10 years or until puberty. Testicle size is often greater than 35–40 mL in adolescents, and fertility is not typically affected (Hagerman 2002). The sperm of males with FXS contains the *FMR1* alleles in the premutation range. Because of this, sons are unaffected and daughters inherit the premutation.

Approximately 10% of males with FXS and an occasional female develop the Prader-Willi phenotype of FXS. Similar to Prader-Willi syndrome, individuals with the Prader-Willi phenotype have obesity, a round face, small hands, and hyperphagia. The phenotype is associated with a decrease in cytoplasmic interacting FMR1 protein mRNA, and not with the typical chromosome 15q11–q13 methylation or cytogenetic abnormalities that occur in Prader-Willi syndrome (Nowicki et al. 2007).

Behaviors commonly seen in individuals with FXS include stereotypies, such as hand flapping and finger or hand biting. Hand calluses may be present as the sequelae of hand biting. Anxiety is a common feature of the behavioral phenotype of FXS, and some of the behaviors such as decreased eye contact can be related to this. Physical aggression and tantrums are also common in adolescents and younger men with FXS. The aggression usually abates after the middle part of life. Individuals with FXS are typically shy in temperament, and when shaking hands they will often avert their gaze and not grip firmly (Hagerman 2002).

Autism spectrum disorders (ASDs) are comorbid conditions in a majority of males with FXS and in a significant proportion of females with FXS. Autistic disorder is found in approximately one-third of males with FXS, and pervasive developmental disorder not otherwise specified is found in another 30% of males with FXS (Harris et al. 2008). In females with FXS, autistic disorder has been found in 3%–10%, whereas pervasive developmental disorder not otherwise specified has been found in around 20% (Leigh et al. 2010; Mazzocco et al. 1997). FXS is considered to be the most common known single-gene cause of autism. Of individuals with autism, approximately 2%–8% will be found to have FXS (Hagerman et al. 2008b).

Individuals with FXS often have problems with impulsivity, inattention, and hyperactivity. Attention-deficit/hyperactivity disorder (ADHD) has been diagnosed in approximately 54%–70% of males with FXS (Roberts et al. 2011; Sullivan et al. 2006). Hyperarousal to sensory stimuli, including auditory, visual, and tactile stimuli, often occurs. Hyperactivity is seen less frequently in girls with FXS than in boys (Sullivan et al. 2006).

Intellectual disability is a hallmark aspect of FXS. Approximately 85% of males and 20%–30% of females with FXS have IQs less than 70 (Hagerman 2006; Hessl et al. 2009). Even individuals with FXS who have a normal or borderline IQ often have learning disabilities, usually in math. Executive function deficits are common and can lead to problems with attention and impulsivity. Individuals with FXS have difficulty with working memory, short-term memory, sustained attention, coordination, and processing of sequential information. Males with FXS experience a slower developmental course, about 50% of normal; as a result, their overall IQ tends to decline as they age (Chonchaiya et al. 2009).

Individuals with FXS have delayed developmental milestones, diagnosed at an average age of 19 months (Bailey et al. 2009). Language delays are frequent in individuals with FXS, and the age of first words is often around 2–3 years. Although most males with FXS will speak, their speech tends to be abnormal. They may have tangential or "cluttered" speech, in which words are spoken fast with long pauses between phrases, or may have repeated stuttering and dysfluency, which interferes with understanding of speech (Abbeduto et al. 2007). Motor delays can occur as well. Gross motor delays may be seen as "clumsiness," and fine motor problems may manifest as poor handwriting.

Seizures occur in approximately 10%–30% of individuals with FXS (Chonchaiya et al. 2009). Without clinical seizures, central temporal spikes can be seen on electroencephalography (EEG). Partial complex seizures are the most common type of seizures co-occurring with FXS.

Although otitis media is not an uncommon occurrence in childhood, children with FXS often have more than the typical number of middle ear infections, and myringotomy tube placement is usually necessary. Repeated occurrences of otitis media, as well as fluid behind the tympanic membranes, are seen in the majority of patients (Hagerman 2002) and may add to the language deficits; thus, aggressive treatment with either antibiotics or myringotomy tubes is important.

Strabismus is seen in 8%–20% of children with FXS and may require surgery or patching. Sleep apnea may also co-occur, and a history of snoring combined with prolonged pauses in breathing during sleep should be addressed in the medical workup. Hernias and joint dislocations may be present in individuals with FXS, and these appear to be related to connective tissue abnormalities (Hagerman 2002). The life span of individuals with FXS is typically not decreased.

Premutation

Most individuals with the fragile X premutation (55–200 CGG repeats) are normal in their early development, although a subgroup of them have developmental problems that may include social deficits such as ASDs, ADHD, seizures, or intellectual disability (Farzin et al. 2006). Individuals with larger CGG repeats (140–200) may have some features of FXS, even though they do not have a full mutation, if there are deficits in the fragile X mental retardation protein (FMRP) (see section "Etiology" below). Symptoms may include prominent ears or hyperextensible finger joints. Because their IQs may be in the borderline range or lower, these individuals may present with learning difficulties. Children with the premutation may also experience anxiety even when they do not have developmental problems (Chonchaiya et al. 2009). Several clinical studies have shown high rates of ADHD and/or ASDs among males with the premutation (Chonchaiya et al. 2011; Farzin et al. 2006). The rates appear to be higher among probands (i.e., carriers first identified in the pedigree with clinical concerns) than among nonprobands identified through family genetic testing.

These probands have been restricted primarily to clinic-referred individuals; therefore, concerns have been raised regarding whether these rates are reflective of the overall population of youth with the premutation. It is noteworthy, however, that Bailey et al. (2008), in a large national survey of 2,964 children from 1,250 families affected by fragile X, including 276 with the premutation, found that males with the premutation were significantly more likely than sibling controls without a mutation to have been diagnosed with or treated for attention problems (41%), anxiety (33%), autism (19%), and aggression (19%). Females with the premutation were significantly more likely than controls without a mutation to have been diagnosed with or treated for anxiety (36%), depression (34%), attention problems (19%), and developmental delay (9%).

Premutation cells are thought to be more sensitive to environmental toxicity because of early cell death (Chen et al. 2010; Paul et al. 2010). Therefore, early environmental toxicity would be more likely to lead to developmental problems in premutation carriers. Chonchaiya et al. (2011) reported that boys with the premutation and a history of seizures are more likely to have an ASD or low IQ. Seizures occur in approximately 7%–13% of those with a premutation (Bailey et al. 2008).

In adulthood, premutation carriers have a variety of psychiatric and medical problems, as described in the following subsections.

Neurological and Rheumatological Problems, Including Tremor-Ataxia Syndrome

FXTAS is characterized by tremors and ataxia in older premutation carriers. As an adult ages, the RNA toxicity of elevated mRNA can lead to a variety of neurological problems that eventually may turn into FXTAS. Mild symptoms of numbness and tingling that are typical of a neuropathy are commonly seen in premutation carriers (Coffey et al. 2008). Often, carriers experience pain in their extremities, particularly in the feet. However, pain symptoms upon touching of the arms, legs, and torso are common in female carriers, and approximately 43% of female carriers who have FXTAS will also have been diagnosed with fibromyalgia. Other rheumatological problems, including chronic fatigue, lupus, Sjögren syndrome, multiple sclerosis, and mixed connective tissue disorder, are also seen in 2%–10% of carriers (Leehey et al. 2011; Zhang et al. 2009).

Before the onset of tremor and ataxia that characterize FXTAS, patients often experience autonomic dysfunction, including hypertension (Coffey et al. 2008), orthostatic hypotension, erectile dysfunction, constipation, episodes of dizziness or vertigo, and then episodic imbalance. Sometimes, an internal tremor is experienced before a visible tremor is seen. A head tremor is common and can predate an intention tremor in the hands. Balance problems typically follow the tremor, and frequent falling is seen in these patients. On magnetic resonance imaging (MRI), the patient typically has global brain atrophy and white matter disease that usually involves the middle cerebellar peduncles (MCP sign), periventricular regions, and insula (Adams et al. 2007). The MRI findings are less severe in women, with only 13% demonstrating the MCP sign, whereas 60% of men with FXTAS have this sign (Adams et al. 2007). Overall, about 8%–13% of females with the premutation develop FXTAS (Coffey et al. 2008), whereas up to 75% of men develop FXTAS as they age into their 80s (Jacquemont et al. 2004).

Typically, the course of FXTAS includes onset in the early 60s, although on rare occasions symptoms can begin in the late 30s. Symptoms gradually worsen, and after about 15 years a person needs a cane or wheelchair because of severe ataxia (Leehey et al. 2007).

Fragile X Premature Ovarian Insufficiency

FXPOI affects approximately 20% of female premutation carriers and is marked by menstrual periods stopping before age 40. This was previously described as premature ovarian failure (POF) but has been changed to "insufficiency" due to reported cases of pregnancy in women diagnosed with POF. This problem is more common in carriers with CGG repeats ranging from 70 to 100 (Sullivan et al. 2005).

The signs of FXPOI include initially irregular periods and eventually the elevation of follicle-stimulating hormone. Another sign of ovarian failure is that a woman's antimüllerian hormone level may be low. The cause of FXPOI is RNA toxicity that affects the viability of the granulosa cells that support the ova and toxicity to the ova themselves. Women with the premutation have fewer viable eggs. Eventually menopause sets in, often accompanied in these women by psychiatric conditions, including anxiety and depression.

Psychopathology and Neuropsychological Profile

Individuals with the premutation were initially thought to be cognitively and emotionally unaffected, but studies over the past decade have provided evidence that at least a subgroup of them have increased rates of psychiatric disorders, including mood and anxiety disorders, ADHD, and ASDs. The rate of mood and anxiety disorders in older premutation carriers is clearly dependent on the presence of FXTAS. Bourgeois et al. (2011) reported that 65% and 52% of older carriers with FXTAS had increased rates of lifetime DSM-IV mood and anxiety disorders, respectively; non-FXTAS carriers had a significantly higher rate of social phobia (34% of the sample) than the national average for age. With the onset of FXTAS, symptoms of anxiety and depression may develop or previously recognized symptoms may become more severe.

Dementia may also be present, with frontal lobe features such as inappropriate social behavior, disinhibition, poor executive functioning, and mood disturbances. Higher rates of mood disorder have also been reported in women with the premutation without FXTAS (Roberts et al. 2009), although it must be acknowledged that most female premutation carriers involved in such studies are raising or have raised one or more children affected by FXS, which has been shown to be associated with elevated parenting stress and increased risk for mood and anxiety symptoms. Notably, however, Roberts et al. found that almost half of the women with a history of major depression had their first episode prior to the birth of their first child with FXS. Franke et al. (1998) reported a lifetime prevalence of anxiety disorder of 41% in premutation carrier mothers of children with FXS and also a high rate of social phobia in their premutation carrier sisters who did not have children with FXS.

Several studies comparing neuropsychological performance in adult premutation carriers without FXTAS and control subjects have been completed. Some studies revealed no significant differences or associations with repeat length across a range of tasks, including memory, executive function, and attention, in males with the premutation under age 50 (Hunter et al. 2008), whereas other studies showed clear weaknesses in executive function (Grigsby et al. 2008) and age-dependent deficits in attention (Cornish et al. 2008) in males with the premutation.

A limited number of recent studies have addressed the association between *FMR1*-specific molecular genetic factors, brain structure and function, and a range of psychiatric and behavior problems, in order to elucidate plausible mechanisms by which the mutation might lead to increased risk of psychiatric disorder. Hessl et al. (2005) reported an association between *FMR1* mRNA and psychological symptoms in men with the premutation, including men with and without FXTAS. This, in combination with reports of effects of increased CGG length and decreased FMRP related to morphology of the amygdala and hippocampus (Moore et al. 2004), led to a hypothesis that the premutation leads to alterations of limbic function and subsequent risk for expression of psychiatric symptoms and memory problems. Subsequent functional MRI studies in young to middle-aged men with the premutation have shown abnormal reduction of amygdala responsiveness to social stimuli associated with both elevated mRNA and decreased FMRP, known to occur even among carriers without detectable methylation at the *FMR1* site (Hessl et al. 2007, 2011). This altered amygdala response is correlated with a range of psychiatric symptoms as well as features of the broad autism phenotype.

The onset of psychopathology in premutation carriers has not been adequately studied to provide a clear view of the developmental course over time, and no longitudinal studies have been published. It is clear from the FXTAS studies that at least some individuals with the premutation either develop mood and anxiety disorders concurrent with the progressive course of the disease or manifest some of these symptoms in middle age to late adulthood before FXTAS develops.

Epidemiology

Estimates of FXS in the general population are approximately 1 in 2,500–4,000 (Hagerman 2008). Studies have identified the premutation in 1 in 250–810 males and in 1 in 130–260 females (Wang et al. 2010).

Etiology

The usual etiology of FXS is an unstable CGG trinucleotide expansion near the promoter region of the fragile X mental retardation-1 gene *FMR1* on the X chromosome. *FMR1* and its surrounding sequence are hypermethylated, usually completely, although methylation may vary. This leads to decreased transcription of *FMR1* mRNA by preventing the binding of transcription factors and results in decreased levels of the fragile X mental retardation protein, FMRP. In the unaffected population, the number of CGG repeats ranges from 5 to 44. One is categorized as having a full mutation with greater than 200 repeats. An individual with the premutation has from 55 to 200 repeats. The range from 45 to 54 repeats is referred to as the "gray zone," and clinical involvement is currently under study. FXS can infrequently be caused by a deletion in or including *FMR1*, leading to a deficit of FMRP (Hagerman 2002).

Molecular measures, including the level of FMRP, can be used to quantify degree of affectedness in FXS. However, in the premutation, *FMR1* mRNA is increased because there is usually no abnormal methylation. Increases in *FMR1* mRNA lead to the toxicity in premutation carriers described above (see "Neurological and Rheumatological Problems, Including Tremor-Ataxia Syndrome"). FMRP is a key protein that is involved in a variety of cellular processes. Levels of FMRP in blood can be measured through research laboratories, and these levels correlate with IQ and degree of physical involvement in FXS (Loesch et al. 2004).

Diagnostic Evaluation and Differential Diagnosis

Diagnostic Evaluation

Based on the responses of over 1,000 families of children with FXS who participated in a national survey, the average age at diagnosis of boys with

FXS was 35–37 months. The average age at diagnosis of girls was around 41 months. Despite a trend toward increasingly earlier diagnosis in boys, from 2001 to 2007 the age at diagnosis in boys remained fairly stable (Bailey et al. 2009). Early methods of testing included cytogenetic testing, which is no longer considered sufficient for evaluation of the fragile X family of disorders. Molecular testing is far more sensitive; it involves fragile X DNA testing, which includes first a polymerase chain reaction and then a Southern blot. Testing is commonly available and is usually covered by insurance.

Due to the frequent co-occurrence of ASDs with FXS, individuals with FXS should at least be systematically screened for ASD and undergo diagnostic evaluation for autism if indicated. Diagnostic evaluation should be done using standardized behavioral assessments, such as the Autism Diagnostic Observation Schedule (Lord et al. 2000) and the Autism Diagnostic Interview, Revised (Lord et al. 1994) or Social Communication Questionnaire (Rutter et al. 2003), to elicit relevant historical information from parents or primary caregivers.

The unique phenotype of FXS calls for attention to several critical factors in psychological assessment practice. First, persons with FXS demonstrate prominent symptoms of anxiety, social phobia, hyperarousal, hyperactivity, and inattention/distractibility that often affect the assessment process. Although always important, establishing rapport is critical in this case because speech and communication, social reciprocity, and coping with the adjustment of a novel testing environment are often affected by anxiety and hyperarousal. In our experience, humor, a casual interpersonal style, an increased warm-up period, and limited direct eye contact can be helpful. Aggression can occur during testing, often prompted by overwhelming anxiety or arousal, and the examiner should obtain information about the potential for such outbursts prior to the evaluation and establish a plan for identifying red flags and appropriate responses to aggression.

Regarding cognitive testing, a very high percentage of males and a substantial number of females with FXS score at the floor of many standardized tests, and their true abilities, strengths, and weaknesses are typically obscured when raw scores are converted to standardized scores (Hessl et al. 2009). Individuals in the intellectually disabled range should be assessed using standardized tests with a low floor (ideally at least five standard deviations below the mean of the standardization sample) and with some items targeting a mental age down to 2 years for school-age children through adults. A test with a floor IQ of 40, for example, is unlikely to be sensitive in a large proportion of males. Choosing a test that is designed for infants and toddlers, and that can generate an age equivalent even if a patient's age exceeds the norms, may be necessary for individuals of very low functioning in clinical settings. Individuals with the premutation, unless they present with very low functioning, can generally be assessed with a wider variety of standardized tests, following general practice guidelines no different from those used for assessing other conditions.

When possible, adaptive behavior should be assessed using a standardized interview, such as the Vineland Adaptive Behavior Scales, 2nd Edition (Sparrow and Cicchetti 1985). Several studies have documented this tool's validity and reliability in patients with FXS (Glaser et al. 2003; Hessl et al. 2009). Other adaptive behavior assessment tools are available but have not been applied to FXS as frequently, so less information and clinical experience have been reported.

Assessment for mood and anxiety disorders in individuals with FXS is challenging and is limited by several key factors, most notably language, communication, and insight deficits that often prevent valid self-reporting of symptoms. Even higher-functioning males and females with FXS appear to have significant limitations in self-assessment, a fact that is not well understood but can be related to executive functioning and social problems. For these reasons, it is important to choose a psychiatric assessment tool that is designed or modified and validated for persons with intellectual disability; to obtain impressions from multiple informants who know the patient well in several settings; and, often, to rely on observations of direct behavior to infer mood and anxiety states when self-report is not possible. When report of mood and anhedonia is not possible, an individual's depression may manifest as irritability, aggression, withdrawal, psychomotor retardation, and sleep and appetite disturbance. When report of worry, apprehension, or nervousness cannot be elicited verbally, anxiety may manifest as fearful behavior, avoidance, comments of feeling "scared," somatic complaints, sympathetic nervous system activation signs such as flushing and increased sweating/heart rate, and pupillary dilatation. Aggression does seem to occur as a result of anxiety in some cases as well. Assessment of mood and anxiety disorders in most premutation carriers can proceed with standardized psychiatric interviews used in both research and clinical practice, such as the Structured Clinical Interview for DSM-IV-TR Axis I Disorders, Research Version, Patient Edition (SCID-I/P; First et al. 2002), or the Schedule for Affective Disorders and Schizophrenia for School-Age Children, Present and Lifetime Version (Kiddie SADS; Kaufman et al. 1997), along with other well-validated rating scales used in general practice.

Obtaining a family history is a key aspect of the diagnostic evaluation of individuals with FXS or the premutation, given the etiology of FXS as a genetic disorder that affects multiple members of a family. A thorough three-generation pedigree should be obtained, seeking information on relatives with features of the fragile X family of disorders, including intellectual disability, tremor, balance problems, early menopause, mood or anxiety disorders, and Parkinson disease.

Differential Diagnosis for Full Mutation

The differential diagnosis for fragile X syndrome may be quite broad given the heterogeneity of the phenotype. For example, individuals with FXS have sometimes been diagnosed with Sotos syndrome due to the presence of macrocephaly; general overgrowth, which can be more commonly seen in childhood; and developmental delays. Table 3–2 describes other syndromes to consider in a differential diagnosis. Individuals with FXS may also have comorbid syndromes, such as Down syndrome, and sex chromosome abnormalities.

Table 3–2. Differential diagnosis for fragile X syndrome

Syndrome	Key features
Angelman	Severe intellectual disability, episodic laughter, absent/minimal speech, ataxia and jerky arm movements resembling those of a puppet on a string
Atkin-Flaitz	Intellectual disability, short stature, macrocephaly, coarse facial features, hypertelorism, macro-orchidism
Coffin-Lowry	Usually severe intellectual disability, hypotonia, coarse facies, soft hands with tapering fingers
FG	Intellectual disability, delayed motor development, hypotonia, seizures, prominent forehead, anal anomalies, small ears
Lujan-Fryns	Intellectual disability, hypotonia, tall thin body habitus, long face, high palate, short philtrum, large head
Prader-Willi	Intellectual disability, hypotonia, obesity, small hands and feet, almond-shaped eyes, hypogonadism
Sotos	Variable IQ, overgrowth including large hands and feet, macrocephaly, poor coordination, gross motor delays

Note. FG=the surname initials of the first family diagnosed with the disorder.

Source. Adapted from Jones KL (ed): *Smith's Recognizable Patterns of Human Malformation,* 6th Edition. Philadelphia, PA, Elsevier Saunders, 2005: "Angelman Syndrome," pp. 220–221, "Coffin-Lowry Syndrome," pp. 312–313, "Prader-Willi Syndrome," pp. 223–224, "Sotos Syndrome," pp. 163–164"; Online Mendelian Inheritance in Man: "Atkin-Flaitz Syndrome." November 27, 2006. Available at: http://omim.org/entry/300431. Accessed April 12, 2012; Lyons MJ: "*MED12*-Related Disorders," in *GeneReviews.* Edited by Pagon RA, Bird TD, Dolan CR, et al. July 14, 2009. Available at: http://www.ncbi.nlm.nih.gov/books/NBK1676/. Accessed April 12, 2012.

Differential Diagnosis for Premutation

The differential diagnosis for young children with the premutation and developmental or behavior problems includes idiopathic autism, ADHD, anxiety disorders, learning disabilities, microdeletion or duplication syndromes such as 15q11–q13 duplication, fetal alcohol syndrome, and sex chromosomal abnormalities. Therefore, in children with a family history of intellectual disability, ASD, fragile X, or neurodegenerative problems, the DNA testing for a fragile X mutation should be done. In adults who present with neurological problems typical of premutation carriers, including neuropathy, tremor, or ataxia, the differential diagnosis includes Parkinson disease, cerebellar ataxia, multiple system atrophy, Alzheimer disease, and spinocerebellar atrophy.

Interventions

Evidence-Based Behavioral or Psychological Treatments

There are very few empirical studies on the efficacy of behavioral treatments in patients with FXS, and the lack of treatment studies severely restricts the specificity of treatment recommendations that can be made to patients with FXS and their families. Providers have therefore generally relied on their own clinical experience in combination with an understanding of the factors shown to be associated with behavior problems in phenotype studies (see earlier section "Signs and Symptoms") to guide the treatment approach. Clinical reports show that individuals with FXS, depending on their individual profiles, benefit from medication, speech and language intervention, occupational therapy, behavioral interventions, and special education services. Beginning interventions early, when developmental delays are first identified, is important for a child with FXS; particularly important are physical, speech, and sensory interventions, along with the promotion of a daily routine for the child that helps to reduce anxiety. Supporting parents and siblings with family education and genetic counseling is important to facilitate the acceptance and understanding of individuals with FXS.

Evidence that children with FXS have heightened autonomic responses to sensory stimuli (Miller et al. 1999) and social stimuli, as well as elevated stress hormone levels related to severity of behavior and social problems (Hessl et al. 2006), suggests that interventions aimed at reducing stress and teaching better strategies to cope with stress and sensory input should result in better outcomes; however, no treatment studies have been done to document this. The findings that children with FXS have heightened autonomic

Reiss and Hall (2007), in their review of assessment and treatment of FXS, provide examples of novel behavior modification interventions, aimed at improving social eye contact and stress reduction, and support treatment models that combine behavioral intervention with experimental pharmacological or hormonal treatments supported by laboratory monitoring.

Large behavioral treatment studies of individuals with FXS are challenging. As an alternative, well-designed multiple-baseline individual-subject studies are quite feasible and can yield convincing accounts of efficacy with relatively few participants. Weiskop et al. (2005) used such a design to investigate a parent training program to reduce sleep problems in children with autism ($N=6$) or FXS ($N=5$). Although the study was small, the program seemed generally successful and provides a good model for other multiple-baseline studies that could be performed focusing on such maladaptive behaviors as aggression and self-injury.

The state of the science in psychosocial treatment through behavioral interventions in autism has been comprehensively reviewed by a panel of national experts sponsored by the National Institutes of Health (Lord and Bishop 2009; Lord et al. 2005). These reviews offer important insights and recommendations, which are applicable to behavioral treatment of individuals with FXS because of their very high rates of ASD and autistic-like behaviors. The authors emphasize that the traditional 1-hour weekly treatments for language, social skills, or behavior used in the U.S. mental health and educational systems are rarely sufficient to lead to generalized improvements in children with autism. This statement probably reflects the needs of children with FXS who have autism as well, although no empirical data are currently available to support this conclusion. The unique factors likely to be contributing to maladaptive behaviors in FXS (i.e., anxiety, sensory overload, and inattention/impulsivity) would need to be fully appreciated by an equivalently trained behavioral intervention team. Lastly, several treatment models, including the Early Start Denver Model (Dawson et al. 2010) and applied behavior analysis (Smith et al. 2007), are well established in autism treatment. These models, or features of these models, should be applied to individuals with FXS, or perhaps more ideally to those with FXS and autism, to test their efficacy. In our clinical experience, these treatment programs have been helpful for many children with FXS and ASD. The use of assistive technology, particularly for nonverbal children with FXS, is essential (Greiss Hess et al. 2009). iPad technology is also emerging to enhance the educational intervention with easily obtained apps (www.kindergarten.com, www.autismspeaks.org/family-services/autism-apps).

Higher-functioning individuals with FXS can benefit from psychotherapy or counseling (Braden 2000b; Hills-Epstein et al. 2002), although many may lack the insight, social skills, or executive function necessary to fully benefit from this type of treatment. This therapy can focus on anxiety reduction through desensitization, sexuality issues, management of depression through cognitive-behavioral approaches, and socialization. Structured and behavioral or cognitive-behavioral approaches are likely to lead to better outcomes than exploratory, patient-guided, or psychodynamic approaches. Many individuals with FXS who have autistic symptoms and social anxiety also can benefit from social skills–oriented group therapy (Braden 2000a). A program to help behavior problems and address sexuality issues in adolescence and young adulthood was developed by the National Fragile X Foundation to guide professionals and the family (www.fragilex.org/treatment-intervention/adults-life-planning/adolescent-and-adult-project).

Psychopharmacological Treatments

Full Mutation

Many of the current medications used by individuals with FXS treat symptomatic problems. Selective serotonin reuptake inhibitors (SSRIs) can be helpful for treatment of anxiety symptoms (Hagerman et al. 2009). For aggression and irritability, the atypical antipsychotic class of medications can be helpful for behavior and mood stabilization. Aripiprazole was associated with a decrease in irritable behavior in an open-label 12-week trial in individuals with FXS ages 6–25 years (Erickson et al. 2011). Melatonin has been found to be useful for sleep problems in children with FXS and autism. In a 4-week randomized, double-blind, crossover trial of melatonin in children ages 2–15 years, mean sleep onset time was earlier, mean sleep onset latency was shorter, and mean duration of sleep was longer for those given melatonin than those given placebo (Wirojanan et al. 2009). For ADHD, modifications in the classroom, such as having the student sit at the front of the room, may be helpful. After children with FXS and attention problems reach age 5, medications such as stimulants or atomoxetine may be helpful (Hagerman et al. 2009). It is important to fully evaluate with EEG for any seizure activity in children, including staring spells, and to treat seizures if present.

Premutation

Premutation disorders that present in childhood typically include anxiety and social deficits. Individuals with premutation disorders usually respond well to an SSRI. If autism is seen in a premutation carrier or if clinical symptoms of staring spells or other seizures are seen, EEG should be performed and abnormalities should be treated as in individuals with full mutation. Once the child reaches age 5 years, ADHD symptoms are usually easily treated with a stimulant medication, as described in the preceding subsection, "Full Mutation." If low levels of FMRP are documented, then targeted treatments for FXS can be tried as described below.

Various treatments are available for the tremor, ataxia, and other neurological symptoms of aging carriers with and without FXTAS, and these have been detailed elsewhere (Hagerman et al. 2008a). The treatment of FXPOI is estrogen replacement, typically prescribed by a gynecologist or a reproductive endocrinologist. Preliminary evidence of glutamate toxicity in FXTAS suggests that memantine, a medication for Alzheimer's disease that blocks glutamate toxicity, might be helpful for the progression of the disease (Ortigas et al. 2010), and a controlled trial of memantine in the treatment of FXS is under way.

Other Supports Needed

Genetic counseling is essential throughout all steps of fragile X testing and diagnosis, since the results of testing have implications for both the individual being tested and his or her family. An experienced genetic counselor should review the different ranges of CGG repeats and their implications, as well as provide further resources for the family.

Community organizations, both in person and online, can be important sources of information and support. The National Fragile X Foundation offers families and medical professionals guidance for care and connects families across the nation as well as locally (www.fragilex.org). The FRAXA Research Foundation also provides information to families and professionals (www.fraxa.org).

Because an individual with FXS may have a number of comorbid conditions, a team of numerous professionals is often necessary to ensure proper comprehensive care.

Outcomes

A large range of issues may be present in individuals with FXS. Factors that seem to contribute to better outcomes include lower severity of comorbid conditions. Often a diagnosis of FXS and ASD leads to a less promising prognosis because cognitive, adaptive, and language skills are decreased in those with FXS and ASD (Rogers et al. 2001). In a study by Chonchaiya et al. (2009), academic skills of boys were predicted by the presence of autistic behaviors and the level of maternal education.

A child with FXS may have a significant effect on family life, and thought should be given to planning the future care of individuals with FXS while they are still children. Females with FXS are more often able to live independently than are males with FXS. As adults, most males with FXS live in group homes or with their families. Other children in the family may need help understanding the extra attention and care their sibling requires and may face questions about why their sibling is different. Please see Heyman (2003) and Stieger (1998) in "Recommended Readings" at the end of the chapter for helpful resources for siblings.

New Research Directions

Progress in understanding the etiology and neurobiology of FXS has led to new targeted treatments for this condition. It is important to understand that the etiology of FXS, secondary to the full mutation and deficit of mRNA and FMRP, is very different from the etiology of premutation disorders, which are caused by too much *FMR1* mRNA and RNA toxicity, as described in the earlier section "Etiology."

FMRP is an RNA binding protein that carries hundreds of other mRNAs to the neuronal synapse and regulates translation of these messages there. Therefore, a deficit or lack of FMRP dysregulates many other proteins. Enhancement of the metabotropic glutamate receptor 5 (mGluR5) pathway leads to long-term depression (weakening of the synaptic connections), and reversal of this with mGluR5 antagonists is being studied now. The lack of FMRP also leads to downregulation of γ-aminobutyric acid type A ($GABA_A$) systems, so $GABA_A$ agonists are currently being studied as a targeted intervention.

This is an exciting age of targeted treatments in FXS, and a number of such treatments are currently being studied nationally and internationally. The first targeted treatment for FXS was an ampakine, CX516, to enhance α-amino-3-hydroxy-5-methyl-4-isoxazolepropionic acid (AMPA) receptors; in FXS, AMPA receptors are internalized instead of being active on the surface, which is related to the long-term depression (a lasting decrease in synaptic strength) that occurs in FXS. However, this controlled trial was not found to be beneficial in adults with FXS, perhaps because CX516 is too weak an ampakine (Berry-Kravis et al. 2006). A subsequent study of an mGluR5 antagonist, fenobam, given as a single dose in 12 adults with FXS showed beneficial effects in behavior and in prepulse inhibition measures (Berry-Kravis et al. 2009). This was a landmark study, although only a single dose was involved, because it gave hope that improvements would be seen with continuous dosing. Currently, two additional studies of mGluR5 antagonists are taking place at multiple centers throughout the United States and internationally. The results of the Novartis mGluR5 antagonist AFQ056 trial demonstrated improvements in those with a fully methylated full mutation, whereas those who were mosaic had a variable response (Jacquemont et al. 2011).

Another targeted treatment for FXS is R-baclofen (arbaclofen; the right isomer of baclofen). Baclofen has been used for years in the treatment of cerebral palsy and has been shown to be safe in children. Arbaclofen is more potent as a $GABA_B$ agonist, which lowers glutamate at the synapse and therefore down-regulates the mGluR5 pathway. An initial study of 60 patients with FXS demonstrated efficacy in those with autism or significant social deficits (Berry-Kravis et al. 2010). In addition, arbaclofen was helpful in an open trial in those with idiopathic autism. Therefore, controlled studies have been initiated both in children and young adults with FXS and in children and adults with idiopathic autism.

Currently, ganaxolone, a $GABA_A$ agonist, is being studied in a controlled trial in children with FXS. Hopes are that the medication will be helpful both for behavior and for seizures in those with FXS. It is too early to speculate as to whether ganaxolone may be helpful for cognition as well, but that is the hope for these targeted treatments.

Minocycline is also a targeted treatment for FXS because it lowers matrix metalloproteinase 9 (MMP9) levels, which are elevated in the FXS knockout mouse model (Bilousova et al. 2009). A survey of 50 individuals with FXS showed a beneficial effect in 70%, particularly in language and attention (Utari et al. 2010), and an open trial in adolescents and young adults with FXS demonstrated efficacy on multiple measures (Paribello et al. 2010). A controlled trial of minocycline is being carried out in young children and adolescents with FXS.

Newborn screening programs have been piloted in California, Illinois, and North Carolina. One of the great benefits of such a program, if parents consent to be contacted, is that it provides early identification so that early interventions can begin. For individuals with the full mutation, earlier treatments, both symptomatic and experimental targeted treatments, may be offered. Babies identified with the premutation can be monitored longitudinally, with interventions as necessary. Cascade testing can be performed to identify other affected members of the individual's family. Although newborn screening can be beneficial to identify affected individuals and provide early intervention, it is important also to recognize that individuals with the premutation may be identified who may not manifest associated problems, or at least not until much later in adulthood. More research is needed to better understand the benefits and risks of newborn screening for FXS, especially in the context of identification of carriers of premutation and intermediate-sized alleles.

Genetic counseling is essential to help families understand the implications of any positive test, as well as to discuss options for further family planning, because prenatal diagnosis of FXS is available. Continuing a healthful lifestyle, including exercise, a balanced diet, use of antioxidants, and avoidance of toxins, is also suggested for carriers of the premutation.

The future looks brighter for individuals diagnosed with FXS or pre-mutation disorders because of recent progress on development of targeted treatments. *FMR1* mutations have provided much information regarding a variety of disorders because FMRP is a key protein for many cellular functions. The future may also confirm that FMRP deficits are associated with other disorders without a known fragile X mutation, including schizophrenia, bipolar disorder, depression, and autism (Fatemi et al. 2010, 2011). Therefore, understanding the regulation of FMRP may help with many disorders, not only FXS.

Key Points

- Fragile X syndrome (FXS) is the most common inherited cause of intellectual disability and the most common known single-gene cause of autism.
- The best diagnostic testing for the fragile X family of disorders is the fragile X DNA test, which includes polymerase chain reaction and Southern blot.
- Key physical features of FXS are large and prominent ears, hyperextensible finger joints, and macro-orchidism.
- Key intellectual and behavioral features of FXS are intellectual disability, hyperarousal to sensory stimuli, autism, anxiety, hyperactivity, and inattention.
- The premutation may be associated with premature ovarian insufficiency (FXPOI), fragile X–associated tremor ataxia syndrome (FXTAS), neuropathy, fibromyalgia, hypothyroidism, anxiety, depression, and attention problems.

Recommended Readings

Hagerman RJ, Hagerman PJ (eds): Fragile X Syndrome: Diagnosis, Treatment and Research. Baltimore, MD, Johns Hopkins University Press, 2002

Heyman C: My eXtra Special Brother: How to Love, Understand, and Celebrate Your Sibling With Special Needs. Marietta, GA, Fragile X Association of Georgia, 2003

Stieger C: My Brother Has Fragile X. Chapel Hill, NC, Avanta Media, 1998

Tassone F, Berry-Kravis (eds): Fragile X–Associated Tremor Ataxia Syndrome (FXTAS). New York, Springer-Verlag, 2011

Recommended Web Sites

Fragile X Research and Treatment Center, UC Davis MIND Institute: http://www.ucdmc.ucdavis.edu/mindinstitute/research/fxrtc.html

FRAXA Research Foundation: http://www.fraxa.org

Kindergarten.com learning applications: http://www.kindergarten.com

Autism Speaks learning applications: http://www.autismspeaks.org/family-services/autism-apps

National Fragile X Foundation: http://www.fragilex.org/html/home.shtml

National Fragile X Foundation Adolescent and Adult Project: http://www.fragilex.org/treatment-intervention/adults-life-planning/adolescent-and-adult-project

References

Abbeduto L, Brady N, Kover ST: Language development and fragile X syndrome: profiles, syndrome-specificity, and within-syndrome differences. Ment Retard Dev Disabil Res Rev 13:36–46, 2007

Adams JS, Adams PE, Nguyen D, et al: Volumetric brain changes in females with fragile X–associated tremor/ataxia syndrome (FXTAS). Neurology 69:851–859, 2007

Bailey DB Jr, Raspa M, Olmsted M, et al: Co-occurring conditions associated with FMR1 gene variations: findings from a national parent survey. Am J Med Genet A 146A:2060–2069, 2008

Bailey DB Jr, Raspa M, Bishop E, et al: No change in the age of diagnosis for fragile X syndrome: findings from a national parent survey. Pediatrics 124:527–533, 2009

Berry-Kravis E, Krause SE, Block SS, et al: Effect of CX516, an AMPA-modulating compound, on cognition and behavior in fragile X syndrome: a controlled trial. J Child Adolesc Psychopharmacol 16:525–540, 2006

Berry-Kravis E, Hessl D, Coffey S, et al: A pilot open label, single dose trial of fenobam in adults with fragile X syndrome. J Med Genet 46:266–271, 2009

Berry-Kravis E, Cherubini M, Zarevics P, et al: Arbaclofen for the treatment of children and adults with fragile X syndrome: results of a phase 2, randomized, double-blind, placebo-controlled, crossover study. Abstract presented at the International Meeting for Autism Research, Philadelphia, PA, May 20–22, 2010, p 741

Bilousova TV, Dansie L, Ngo M, et al: Minocycline promotes dendritic spine maturation and improves behavioural performance in the fragile X mouse model. J Med Genet 46:94–102, 2009

Bourgeois JA, Seritan AL, Casillas EM, et al: Lifetime prevalence of mood and anxiety disorders in fragile X premutation carriers. J Clin Psychiatry 72:175–182, 2011

Braden ML: Education, in Children With Fragile X Syndrome: A Parent's Guide. Edited by Weber J. Bethesda, MD, Woodbine House, 2000a, pp 243–305

Braden ML: Fragile, Handle With Care: More About Fragile X Syndrome, Adolescents, and Adults. Dillon, CO, Spectra Publishing, 2000b

Chen Y, Tassone F, Berman RF, et al: Murine hippocampal neurons expressing FMR1 gene premutations show early developmental deficits and late degeneration. Hum Mol Genet 19:196–208, 2010

Chonchaiya W, Schneider A, Hagerman RJ: Fragile X: a family of disorders. Adv Pediatr 56:165–186, 2009

Chonchaiya W, Au J, Schneider A, et al: Increased prevalence of seizures in boys who were probands with the FMR1 premutation and co-morbid autism spectrum disorder. Hum Genet 13:581–589, 2011

Coffey SM, Cook K, Tartaglia N, et al: Expanded clinical phenotype of women with the FMR1 premutation. Am J Med Genet A 146A:1009–1016, 2008

Cornish KM, Li L, Kogan CS, et al: Age-dependent cognitive changes in carriers of the fragile X syndrome. Cortex 44:628–636, 2008

Dawson G, Rogers S, Munson J, et al: Randomized, controlled trial of an intervention for toddlers with autism: the Early Start Denver Model. Pediatrics 125:e17–e23, 2010

Erickson CA, Stigler KA, Wink LK, et al: A prospective open-label study of aripiprazole in fragile X syndrome. Psychopharmacology (Berl) 216:85–90, 2011

Farzin F, Perry H, Hessl D, et al: Autism spectrum disorders and attention-deficit/hyperactivity disorder in boys with the fragile X premutation. J Dev Behav Pediatr 27(suppl):S137–S144, 2006

Fatemi SH, Kneeland RE, Liesch SB, et al: Fragile X mental retardation protein levels are decreased in major psychiatric disorders. Schizophr Res 124:246–247, 2010

Fatemi SH, Folsom TD, Kneeland RE, et al: Metabotropic glutamate receptor 5 upregulation in children with autism is associated with underexpression of both Fragile X mental retardation protein and GABAA receptor beta 3 in adults with autism. Anat Rec (Hoboken) 294:1635–1645, 2011

First MB, Spitzer RL, Gibbon M, et al: Structured Clinical Interview for DSM-IV-TR Axis I Disorders, Research Version, Patient Edition (SCID-I/P). New York, Biometrics Research, New York State Psychiatric Institute, 2002

Franke P, Leboyer M, Gänsicke M, et al: Genotype-phenotype relationship in female carriers of the premutation and full mutation of FMR-1. Psychiatry Res 80:113–127, 1998

Glaser B, Hessl D, Dyer-Friedman J, et al: Biological and environmental contributions to adaptive behavior in fragile X syndrome. Am J Med Genet A 117A:21–29, 2003

Greiss Hess L, Lemons-Chitwood K, Harris S, et al: Assistive technology use by persons with fragile X syndrome: three case reports. AOTA: Special Interest Section Quarterly: Technology 19:1–4, 2009

Grigsby J, Brega AG, Engle K, et al: Cognitive profile of fragile X premutation carriers with and without fragile X–associated tremor/ataxia syndrome. Neuropsychology 22:48–60, 2008

Hagerman PJ: The fragile X prevalence paradox. J Med Genet 45:498–499, 2008

Hagerman RJ: The physical and behavioral phenotype, in Fragile X Syndrome: Diagnosis, Treatment and Research. Edited by Hagerman RJ, Hagerman PJ. Baltimore, MD, Johns Hopkins University Press, 2002, pp 3–109

Hagerman RJ: Lessons from fragile X regarding neurobiology, autism, and neurodegeneration. J Dev Behav Pediatr 27:63–74, 2006

Hagerman RJ, Hall DA, Coffey S, et al: Treatment of fragile X–associated tremor ataxia syndrome (FXTAS) and related neurological problems. Clin Interv Aging 3:251–262, 2008a

Hagerman RJ, Rivera SM, Hagerman PJ: The fragile X family of disorders: a model for autism and targeted treatments. Curr Pediatr Rev 4:40–52, 2008b

Hagerman RJ, Berry-Kravis E, Kaufmann WE, et al: Advances in the treatment of fragile X syndrome. Pediatrics 123:378–390, 2009

Harris SW, Hessl D, Goodlin-Jones B, et al: Autism profiles of males with fragile X syndrome. Am J Ment Retard 113:427–438, 2008

Hessl D, Tassone F, Loesch DZ, et al: Abnormal elevation of FMR1 mRNA is associated with psychological symptoms in individuals with the fragile X premutation. Am J Med Genet B Neuropsychiatr Genet 139B:115–121, 2005

Hessl D, Glaser B, Dyer-Friedman J, et al: Social behavior and cortisol reactivity in children with fragile X syndrome. J Child Psychol Psychiatry 47:602–610, 2006

Hessl D, Rivera S, Koldewyn K, et al: Amygdala dysfunction in men with the fragile X premutation. Brain 130:404–416, 2007

Hessl D, Nguyen DV, Green C, et al: A solution to limitations of cognitive testing in children with intellectual disabilities: the case of fragile X syndrome. J Neurodev Disord 1:33–45, 2009

Hessl D, Wang JM, Schneider A, et al: Decreased fragile X mental retardation protein expression underlies amygdala dysfunction in carriers of the fragile X premutation. Biol Psychiatry 70:859–865, 2011

Hills-Epstein J, Riley K, Sobesky W: The treatment of emotional and behavioral problems, in Fragile X Syndrome: Diagnosis, Treatment, and Research, 3rd Edition. Edited by Hagerman RJ, Hagerman PJ. Baltimore, MD, Johns Hopkins University Press, 2002, pp 339–362

Hunter JE, Allen EG, Abramowitz A, et al: No evidence for a difference in neuropsychological profile among carriers and noncarriers of the FMR1 premutation in adults under the age of 50. Am J Hum Genet 83:692–702, 2008

Jacquemont S, Hagerman RJ, Leehey MA, et al: Penetrance of the fragile X–associated tremor/ataxia syndrome in a premutation carrier population. JAMA 291:460–469, 2004

Jacquemont S, Curie A, des Portes V, et al: Epigenetic modification of the FMR1 gene in fragile X syndrome is associated with differential response to the mGluR5 antagonist AFQ056. Sci Transl Med 3:64ra1, 2011

Kaufman J, Birmaher B, Brent D, et al: Schedule for Affective Disorders and Schizophrenia for School-Age Children—Present and Lifetime Version (K-SADS-PL): initial reliability and validity data. J Am Acad Child Adolesc Psychiatry 36:980–988, 1997

Leehey MA, Berry-Kravis E, Min SJ, et al: Progression of tremor and ataxia in male carriers of the FMR1 premutation. Mov Disord 22:203–206, 2007

Leehey MA, Legg W, Tassone F, et al: Fibromyalgia in fragile X mental retardation 1 gene premutation carriers. Rheumatology (Oxford) 50:2233–2236, 2011

Leigh MJ, Tassone F, Mendoza-Morales G, et al: Evaluation of autism spectrum disorders in females with fragile X syndrome. Abstract presented at the International Meeting for Autism Research, Philadelphia, PA, May 20–22, 2010, pp 375–376

Loesch DZ, Huggins RM, Hagerman RJ: Phenotypic variation and FMRP levels in fragile X. Ment Retard Dev Disabil Res Rev 10:31–41, 2004

Lord C, Bishop SL: The autism spectrum: definitions, assessment and diagnoses. Br J Hosp Med (Lond) 70:132–135, 2009

Lord C, Rutter M, Le Couteur A: Autism Diagnostic Interview—Revised: a revised version of a diagnostic interview for caregivers of individuals with possible pervasive developmental disorders. J Autism Dev Disord 24:659–685, 1994

Lord C, Risi S, Lambrecht L, et al: The Autism Diagnostic Observation Schedule—generic: a standard measure of social and communication deficits associated with the spectrum of autism. J Autism Dev Disord 30:205–223, 2000

Lord C, Wagner A, Rogers S, et al: Challenges in evaluating psychosocial interventions for autistic spectrum disorders. J Autism Dev Disord 35:695–708; discussion 709–711, 2005

Mazzocco MM, Kates WR, Baumgardner TL, et al: Autistic behaviors among girls with fragile X syndrome. J Autism Dev Disord 27:415–435, 1997

Miller LJ, McIntosh DN, McGrath J, et al: Electrodermal responses to sensory stimuli in individuals with fragile X syndrome: a preliminary report. Am J Med Genet 83:268–279, 1999

Moore CJ, Daly EM, Tassone F, et al: The effect of pre-mutation of X chromosome CGG trinucleotide repeats on brain anatomy. Brain 127:2672–2681, 2004

Nowicki ST, Tassone F, Ono MY, et al: The Prader-Willi phenotype of fragile X syndrome. J Dev Behav Pediatr 28:133–138, 2007

Ortigas MC, Bourgeois JA, Schneider A, et al: Improving fragile X–associated tremor/ataxia syndrome symptoms with memantine and venlafaxine. J Clin Psychopharmacol 30:642–644, 2010

Paribello C, Tao L, Folino A, et al: Open-label add-on treatment trial of minocycline in fragile X syndrome. BMC Neurol 10:91, 2010

Paul R, Pessah IN, Gane L, et al: Early onset of neurological symptoms in fragile X premutation carriers exposed to neurotoxins. Neurotoxicology 31:399–402, 2010

Reiss AL, Hall SS: Fragile X syndrome: assessment and treatment implications. Child Adolesc Psychiatr Clin N Am 16:663–675, 2007

Roberts JE, Bailey DB Jr, Mankowski J, et al: Mood and anxiety disorders in females with the FMR1 premutation. Am J Med Genet B Neuropsychiatr Genet 150B:130–139, 2009

Roberts JE, Miranda M, Boccia M, et al: Treatment effects of stimulant medication in young boys with fragile X syndrome. J Neurodev Disord 3:175–184, 2011

Rogers SJ, Wehner DE, Hagerman R: The behavioral phenotype in fragile X: symptoms of autism in very young children with fragile X syndrome, idiopathic autism, and other developmental disorders. J Dev Behav Pediatr 22:409–417, 2001

Rutter M, Bailey A, Lord C: Social Communication Questionnaire. Los Angeles, CA, Western Psychological Services, 2003

Smith T, Mozingo D, Mruzek DW, et al: Applied behavior analysis in the treatment of autism, in Clinical Manual for the Treatment of Autism. Edited by Hollander E, Anagnostou E. Washington, DC, American Psychiatric Publishing, 2007, pp 153–177

Sparrow SS, Cicchetti DV: Diagnostic uses of the Vineland Adaptive Behavior Scales. J Pediatr Psychol 10:215–225, 1985

Sullivan AK, Marcus M, Epstein MP, et al: Association of FMR1 repeat size with ovarian dysfunction. Hum Reprod 20:402–412, 2005

Sullivan K, Hatton D, Hammer J, et al: ADHD symptoms in children with FXS. Am J Med Genet A 140:2275–2288, 2006

Utari A, Chonchaiya W, Rivera SM, et al: Side effects of minocycline treatment in patients with fragile X syndrome and exploration of outcome measures. Am J Intellect Dev Disabil 115:433–443, 2010

Wang LW, Berry-Kravis E, Hagerman RJ: Fragile X: leading the way for targeted treatments in autism. Neurotherapeutics 7:264–274, 2010

Weiskop S, Richdale A, Matthews J: Behavioural treatment to reduce sleep problems in children with autism or fragile X syndrome. Dev Med Child Neurol 47:94–104, 2005

Wirojanan J, Jacquemont S, Diaz R, et al: The efficacy of melatonin for sleep problems in children with autism, fragile X syndrome, or autism and fragile X syndrome. J Clin Sleep Med 5:145–150, 2009

Zhang L, Coffey S, Lua LL, et al: FMR1 premutation in females diagnosed with multiple sclerosis. J Neurol Neurosurg Psychiatry 80:812–814, 2009

CHAPTER 4

CHROMOSOME 22q11.2 DELETION SYNDROME

Kathleen Angkustsiri, M.D.
Tony J. Simon, Ph.D.

Chromosome 22q11.2 deletion syndrome (22q11.2DS) is the most common microdeletion syndrome in humans (Botto et al. 2003). Aspects of the currently recognized syndrome were separately described, first in the 1960s by Angelo DiGeorge (Kirkpatrick and DiGeorge 1968) and then in the 1970s by Robert Shprintzen (Shprintzen et al. 1978). DiGeorge sequence is characterized by immune deficiency from thymic hypoplasia, hypocalcemia secondary to hypoparathyroidism, and congenital heart anomalies (Kirkpatrick and DiGeorge 1968). Pertinent features of velocardiofacial syndrome (VCFS) described by Shprintzen include velopharyngeal or palatal anomalies ("velo"), congenital cardiovascular defects ("cardio"), and mild facial dysmorphisms ("facial") (Shprintzen et al. 1978). In the early 1990s, a common cause for almost all cases of both DiGeorge sequence and VCFS was identified in the form of a microdeletion on the long arm (band q11.2) of chromosome 22 (Driscoll et al. 1993). This same microdeletion is responsible for symptoms of other previously identified disorders, such as conotruncal anomaly face syndrome, Cayler cardiofacial syndrome, and Opitz G/BBB syndrome. The overlap in these multiple syndromes has led to confusion about proper terminology when the deletion is present. In this chapter, we use the most inclusive label: chromosome 22q11.2 deletion syndrome. Symptoms of 22q11.2DS are highly variable and include high risk for physical anomalies, learning difficulties, and psychiatric disorders.

Epidemiology

Due to variations in ascertainment sources, estimates of 22q11.2DS prevalence have a wide range, spanning from 1 in 2,000 to 1 in 7,000 (Botto et al. 2003; Shprintzen 2008). Estimates are based on diagnoses made through subspecialty referrals and not on population-based screening, so the true prevalence is unknown. The broadly accepted prevalence is approximately 1 in 4,000 (Oskarsdóttir et al. 2004), although this may be considered a minimum estimate given variability of symptoms and missed diagnosis of individuals without cardiac or palatal lesions. Clinicians are less likely to suspect the diagnosis of 22q11.2DS in the context of characteristic behavioral and learning difficulties in the absence of medical problems, so increasing awareness of the phenotypic variability across disciplines is greatly needed.

Signs and Symptoms

Over 180 possible physical manifestations of 22q11.2DS have been described, with highly variable expression. No single clinical feature is present in 100% of cases, and no individual exhibits all possible findings (Shprintzen 2008). Table 4–1 lists the prevalences of conditions that are suggestive of 22q11.2DS, along with how common 22q11.2DS is among individuals with these conditions. For example, cardiac defects are common, occurring in 75% of individuals with 22q11.2DS, although the deletion is responsible for causing congenital heart disease in only a minority (7%) of congenital heart disease cases. This estimate is derived from the results of universal screening for 22q11.2DS in all infants with certain heart defects, whereas testing may be done less frequently in the context of developmental delay or psychiatric problems. Recognition of facial characteristics can increase identification, especially in the presence of hypernasal voice quality or nasal regurgitation.

Physical Symptoms

Cardiovascular

Structural heart defects, specifically conotruncal anomalies, are common in 22q11.2DS. Genetic testing for 22q11.2 is often requested automatically when certain cardiac conditions are present. Tetralogy of Fallot (TOF) is most common, followed by ventricular septal defects (VSD) with pulmonary atresia (PA), aortic arch abnormalities, and truncus arteriosus (TA). Other lesions include isolated atrial septal defects (ASD) and transposition of the great arteries (TGA). Recent advances in cardiac surgery have al-

Table 4–1. Common signs and symptoms in 22q11.2DS

	% with 22q11.2DS who have condition	% with condition who have 22q11.2DS[a]
Conotruncal heart disease	75	7
Tetralogy of Fallot	15–35	10–15
VSD with pulmonary atresia	15–30	20–50
Interrupted aortic arch type B	5–20	60–80
Truncus arteriosus	5–10	30–35
Palatal anomalies		
Hypernasality	75	
Velopharyngeal insufficiency[b]	30	
Submucous cleft palate	15	
Overt cleft palate	10	
Bifid uvula	5	
Facial dysmorphism	75	
Hypocalcemia	10–30	

Note. 22q11.1DS=chromosome 22q11.2 deletion syndrome; VSD=ventricular septal defect.
[a]Percentage with palatal anomalies and hypocalcemia who have 22q11.2DS not included because not reliable due to ascertainment bias and small sample size.
[b]Including nasal regurgitation.
Source. Adapted from Mazzocco MM, Ross J (eds.), *Neurogenetic Developmental Disorders: Variation of Manifestation in Childhood*, Table 6–1, © 2007 Massachusetts Institute of Technology, by permission of the MIT Press.

lowed many individuals with 22q11.2DS to survive into adulthood, and every person with 22q11.2DS should be evaluated by a cardiologist.

Ear, Nose, and Throat

Velopharyngeal insufficiency, or VPI (also known as velopharyngeal dysfunction, or VPD), is another common presenting feature of 22q11.2DS. Speech therapists may be the first to detect 22q11.2DS in individuals with VPI. This condition usually results in hypernasal speech due to improper movement of the velum (soft palate) and pharyngeal (throat) muscles. VPI is often but not always present in combination with a cleft palate. Submucous cleft palates are more common, although less obvious due to overlying mucous membrane covering of the palate, and are often associated with a bifid (split) uvula. They are often visualized only through nasendoscopy (Shprintzen and Golding-Kushner 1989). Clefts of the hard palate involve a defect in bone and are usually more obvious. Nasal regurgitation (escape of liquid or food through the nasal passages) is highly associated with VPI and is an important symptom to elicit in the patient's history.

Facial

A distinct physical phenotype is present in over 75% of people with 22q11.2DS (Cohen et al. 1999; Lipson et al. 1991) (Figure 4–1). Although the facial characteristics are sometimes subtle in appearance, individuals usually have long and narrow faces, hypertelorism (widely spaced eyes), narrow palpebral fissures (vertical distance of the ocular opening), and "hooded" eyelids. Noses tend to be long and bulbous or square, and ears are often small and sometimes misfolded. Individuals often have short philtrums (ridge between nose and mouth). Greater awareness of the facial features, especially in combination with congenital heart disease, VPI, or nasal regurgitation, can increase detection of 22q11.2DS.

Endocrine

Hormone abnormalities are also frequently part of 22q11.2DS. The deletion affects structures of the third and fourth pharyngeal arches, the embryonic structures that ultimately develop into the palate, thymus, and aortic arch. The thyroid and parathyroid glands also arise from these structures, and hypocalcemia from parathyroid dysfunction may be a presenting feature. Hypocalcemia can cause seizures, muscle spasms/cramps, a tingling sensation (paresthesia), osteoporosis, or arrhythmia. Hypocalcemia is easily treatable, and calcium levels in individuals with the deletion should be screened regularly.

Thyroid hormone levels may be abnormal (mostly low), and this abnormality can cause developmental and/or growth delay if present and not treated at birth. Symptoms may include constipation, cold intolerance, fatigue, brittle hair, dry skin, and weight gain. Although feeding difficulties may lead to growth delay, growth hormone deficiency has also been reported. Therefore, endocrinology referral should be considered in children with height and/or weight below the 5th percentile, although up to 40% of children with 22q11.2DS have poor growth, usually with normal growth hormone levels (Weinzimer et al. 1998). Adult height is often in the normal range. Growth charts specific for 22q11.2DS have been developed and may be useful in evaluating growth (Shprintzen 2009).

Immune

Thymic hypoplasia (underdevelopment) is responsible for poor immune response and frequent ear and/or respiratory infections during infancy and childhood. Live vaccines should not be administered unless an immunolo-

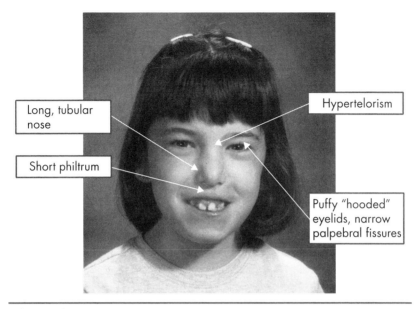

FIGURE 4-1. Characteristic facial features in chromosome 22q11.2 deletion syndrome.

Source.   Image used with parental permission.

gist determines that a child's immune function is adequate. Vaccine titers may be checked to confirm immunity. Individuals with 22q11.2DS are at higher risk for autoimmune diseases (e.g., hypothyroidism, celiac disease), likely due to poor T-cell function. T-cell dysfunction and loss of tolerance may also contribute to increased cancer risk, although this has not been confirmed in the literature.

Gastrointestinal

Common gastrointestinal problems include constipation, gastroesophageal reflux disease (GERD), which may also manifest as nasal regurgitation if an individual has VPI, and feeding dysfunction due to hypotonia and poor coordination of the swallowing muscles. Some children require surgical intervention for GERD and/or gastrostomy or nasogastric tube placement for failure to thrive.

Ophthalmological

Strabismus, posterior embryotoxon (a thick ring around the cornea), and refraction errors are common and should be screened for yearly. Examination with dilation may identify tortuous retinal vessels (Forbes et al. 2007).

Musculoskeletal

Scoliosis is common in 22q11.2DS. Many children complain of leg pain similar to growing pains. If caused by flat feet, this pain can often be treated with insoles and muscle stretching (Al-Khattat and Campbell 2000). Fingers tend to be long and thin. Sprengel deformity (uneven scapula placement due to failure of one shoulder blade to descend to its proper position) may also be seen.

Brain/Neurological

As stated in the earlier "Endocrine" subsection, seizures may occur secondary to hypocalcemia. Characteristic structural brain abnormalities have been reported in 22q11.2DS. Their significance is unclear because only a loose relationship appears to exist between these structural anomalies and their functional implications, and the impact of environmental and experiential factors during prenatal and postnatal development remains poorly understood. However, investigation into these differences is accelerating and will likely provide valuable insight into mechanisms involved in the specific cognitive impairments seen in 22q11.2DS. Recognition of these differences is important to avoid misdiagnosis or unnecessary invasive interventions.

Compared to typical but not IQ-matched controls of the same age, children and adolescents with 22q11.2DS have decreased brain volumes and reductions in white matter volume (Karayiorgou et al. 2010). Enlarged lateral ventricles are also commonly seen on imaging (Campbell et al. 2006; Simon et al. 2005c), and these characteristics seem to parallel structural abnormalities reported commonly in schizophrenia. Additionally, it is important to distinguish these findings from hydrocephalus to avoid unnecessary intervention.

Other structural brain differences include enlarged cavum septi pellucidi (Beaton et al. 2010; Campbell et al. 2006) and other midline defects, particularly involving the cerebellum (Bish et al. 2006; Eliez et al. 2001), subcortical regions (Eliez et al. 2002), and limbic system (Campbell et al. 2006). Rarely, individuals with 22q11.2DS have polymicrogyria (Robin et al. 2006), which may be accompanied by neurological symptoms such as seizures and spasticity. If polymicrogyria in the perisylvian region is found, the individual should be tested for 22q11.2DS through fluorescence in situ hybridization (FISH) (Gerkes et al. 2010).

Genitourinary

Structural urinary tract anomalies, present in up to 30% of individuals with 22q11.2DS (Wu et al. 2002), may affect the kidneys or genitals and predispose to urinary tract infections. Kidney involvement includes agenesis (underdevelopment) or dysplasia (abnormal shape), such as horseshoe or single kidney. Hydronephrosis and/or vesicoureteral reflux may also be seen.

Males may have undescended testes or hypospadias in frequencies greater than those seen in the general population.

Summary

Multiple organ systems may be affected in 22q11.2DS. Testing to confirm 22q11.2DS should be considered if one of the typical cardiac lesions (TOF, interrupted aortic arch, TA, VSD+PA, or VSD+arch anomaly) is present or if two or more of the following are involved: cardiac defects other than those mentioned above (e.g., isolated ASD/VSD, pulmonary stenosis, TGA, double outlet right ventricle), immunodeficiency/hypoplastic thymus, hypocalcemia, feeding problems, cleft palate, developmental delay, other malformation (skeletal, renal, hernia, central nervous system), or facial dysmorphism (Oskarsdóttir et al. 2004). Because recognition of the facial characteristics in the presence of congenital heart disease, VPI, or developmental delay can increase identification of the syndrome, physicians, speech therapists, occupational therapists, psychologists, and educators who are aware of these characteristics may be the first to suspect 22q11.2DS.

Development

Motor

Most children with 22q11.2DS have early hypotonia (low muscle tone) and gross motor delays, walking at a mean age of 18 months (Sobin et al. 2005a). Fine motor delays are also common, with poor coordination and balance problems (Roizen et al. 2010). Physical and occupational therapy are often beneficial.

Speech and Language

Despite relative strength in verbal skills when compared with visuospatial abilities, early delays in language, particularly expressive language skills, are common for children with 22q11.2DS. Pragmatic language is also commonly an area of weakness (Glaser et al. 2002), and communication tends to be concrete and literal. This finding is consistent with difficulties in abstraction and more complex use of language.

Cognitive Function

For children with 22q11.2DS, mean Full Scale IQ (FSIQ) is usually in the borderline range, although individual variability exists (De Smedt et al. 2007). FSIQ can be misleading due to higher verbal IQ (usually 75–80) than nonverbal IQ (usually 70–75), although this pattern can be reversed in some individuals (Wang et al. 2000). For most individuals, reading and spelling are relative strengths (Woodin et al. 2001), and rote verbal memory is often unimpaired (Woodin et al. 2001). Reading comprehension (Woodin et al. 2001) and math (De Smedt et al. 2009) are often problematic. Some practitioners describe the presence of a nonverbal learning disorder, given some of the visuospatial difficulties, although this label may not be a good fit for children with 22q11.2DS because many have language delay and considerable weaknesses in comprehension and other verbal domains. For further discussion of nonverbal learning disorder, see Chapter 10, "Disorders of Learning."

Individuals with 22q11.2DS often have a specific neurocognitive profile characterized by visuospatial impairments (Simon et al. 2005a), most significantly involving spatial attention. Their problems selecting among competing salient visual inputs can further affect their development of spatial and numerical processing (Simon 2008). Children with 22q11.2DS frequently have a specific impairment with volitional, rather than reflexive, control of attention, and impairments are reduced when attention can be directed to objects rather than to locations in space (Bish et al. 2007; Simon and Luck 2011). These spatial difficulties likely contribute during development to problems with counting/enumeration (Simon et al. 2005a) and with magnitude estimation, which involves mapping quantity and space (Simon 2008). Children with 22q11.2DS also show clear impairments in inhibitory aspects of attention, and these, along with other weaknesses in attention and executive control, may possibly relate to later psychosis risk (Bish et al. 2005; Sobin et al. 2004; Stoddard et al. 2010).

Behavioral and Psychiatric Disorders

Although early behavioral symptoms of children with 22q11.2DS are often related to medical problems and interventions, learning and mental health problems typically arise during primary and secondary school years.

Attention-Deficit/Hyperactivity Disorder

Approximately 40% of children with 22q11.2DS have attention-deficit/ hyperactivity disorder (ADHD) with impairments in working memory and attention that are related to the visuospatial deficits described previously in the section on cognitive function (Sobin et al. 2005b; Woodin et al. 2001). The inattentive or combined subtype of ADHD, rather than the hyperactive subtype, is more commonly seen in 22q11.22DS. Individuals are "less able to inhibit the processing of irrelevant information" (Simon et al. 2005b, p. 765) due to attentional and executive function problems. As a result, they have difficulty narrowing their focus of attention and adjusting their attentional resources in the context of conflicting or competing information, and this difficulty is likely exacerbated by common high levels of anxiety as discussed in the subsection on anxiety below.

Oppositional Defiant Disorder

Oppositional defiant disorder is a common comorbidity of ADHD. Prevalence of oppositional defiant disorder in 22q11.2DS is similar to that in cognitively matched control children (Feinstein et al. 2002).

Anxiety

Anxiety disorders affect 20%–60% of children with 22q11.2DS (Feinstein et al. 2002). A meta-analysis estimated that 39% of children with 22q11.2DS have some type of anxiety disorder (Jolin et al. 2011). Most frequent are specific phobias (31%–60%), generalized anxiety disorder (13%–29%), separation anxiety (9%–21%), and obsessive-compulsive disorder (8%–32%) (Feinstein et al. 2002; Jolin et al. 2011). Despite this known risk for anxiety in individuals with 22q11.2DS, our clinical experience is that anxiety is still underidentified and may be misdiagnosed as inattention, avoidance, or shyness. Treatment of anxiety symptoms is important because severity seems to affect adaptive functioning in this population (Angkustsiri et al. 2010). Evidence-based interventions are readily available.

Childhood disorders may contribute to the development of psychiatric disorders in adulthood, and early anxiety and chronic stress may increase the risk for psychosis in individuals with 22q11.2DS (Beaton and Simon 2011). Anxiety, specifically obsessive-compulsive disorder, was strongly associated with later development of a psychotic disorder in longitudinal follow-up of adolescents with 22q11.2DS (Gothelf et al. 2007).

Schizophrenia/Psychosis

By late adolescence and early adulthood, individuals with 22q11.2DS have a 25%–30% risk of schizophrenia-like psychotic disorders (Bassett et al. 2003). This deletion syndrome is the third highest genetic risk factor, preceded in degree of risk only by having both parents or an identical twin with schizophrenia. Up to 50% of adolescents with 22q11.2DS may have subclinical symptoms (Stoddard et al. 2010), indicating that not all individuals convert to full-blown disease and that protective factors are important to identify. Risk factors for later development of schizophrenia include baseline anxiety (particularly obsessive-compulsive disorder) and declining verbal IQ (Gothelf et al. 2007).

Autism Spectrum Disorders

Autism spectrum disorders have been reported in 30% of individuals with 22q11.2DS, with greater representation of pervasive developmental disorder not otherwise specified than of autistic disorder meeting full DSM-IV criteria (Kates et al. 2007; Vorstman et al. 2006). These studies, however, may overestimate the prevalence of autism spectrum disorders because they were based on interviews relying on parent report (Autism Diagnostic Interview—Revised) rather than direct assessment with the Autism Diagnostic Observation Schedule. In addition, social communication deficits during childhood for individuals with 22q11.2DS may be complicated by developmental delay and pragmatic language difficulties.

Etiologies

Chromosome 22q11.2 deletion syndrome is caused by a deletion on the long arm of chromosome 22. Most individuals (90%) with 22q11.2DS have a common 3-megabase (Mb) deletion in the DiGeorge critical region (DGCR), and over 90% of cases are de novo (sporadic) rather than inherited. It is an autosomal dominant disease, so individuals have a 50% chance of passing the deletion to offspring. Genes of interest in the DGCR include the T-box 1 gene *TBX1*, which is responsible for transcription factors in the formation of embryonic heart, parathyroid, and thymic tissue, and the catechol O-methyltransferase gene *COMT*, which is important in the metabolism of catecholamine neurotransmitters such as dopamine and norepinephrine. However, the association between *COMT* alleles and psychiatric disease is unclear, with variation in findings across studies.

Differential Diagnosis and Diagnostic Evaluation

Symptoms of 22q11.2DS are highly variable; more than 180 possible manifestations exist, although typical presentations seem to relate to age, with early diagnosis associated with cardiac problems and later diagnosis confirmed due to speech delay, developmental delay, learning difficulties, or recurrent infections (Oskarsdóttir et al. 2004). Opitz G/BBB syndrome affects midline structures, such as the trachea and larynx, and also may involve cleft lip/palate along with heart defects. There are two forms of Opitz G/BBB syndrome with similar phenotypic expression; the autosomal dominant form is caused by deletion of the chromosome 22q11.2 region, and the X-linked form is associated with the *MID1* gene on the X chromosome. Deletion of chromosome 10p13–p14 is also responsible for conotruncal heart disease and has clinical overlap with 22q11.2DS.

All individuals suspected of having 22q11.2DS should have confirmatory genetic testing through FISH, which incorporates the use of fluorescent probes to identify the presence of only one copy (normally there are two) of the 22q11.2 chromosomal region. The growing availability of chromosomal microarray analysis is likely to increase detection of more unusual presentations of the 22q11.2 deletion, and chromosomal microarray may be the test of choice if features are not classic for 22q11.2DS.

Once 22q11.2DS is identified, important evaluations include developmental and educational assessment for cognitive and learning difficulties; psychological assessment for ADHD, anxiety, and other mental health issues; and medical surveillance related to the topics discussed in the section "Signs and Symptoms." (For a review of practical management guidelines, see Bassett et al. 2011.)

Management and Intervention

Educational and Behavioral Treatments

Very few intervention studies of 22q11.2DS have been reported. This lack of research is especially unfortunate because for most domains of cognitive and behavioral functioning, it is likely that disorder-specific responses will be necessary. In the absence of such data, we recommend the use of available evidence-based treatments for the general underlying conditions identified (e.g., anxiety, ADHD, dyslexia). Although the deletion may predispose individuals to develop ADHD and learning difficulties, the underlying dysfunction is almost certainly no different from that in individuals without the deletion, and careful treatment is warranted if there is impairment in functioning. Appropriate educational intervention through the local school district (usually in the form of an Individualized Education Program, or IEP) is recommended as a starting point. Other modalities that may complement or supplement these interventions include center-based instructional programs and home interactive software. Neuropsychological assessment is indicated to identify an individual's strengths and weaknesses, which are important when choosing appropriate interventions. Many interventions require a considerable commitment of time and financial resources, so consideration only of treatments that have validated results helps when sorting through the numerous options currently available. Please see Chapter 10, "Disorders of Learning," for a discussion of how to choose evidenced-based interventions for learning disorders.

For treatment of anxiety, cognitive-behavioral therapy (with or without medication) has an established evidence base (Compton et al. 2004) and is the desired intervention modality. It is usually appropriate as long as the individual has adequate cognitive and verbal abilities. For those with more limited capacities, a behavioral approach focused on relaxation and coping skills may be helpful.

Psychopharmacological Treatments

Medications are available for the treatment of associated behavioral symptoms, such as ADHD and anxiety. Although child psychiatrists and developmental pediatricians may have more expertise with different medication classes, primary care providers can manage pharmacological treatments if they have access to specialists, a sufficient comfort level, and appropriate experience. In general, children with 22q11.2DS take the same medications as other children do, although more cautious monitoring of dosing is necessary because of potential differences in metabolism related to deletion of the 22q11.2 region. As with any intervention, the risks and benefits of treatment should be carefully considered before initiation. Any medication treatments should be complemented with other environmental supports, including family supports, IEPs, and community programs.

Attention-Deficit/Hyperactivity Disorder

Particular concerns have been expressed about the use of stimulant medications in individuals with 22q11.2DS due to the presumed effect of homozygosity in the COMT allele that regulates the degradation of dopamine in the prefrontal cortex. The Met/Val alleles have been studied most extensively, although there are other allelic variants in the COMT polymorphism. Compared with the Val allele, the Met allele has an approximately fourfold lower activity level in degrading dopamine, so individuals with 22q11.2DS who have one copy of the Met allele presumably have higher levels of synaptic dopamine than do those with the Val allele. Many practitioners avoid the use of stimulant medications for fear of inducing psychotic symptoms (through increased synaptic dopamine) in such a high-risk population, as well as from the desire to avoid cardiovascular side effects in children with a history of congenital heart disease. An early study of stimulant treatment for ADHD symptoms in children with 22q11.2DS involved an open-label trial of low-dose methylphenidate in 18 children for 4 weeks (Gothelf et al. 2003). Seventy-five percent of those treated demonstrated significant clinical improvement, and treatment was well tolerated. None of the participants discontinued medication, and no psychotic symptoms were reported. A larger study of 34 children with low-dose methylphenidate demonstrated similar efficacy and tolerability after 6 months (Green et al. 2011). Studies of other pharmacological treatments for ADHD, such as atomoxetine or α-adrenergic agonists, have not been published. Practical clinical guidelines (Bassett et al. 2011) recommend "standard treatment" of childhood neuropsychiatric disorders. If medications are to be used, we recommend starting at lower dosages with slow titration and more frequent monitoring for side effects.

Anxiety and Depression

The most common pharmacological treatments for anxiety and depressive disorders are the selective serotonin reuptake inhibitors (SSRIs). There are no known published studies on the efficacy and side-effect profile of these medications specifically in 22q11.2DS; anecdotally, however, we and others have noted symptomatic improvement and good tolerability of the SSRIs in this population. As always, nonpharmacological treatments and behavioral therapies, many of which have a good evidence base in the non-22q11.2DS population, should be considered as well.

Schizophrenia and Psychotic Disorders

Clinical features of schizophrenia, including age at onset, core symptoms, and severity, do not differ between individuals with or without 22q11.2DS who develop schizophrenia (Bassett et al. 2003). Pharmacological intervention for schizophrenia and psychotic symptoms should be managed by a child and adolescent psychiatrist, although it is not necessary to seek a provider who is an expert in 22q11.2DS. However, awareness of altered dopamine metabolism in individuals with 22q11.2DS is useful in the management of available effective therapies, including atypical antipsychotics and mood stabilizers.

Outcomes

Outcomes are heterogeneous, with a broad range of functioning. These differences are attributable not only to variability in symptom expression but also to improvements in cardiac surgery and medical treatments that have led to greater survival of individuals with serious medical conditions. As a large cohort nears adulthood, there is even greater urgency to identify psychiatric disease early, provide appropriate treatment, and identify protective factors that may mitigate associated morbidity. Expected life span is not thought to be significantly decreased in the absence of cardiac or severe disease, although one study (Bassett et al. 2009) reported decreased survival during adulthood in the 22q11.2DS population compared to sibling control subjects. In that study, 11% of the 22q11.2DS group had died by follow-up, with a mean age of 41.5 years at time of death. None of the sibling controls had died at the end of the follow-up period.

Family and environmental supports are other likely contributors to outcome, underscoring the importance of early intervention for developmental delays. Although most cases of 22q11.2DS are sporadic, approximately 10% are inherited from a parent, and some presentations may be subtle or unrecognized. Children with an inherited deletion may have lower IQ scores compared with individuals with a de novo mutation, although their psychiatric disorders are similar (Gothelf et al. 2007). Challenges related to raising a child with special health care and behavioral needs (including access to services, poor physician and therapist understanding of symptoms, and school challenges) may also add family stress.

New Research Directions

With any disorder, research to identify factors that lead to better outcomes (both prevention and intervention) and improved adult functioning has practical societal and individual implications. In addition, the 22q11.2DS population is a valuable population for research given the known identification of genes in the deletion region and the availability of animal models, both of which may have significance in understanding the underlying etiology of particular medical conditions, learning disabilities, and psychiatric disease in the general population. Intervention for visuospatial difficulties is one area of particular interest, as are a range of potential interventions for the well-known executive function impairments and significant social difficulties that, together, affect a wide range of functioning for the developing individual. Other research is focused on candidate genes in the 22q11.2 deleted region, such as *COMT* and *TBX1*, mentioned earlier in the section "Etiologies." Genes that code for proteins involved in brain function in the 22q11.2 locus include *PRODH* (proline dehydrogenase) and *DGCR8* (DiGeorge syndrome critical region 8).

Summary

The chromosome 22q11.2 deletion syndrome is the most common microdeletion syndrome in humans and has wide symptom variability. Frequent physical manifestations include congenital heart disease, palatal dysfunction, immune difficulties, and hypocalcemia, although other organ systems are often involved as well. Individuals with 22q11.2DS may also have learning and psychiatric involvement, with developmental delay, deficits in visuospatial planning, and mental health disorders such as ADHD, anxiety, and later risk of psychosis. Of course, no individual exhibits every related symptom of 22q11.2DS, and diagnosis is complicated by the relatively recent discovery of a common genetic deletion and by confusion in the labeling of multiple overlapping phenotypic syndromes. Recognition of the broader phenotype by physicians, psychologists, educators, and other providers can increase identification of the syndrome, enabling individuals to receive educational, medical, and behavioral treatments to improve outcomes.

Key Points

- Chromosome 22q11.2 deletion syndrome is the most common micro-deletion syndrome in humans, with an estimated prevalence of 1 in 2,000–4,000 live births.

- There is phenotypic variability, with possible involvement of multiple body systems, including the cardiac, ear nose and throat, endocrine, immune, gastrointestinal, genitourinary, neurological, ophthalmological, and musculoskeletal systems.

- 22q11.2DS is often associated with conotruncal heart disease, including tetralogy of Fallot and aortic arch abnormalities.

- Other common symptoms include velopharyngeal insufficiency, hypocalcemia, and immune dysfunction.

- Most children with 22q11.2DS have developmental delays and borderline IQs, although verbal IQ is often higher than performance IQ.

- A characteristic facial phenotype is present in over 75% of individuals with 22q11.2DS.

- Individuals are at risk for psychiatric disorders, including anxiety disorders, ADHD, social impairments, and schizophrenia.

- Practitioners should screen for and treat medical, educational, and psychiatric disorders in people with 22q11.2DS.

Recommended Readings

Bassett AS, McDonald-McGinn DM, Devriendt K, et al: Practical guidelines for managing patients with 22q11.2 deletion syndrome. J Pediatr 159:332-339, 2011

Cutler-Landsman D: Educating Children With Velo-Cardio-Facial Syndrome. San Diego, CA, Plural Publishing, 2007

De Smedt B, Devriendt K, Fryns JP, et al: Intellectual abilities in a large sample of children with velo-cardio-facial syndrome: an update. J Intellect Disabil Res 51:666-670, 2007

Karayiorgou M, Simon TJ, Gogos JA: 22q11.2 microdeletions: linking DNA structural variation to brain dysfunction and schizophrenia. Nat Rev Neurosci 11: 402-416, 2010

McDonald-McGinn DM, Emanuel BS, Zackai EH: 22q11.2 Deletion syndrome, in GeneReviews™ [Internet]. Edited by Pagon RA, Bird TD, Dolan CR, et al. Seattle, University of Washington, Seattle. Sep 23, 1999 [Updated Dec 16, 2005]. Available at: http://www.ncbi.nlm.nih.gov/books/NBK1523. Accessed September 4, 2012.

Shprintzen RJ: Velo-cardio-facial syndrome: 30 years of study. Dev Disabil Res Revs 14:3-10, 2008

References

Al-Khattat A, Campbell J: Recurrent limb pain in childhood. Foot (Edinb) 10:117–123, 2000

Angkustsiri K, Leckliter I, Beaton EA, et al: Anxiety, not intelligence, predicts adaptive functioning in children with VCFS/22q11.2DS. Abstract presented at the 17th annual International Scientific Meeting of the Velo-Cardio-Facial Syndrome Educational Foundation, Salt Lake City, UT, July 16–18, 2010

Bassett AS, Chow EW, AbdelMalik P, et al: The schizophrenia phenotype in 22q11 deletion syndrome. Am J Psychiatry 160:1580–1586, 2003

Bassett AS, Chow EW, Husted J, et al: Premature death in adults with 22q11.2 deletion syndrome. J Med Genet 46:324–330, 2009

Bassett AS, McDonald-McGinn DM, Devriendt K, et al: Practical guidelines for managing patients with 22q11.2 deletion syndrome. J Pediatr 159:332–339, 2011

Beaton EA, Simon TJ: How might stress contribute to increased risk for schizophrenia in children with chromosome 22q11.2 deletion syndrome? J Neurodev Disord 3:68–75, 2011

Beaton EA, Qin Y, Nguyen V, et al: Increased incidence and size of cavum septum pellucidum in children with chromosome 22q11.2 deletion syndrome. Psychiatry Res 181:108–113, 2010

Bish JP, Ferrante SM, McDonald-McGinn D, et al: Maladaptive conflict monitoring as evidence for executive dysfunction in children with chromosome 22q11.2 deletion syndrome. Dev Sci 8:36–43, 2005

Bish JP, Pendyal A, Ding L, et al: Specific cerebellar reductions in children with chromosome 22q11.2 deletion syndrome. Neurosci Lett 399:245–248, 2006

Bish JP, Chiodo R, Mattei V, et al: Domain specific attentional impairments in children with chromosome 22q11.2 deletion syndrome. Brain Cogn 64:265–273, 2007

Botto LD, May K, Fernhoff PM, et al: A population-based study of the 22q11.2 deletion: phenotype, incidence, and contribution to major birth defects in the population. Pediatrics 112:101–107, 2003

Campbell LE, Daly E, Toal F, et al: Brain and behaviour in children with 22q11.2 deletion syndrome: a volumetric and voxel-based morphometry MRI study. Brain 129:1218–1228, 2006

Cohen E, Chow EW, Weksberg A, et al: Phenotype of adults with the 22q11 deletion syndrome: a review. Am J Med Genet 86:359–365, 1999

Compton SN, March JS, Brent D, et al: Cognitive-behavioral psychotherapy for anxiety and depressive disorders in children and adolescents: an evidence-based medicine review. J Am Acad Child Adolesc Psychiatry 43:930–959, 2004

De Smedt B, Devriendt K, Fryns JP, et al: Intellectual abilities in a large sample of children with velo-cardio-facial syndrome: an update. J Intellect Disabil Res 51:666–670, 2007

De Smedt B, Swillen A, Verschaffel L, et al: Mathematical learning disabilities in children with 22q11.2 deletion syndrome: a review. Dev Disabil Res Rev 15:4–10, 2009

Driscoll DA, Salvin J, Sellinger B, et al: Prevalence of 22q11 microdeletions in DiGeorge and velocardiofacial syndromes: implications for genetic counselling and prenatal diagnosis. J Med Genet 30:813–817, 1993

Eliez S, Blasey CM, Schmitt EJ, et al: Velocardiofacial syndrome: are structural changes in the temporal and mesial temporal regions related to schizophrenia? Am J Psychiatry 158:447–453, 2001

Eliez S, Barnea-Goraly N, Schmitt JE, et al: Increased basal ganglia volumes in velo-cardio-facial syndrome (deletion 22q11.2). Biol Psychiatry 52:68–70, 2002

Feinstein C, Eliez S, Blasey C, et al: Psychiatric disorders and behavioral problems in children with velocardiofacial syndrome: usefulness as phenotypic indicators of schizophrenia risk. Biol Psychiatry 51:312–318, 2002

Forbes BJ, Binenbaum G, Edmond JC, et al: Ocular findings in the chromosome 22q11.2 deletion syndrome. J AAPOS 11:179–182, 2007

Gerkes EH, Hordijk R, Dijkhuizen T, et al: Bilateral polymicrogyria as the indicative feature in a child with a 22q11.2 deletion. Eur J Med Genet 53:344–346, 2010

Glaser B, Mumme DL, Blasey C, et al: Language skills in children with velocardiofacial syndrome (deletion 22q11.2). J Pediatr 140:753–758, 2002

Gothelf D, Gruber R, Presburger G, et al: Methylphenidate treatment for attention-deficit/hyperactivity disorder in children and adolescents with velocardiofacial syndrome: an open-label study. J Clin Psychiatry 64:1163–1169, 2003

Gothelf D, Feinstein C, Thompson T, et al: Risk factors for the emergence of psychotic disorders in adolescents with 22q11.2 deletion syndrome. Am J Psychiatry 164:663–669, 2007

Green T, Weinberger R, Diamond A, et al: The effect of methylphenidate on prefrontal cognitive functioning, inattention, and hyperactivity in velocardiofacial syndrome. J Child Adolesc Psychopharmacol 21:589–595, 2011

Jolin EM, Weller RA, Weller EB: Occurrence of affective disorders compared to other psychiatric disorders in children and adolescents with 22q11.2 deletion syndrome. J Affect Disord 136:222–228, 2011

Karayiorgou M, Simon TJ, Gogos JA: 22q11.2 microdeletions: linking DNA structural variation to brain dysfunction and schizophrenia. Nat Rev Neurosci 11:402–416, 2010

Kates WR, Antshel KM, Fremont WP, et al: Comparing phenotypes in patients with idiopathic autism to patients with velocardiofacial syndrome (22q11 DS) with and without autism. Am J Med Genet A 143A:2642–2650, 2007

Kirkpatrick JA Jr, DiGeorge AM: Congenital absence of the thymus. Am J Roentgenol Radium Ther Nucl Med 103:32–37, 1968

Lipson AH, Yuille D, Angel M, et al: Velocardiofacial (Shprintzen) syndrome: an important syndrome for the dysmorphologist to recognise. J Med Genet 28:596–604, 1991

Oskarsdóttir S, Vujic M, Fasth A: Incidence and prevalence of the 22q11 deletion syndrome: a population-based study in western Sweden. Arch Dis Child 89:148–151, 2004

Robin NH, Taylor CJ, McDonald-McGinn DM, et al: Polymicrogyria and deletion 22q11.2 syndrome: window to the etiology of a common cortical malformation. Am J Med Genet A 140:2416–2425, 2006

Roizen NJ, Higgins AM, Antshel KM, et al: 22q11.2 deletion syndrome: are motor deficits more than expected for IQ level? J Pediatr 157:658–661, 2010

Shprintzen RJ: Velo-cardio-facial syndrome: 30 years of study. Dev Disabil Res Rev 14:3–10, 2008

Shprintzen RJ: Growth Velocity, Weight Gain & Growth Charts for Velo-Cardio-Facial Syndrome: Management of Feeding and Swallowing Problems. San Diego, CA, Plural Publishing, 2009

Shprintzen RJ, Golding-Kushner KJ: Evaluation of velopharyngeal insufficiency. Otolaryngol Clin North Am 22:519–536, 1989

Shprintzen RJ, Goldberg RB, Lewin ML, et al: A new syndrome involving cleft palate, cardiac anomalies, typical facies, and learning disabilities: velo-cardio-facial syndrome. Cleft Palate J 15:56–62, 1978

Simon TJ: A new account of the neurocognitive foundations of impairments in space, time and number processing in children with chromosome 22q11.2 deletion syndrome. Dev Disabil Res Rev 14:52–58, 2008

Simon TJ, Luck SJ: Attentional impairments in children with chromosome 22q11.2 deletion syndrome, in Cognitive Neursocience of Attention. Edited by Posner MI. New York, Guilford, 2011, pp 441–453

Simon TJ, Bearden CE, Mc-Ginn DM, et al: Visuospatial and numerical cognitive deficits in children with chromosome 22q11.2 deletion syndrome. Cortex 41:145–155, 2005a

Simon TJ, Bish JP, Bearden CE, et al: A multilevel analysis of cognitive dysfunction and psychopathology associated with chromosome 22q11.2 deletion syndrome in children. Dev Psychopathol 17:753–784, 2005b

Simon TJ, Ding L, Bish JP, et al: Volumetric, connective, and morphologic changes in the brains of children with chromosome 22q11.2 deletion syndrome: an integrative study. Neuroimage 25:169–180, 2005c

Simon TJ, Burg-Malki M, Gothelf D: Cognitive and behavioral characteristics of children with chromosome 22q11.2 deletion, in Neurogenetic Developmental Disorders: Variation of Manifestation in Childhood. Edited by Mazzocco MM, Ross JL. Cambridge, MA, MIT Press, 2007, pp 297–334

Sobin C, Kiley-Brabeck K, Daniels S, et al: Networks of attention in children with the 22q11 deletion syndrome. Dev Neuropsychol 26:611–626, 2004

Sobin C, Kiley-Brabeck K, Daniels S, et al: Neuropsychological characteristics of children with the 22q11 deletion syndrome: a descriptive analysis. Child Neuropsychol 11:39–53, 2005a

Sobin C, Kiley-Brabeck K, Karayiorgou M: Associations between prepulse inhibition and executive visual attention in children with the 22q11 deletion syndrome. Mol Psychiatry 10:553–562, 2005b

Stoddard J, Niendam T, Hendren R, et al: Attenuated positive symptoms of psychosis in adolescents with chromosome 22q11.2 deletion syndrome. Schizophr Res 118:118–121, 2010

Vorstman JA, Staal WG, van Daalen E, et al: Identification of novel autism candidate regions through analysis of reported cytogenetic abnormalities associated with autism. Mol Psychiatry 11:18–28, 2006

Wang PP, Woodin MF, Kreps-Falk R, et al: Research on behavioral phenotypes: velocardiofacial syndrome (deletion 22q11.2). Dev Med Child Neurol 42:422–427, 2000

Weinzimer SA, McDonald-McGinn DM, Driscoll DA, et al: Growth hormone deficiency in patients with 22q11.2 deletion: expanding the phenotype. Pediatrics 101:929–932, 1998

Woodin M, Wang PP, Aleman D, et al: Neuropsychological profile of children and adolescents with the 22q11.2 microdeletion. Genet Med 3:34–39, 2001

Wu HY, Rusnack SL, Bellah RD, et al: Genitourinary malformations in chromosome 22q11.2 deletion. J Urol 168:2564–2565, 2002

CHAPTER 5

TOURETTE SYNDROME, TIC DISORDERS, AND COMORBIDITIES

Joan R. Gunther, Psy.D.
Frank R. Sharp, M.D.

Gilles de la Tourette syndrome is a neurodevelopmental disorder with symptoms initially appearing in childhood. The disorder may also be called GTS or Tourette's disorder but is most commonly referred to as Tourette syndrome (TS) or Tourette's. The syndrome is named for Georges Gilles de la Tourette, who first characterized the disorder in 1885 (Walusinski and Bogousslavsky 2011).

TS is at one end of the continuum of tic disorders identified in DSM-IV-TR (American Psychiatric Association 2000). DSM-IV-TR differentiates four tic disorders: Tourette's disorder, chronic motor or vocal tic disorder, transient tic disorder, and tic disorder not otherwise specified. Although the occurrence of tics is the major clinical feature of each of these disorders, they are characterized according to the type of tics exhibited as well as their duration. TS is characterized by multiple motor tics and at least one vocal tic beginning before age 18 and persisting for at least 1 year. Chronic tic disorders comprise either motor or vocal tics, appear before age 18, and are present for 1 year or longer. Transient tic disorder involves the presence of either or both motor or vocal tics that begin before age 18 and occur for less than 1 year. Finally, a diagnosis of tic disorder not otherwise specified is indicated when tics do not meet the criteria for other tic disorders, such as those that have adult onset. Full DSM-IV-TR criteria for the three specified disorders are listed in Table 5–1 (American Psychiatric Association 2000).

Table 5–1. DSM-IV-TR diagnostic criteria for tic disorders

Tourette's disorder

A. Both multiple motor and one or more vocal tics have been present at some time during the illness, although not necessarily concurrently. (A *tic* is a sudden, rapid, recurrent, nonrhythmic, stereotyped motor movement or vocalization.)

B. The tics occur many times a day (usually in bouts) nearly every day or intermittently throughout a period of more than 1 year, and during this period there was never a tic-free period of more than 3 consecutive months.

C. The onset is before age 18 years.

D. The disturbance is not due to the direct physiological effects of a substance (e.g., stimulants) or a general medical condition (e.g., Huntington's disease or postviral encephalitis).

Chronic motor or vocal tic disorder

A. Single or multiple motor or vocal tics (i.e., sudden, rapid, recurrent, nonrhythmic, stereotyped motor movements or vocalizations), but not both, have been present at some time during the illness.

B. The tics occur many times a day nearly every day or intermittently throughout a period of more than 1 year, and during this period there was never a tic-free period of more than 3 consecutive months.

C. The onset is before age 18 years.

D. The disturbance is not due to the direct physiological effects of a substance (e.g., stimulants) or a general medical condition (e.g., Huntington's disease or postviral encephalitis).

E. Criteria have never been met for Tourette's disorder.

Transient tic disorder

A. Single or multiple motor and/or vocal tics (i.e., sudden, rapid, recurrent, nonrhythmic, stereotyped motor movements or vocalizations)

B. The tics occur many times a day, nearly every day for at least 4 weeks, but for no longer than 12 consecutive months.

C. The onset is before age 18 years.

D. The disturbance is not due to the direct physiological effects of a substance (e.g., stimulants) or a general medical condition (e.g., Huntington's disease or postviral encephalitis).

E. Criteria have never been met for Tourette's disorder or chronic motor or vocal tic disorder.

Source. Reprinted from *Diagnostic and Statistical Manual of Mental Disorders*, 4th Edition, Text Revision. Washington, DC, American Psychiatric Association, 2000, pp. 114–116. Used with permission. Copyright © 2000 American Psychiatric Association.

Signs and Symptoms, Onset, and Developmental Course

Tics are the distinguishing feature of TS and the related tic disorders. Tics are characterized as sudden, repetitive movements (motor tics) or sounds (vocal tics) that are, at best, only partially controlled by the individual. Vocal tics may more aptly be referred to as phonic tics, because many of the sounds do not involve the vocal cords but instead are made with the tongue (clucking), with the teeth (clicking), or by movement of air through the nose (sniffing) or throat (clearing). Motor and phonic tics are further classified as simple or complex tics.

Simple tics consist of rapid, brief, meaningless movements or sounds that typically involve only one muscle group and are completed within a few seconds. Simple motor tics include actions such as repeatedly blinking the eyes, widely opening the mouth, or jerking the head. Simple motor tics can be further categorized into clonic tics (jerklike movement, such as blinking or thrusting a limb), dystonic tics (slow, briefly sustained movements, such as looking to the side, rotating the shoulder), or tonic tics (tensing the abdomen or buttocks). Simple phonic tics include brief sounds, such as throat clearing, sniffing, or grunting.

Complex motor tics are more elaborate and may appear purposeful, such as jumping, brushing back hair, or touching objects, or may consist of a pattern of movements involving more than one muscle group, such as jerking the head back followed by raising the shoulders. Complex phonic tics may include repetitively saying out-of-context words, phrases, or sentences or may include the involuntary repetition of another person's words or sounds (echolalia), the involuntary mimicking of another's movements (echopraxia), or the repeating of one's own words (palilalia). Palilalia is usually limited to the repetition of the last word, phrase, or syllable (Jankovic and Kurlan 2011).

Although most tics are relatively benign, some individuals exhibit tics that result in dire interpersonal, social, or physical consequences. Individuals with severe tics are at increased risk not only for physical injuries such as bruising, fractures, and dislocations, but also for social isolation, depression, and drug abuse (Cheung et al. 2007). Interpersonal problems range from increased family stress to the loss of relationships. Social consequences extend from mild embarrassment to the misinterpretation of tics as volitional acts requiring legal action (Robertson 2000). Physical consequences span from mild skin picking or hair pulling to potentially life-threatening actions such as forcing objects into the throat or into open wounds. One study found that 5.1% of 332 patients with TS seen in a TS clinic over the course of 3 years met criteria for what the authors described as "malignant TS," defined by either two emergency room visits or one hospitalization due to violent acts, self-injurious behaviors, or suicide attempts related to TS (Cheung et al. 2007).

Among those tics that have the potential to cause socially devastating consequences are coprophenomena, which are complex tics of a markedly unusual nature. Coprophenomena include coprolalia, the involuntary utterance of obscene language; copropraxia, the involuntary production of obscene gestures (Freeman et al. 2009); and nonobscene socially inappropriate behaviors, such as the unintentional use of insulting comments or actions, which may include sexual, religious, racial, or ethnic content (Robertson 2000). Although it is one of the most publicly recognized symptoms of TS, coprolalia is relatively rare, and copropraxia is even rarer. In an extensive study, Freeman et al. (2009) gathered data from the Tourette Syndrome International Database Consortium. Based on data from 597 patients with TS from 15 sites in seven countries, the researchers found the lifetime prevalence rate of coprolalia to be 19.3% for males and 14.6% for females. Copropraxia was found in 5.9% of males and 4.9% of females. Some evidence suggests that coprolalia may be influenced by culture. In Japan, only 4% of individuals exhibit this symptom, whereas higher rates are reported in some other countries than in the United States. Finally, nonobscene socially inappropriate behaviors may have a close association to comorbid conduct disorder or attention-deficit/hyperactivity disorder (ADHD) (Robertson 2000).

Although tics usually manifest in distinct patterns unique to an individual, the breadth of TS symptoms across individuals is extensive. By no means all-inclusive, Table 5–2 delineates examples of simple and complex motor and phonic tics.

Table 5–2.   Simple and complex tics

Simple motor	Complex motor	Simple phonic	Complex phonic
Arm thrusting	Copropraxia	Barking	Breathing patterns
Eye blinking	Echopraxia	Belching	Calling out
Eye opening	Flapping arms	Gasping	Coprolalia
Grimacing	Jumping	Grunting	Echolalia
Head jerking	Pinching	Gurgling	Humming
Mouth opening	Sequential actions	Screeching	Intonation changes
Nose twitching	Smelling objects	Sniffing	Laughing
Pouting	Squatting	Squeaking	Palilalia
Shrugging	Stooping	Throat clearing	Phrases
Stretching fingers	Touching objects	Words	Speech patterns

Tics usually occur in discrete bouts and may change in number, frequency, form, and location, while waxing and waning in severity. Anxiety, stress, and fatigue have the tendency to intensify tics, whereas deliberate focus diminishes them. An increase in tics may be noticed when a holiday approaches, and a reduction may be noticed when the individual is engaged in sports, playing a musical instrument, or involved in fine motor activities (Leckman et al. 2010).

The typical age at tic onset is approximately 4–6 years. TS usually begins with simple tics that involve the face, such as an eyeblink. The typical course of the disorder involves motor and phonic tics evolving from simple to complex. As the disorder progresses, motor tics usually move from the head and neck in a downward direction, to movements of the shoulders; then arm, finger, or leg movements; and then tensing of the abdomen or buttocks. The onset of phonic tics typically follows 1–2 years after motor tics have begun. Phonic tics often begin as simple vocalizations or sounds and progress to full words, phrases, or sentences (Bloch and Leckman 2009).

Tics usually peak in severity during early adolescence (Leckman et al. 2010). If coprolalia manifests, it usually appears around the age of worst tic severity (Freeman et al. 2009). Although childhood tic severity is a poor predictor of severity in adulthood, the intensity of tics in early adolescence is weakly associated with severity in adulthood (Bloch and Leckman 2009). Complex tics tend to decrease during adulthood, but tics of the face, neck, and trunk may persist (Jankovic and Kurlan 2011). Approximately one-third of children diagnosed with tic disorders will be tic free by the time they reach adulthood, and approximately three-quarters will experience only mild tics. The remainder will continue to suffer moderate tic severity, with 5% of individuals reporting worsening tics in adulthood (Bloch and Leckman 2009).

As they grow older, many patients report an ability to suppress their tics or disguise them as purposeful actions. For example, an individual may mask a head-flicking tic by appearing to purposefully flip hair away from his or her face. Unfortunately, the effort of suppression often results in decreased concentration, increased tension, and exhaustion (Conelea and Woods 2008; Du et al. 2010).

Many adolescents and adults with TS experience a sensation associated with tics. This sensation, known as a premonitory urge, is experienced immediately before exhibition of the tic. The premonitory urge is reported as being similar to, but much more powerful than, the feeling experienced just before sneezing or scratching an itch. Although most children under age 10 appear to be unaware of these sensations, 90% of older individuals report a premonitory urge. Individuals who are able to temporarily suppress their tics report that the urges are not as easily squelched (Leckman et al. 2006). When individuals are prevented from performing their tic, 74% report that the urge intensifies. So predominant is the urge that many people with TS describe their tic as a "voluntary motor response to an involuntary sensation" (Kwak et al. 2003).

Comorbid Conditions

Although individuals with chronic or transient tic disorders do not commonly have comorbid psychiatric disorders, individuals with TS often have at least one comorbid condition. A survey carried out by the Health Resources and Services Administration found that 79% of children and adolescents with TS were also diagnosed with a comorbid mental health disorder (Centers for Disease Control and Prevention 2009).

Some evidence suggests that the severity of tics is related to comorbidity (Cheung et al. 2007). However, the symptoms of the comorbid disorders often prove to be more behaviorally, academically, and socially challenging than the tics (Leckman et al. 2006). These findings emphasize the importance of a clinician's knowledge, ongoing monitoring, and treatment of comorbidities, as well as the need for parents to become aware of the symptoms of commonly occurring comorbid disorders.

Attention-Deficit/Hyperactivity Disorder

Individuals with ADHD exhibit age-inappropriate inattention, hyperactivity, and impulsivity evident in two or more settings before age 7 (American Psychiatric Association 2000). According to a 2008 report by the Centers for Disease Control and Prevention, 9.6% of children in the general population between ages 4 and 17 are diagnosed with ADHD (Pastor and Reuben 2008), and the percentage of individuals with TS who have a comorbid ADHD diagnosis is estimated at more than 50% (Bloch and Leckman 2009).

The emergence of ADHD symptoms frequently precedes the onset of tics (Hoekstra et al. 2004). It has been suggested that in TS, it is the comorbid ADHD symptoms rather than tics that are the greatest contributor to school problems, social challenges (Bloch and Leckman 2009), and sleep disturbances (Cohrs et al. 2001).

Obsessive-Compulsive Disorder

Obsessive-compulsive disorder (OCD) is characterized by unpleasant involuntary and repetitive thoughts (obsessions) and actions (compulsions) resulting in impaired functioning (American Psychiatric Association 2000). The prevalence of OCD in the general population is estimated at 1%–3%

(Robertson 2000), and approximately 33% of individuals with TS have comorbid OCD (Bloch and Leckman 2009).

Obsessive-compulsive behaviors usually precede the onset of tics (Bloch and Leckman 2009). However, the worst OCD symptoms often emerge 2 years after the period of worst tics. The tics of individuals with both TS and OCD follow the same general improvement profile as those of persons with TS alone, with tics peaking in early adolescence and decreasing in adulthood (Bloch and Leckman 2009).

The obsessions of individuals with TS often involve concerns with symmetry or have sexual, violent, aggressive, or religious content. This is in contrast to those of individuals who have OCD without TS, whose obsessions often center on contamination, neatness, cleaning, illness, or foreboding. Furthermore, TS-related compulsions often include checking, counting, repeating, touching, arranging, getting things "just right," or self-injurious behaviors, whereas compulsions in individuals with OCD without TS often involve cleaning and washing. One study reported that obsessions and compulsions abruptly emerge in individuals with TS-related OCD; in contrast, in those individuals who suffer from OCD without tics, obsessions and compulsions are preceded by anxious feelings, guilt, or worry (Robertson 2000).

Anxiety

Anxiety disorders are commonly reported comorbid conditions in individuals with TS. Results presented at the 2010 International Congress of Parkinson's Disease and Movement Disorders indicated estimates of anxiety in individuals with TS to be approximately 40.9% (Brooks 2010), compared with 18.1% in the general population (Kessler et al. 2005).

Depression

Several studies have indicated higher rates of depression in both children and adults with TS than in the general population. The etiology of TS-associated depression may be related not only to general factors but also to direct aspects of TS, such as the duration of the symptoms and the experience of being bullied because of the tics (Robertson 2000).

Learning Disabilities and Academic Difficulties

Although estimates are difficult to determine due to the multiple definitions of learning disorders, a large study of 5,450 subjects with TS determined that 22.7% exhibited learning difficulties (Burd et al. 2005). Learning difficulties associated with TS may largely result from the presence of comorbid ADHD (Gorman et al. 2010). However, it is essential to recognize that individuals with TS alone are apt to experience difficulties in learning. For example, visual-motor integration problems likely contribute to the handwriting difficulties that are experienced by many individuals with TS, and tics involving the eyes, head, neck, and upper extremities may interfere with reading. At the very least, the effort to suppress tics makes it more difficult to concentrate on tasks (Packer 2005).

Oppositional Defiant Disorder and Conduct Disorder

A recent study indicated that 28.6% of patients with TS had comorbid oppositional defiant disorder and 5.7% presented with comorbid conduct disorder. Although disruptive behavior disorders are more common in individuals with TS than in the general population, they often co-occur with ADHD and therefore may be due to that comorbidity (Gorman et al. 2010).

Autism Spectrum Disorders

Research indicates that approximately 13% of individuals with tics have a coexisting autism spectrum disorder. A child who exhibits tics but also presents with unusual social challenges and behaviors requires a careful diagnosis to distinguish TS from autism spectrum disorders, especially Asperger disorder (Mejia and Jankovic 2005).

Tourette Syndrome–Related Behaviors

Sensory Sensitivities

Many individuals with TS report extreme sensitivity to sensory stimuli. The National Institute of Neurological Disorders and Stroke (2010) reported the results of a survey indicating that 88% of individuals with TS considered themselves sensitive to smells, in contrast to 27% of those without TS. Additionally, 88% of TS subjects reported hypersensitivity to touch, compared with 40% of those without TS.

Sleep Problems

Sleep disturbances are reported by a number of individuals with TS. Problems include difficulty falling asleep, staying asleep, or resting peacefully (Cohrs et al. 2001). Given that sleep problems are commonly reported among individuals who experience a number of other disorders, including depression and anxiety, it may be important to determine the coexistence of comorbidities (Schmidt et al. 2011).

Self-Injurious Behavior

The estimates of patients with TS who exhibit self-injurious behavior range up to 60%. Mathews et al. (2004b) reported that self-injurious behaviors found in individuals with TS include head banging; self-biting; skin picking; hair pulling; filing of the teeth; and body, face, or eye poking with sharp objects.

Episodic Rage and Aggression

Studies indicate that at least one-third of children with TS exhibit problems with anger control. These angry episodes are sometimes referred to as rage attacks, storms, or meltdowns. The goal of these episodes appears to be the experience of relief from pent-up tension. The aggression associated with TS is impulsive, may be triggered by benign events, and may be directed toward self, others, or property. Feelings of increasing stress and pressure lead to the rage attacks, which are followed by feelings of relief and remorse after the episode has passed. Understandably, such behaviors give rise to family stress, educational challenges, peer conflicts, and increased periods of psychiatric care and hospitalization. Research indicates that those subjects with TS who have explosive outbursts are more likely than those without explosive outbursts to meet DSM-IV-TR criteria for ADHD, OCD, major depressive disorder, depression not otherwise specified, bipolar I disorder, oppositional defiant disorder, or conduct disorder (Tourette Syndrome "Plus" 2009).

Personality Disorders

In a study involving 39 adult patients with moderate TS, 64% were found to have at least one personality disorder, compared with only 16% of age- and gender-matched controls. Moreover, 71% of patients with TS exhibited more than one personality disorder, compared to 15% of the control group. Personality disorders found in patients with TS include borderline, obsessive-compulsive, paranoid, avoidant, schizotypal, and schizoid type, among others (Robertson 2000).

Impulse Control Problems

Some authors consider the socially inappropriate behaviors of TS to be the consequence of poor impulse control, perhaps attributable to comorbid ADHD (Kurlan et al. 1996).

Epidemiology

The estimate of lifetime prevalence of TS in the United States is 0.03%, with a diagnosis three times more likely for males than females and twice as likely for non-Hispanic white as non-Hispanic black individuals (Centers for Disease Control and Prevention 2009). A large study of 1,579 individuals indicated that transient tics occurred in 2.6%, chronic tics in 3.7%, and tic disorder not otherwise specified in 2.9% of the population (Stefanoff et al. 2008).

Etiology

Chromosomes and Genes

Although the genetics of TS are not well understood, various studies have provided evidence of at least some heritability. Consistent findings demonstrate 10- to 100-fold increases in rates of first-degree relatives with TS when compared to the general population. One well-known study demonstrated that monozygotic twins show 53% concordance for TS and approximately 77% for the presence of any tics. Dizygotic twins show 8% concordance for TS and 23% for any evidence of tics (O'Rourke et al. 2009).

A number of recent studies suggest that TS, once thought to be an autosomal dominant disorder, is the complex result of bilineal transmission combined with various environmental factors that affect the phenotype and severity of the disorder (Müller 2007).

Linkage studies of nuclear and multigenerational families have indicated regions on chromosomes 2, 5, and 6 as possible contributors to TS. Additionally, chromosomal anomalies in individual patients with TS have been noted on chromosomes 1, 7, 8, 9, 17, and 18 and, in one instance, XYY chromosome (O'Rourke et al. 2009). Studies conducted in isolated populations have found particular ancestral alleles that are unique to each group (Díaz-Anzaldúa et al. 2004; Mathews et al. 2004a; Simonic et al. 1998).

Partly owing to the success of dopamine antagonists for tic suppression, many studies focus on the dopamine pathway and have identified a number of dopamine-related candidate genes (Díaz-Anzaldúa et al. 2004). Additionally, mutations involving the gene *SLITRK1* have been found in a number of people with TS (O'Rourke et al. 2009). Finally, some genes are of interest due to their suggested involvement in more than one neurodevelopmental disorder. For instance, the gene *NLGN4X* was found associated to TS, autism, learning disabilities, anxiety, and depression in different members of one family (Lawson et al. 2005).

Alternatively Spliced Genes

Alternative splicing is a process that occurs during gene transcription in which the introns of a gene drop out, leaving the exons to reconnect in multiple ways. Alternative splicing is thought to be an important mechanism in human disease (Cáceres and Kornblihtt 2002).

A recent study was the first to show that a number of exons are differently expressed in children with TS compared to children without. Furthermore, the study revealed few changes in gene-level expression. Although the small sample size necessitates replication, this study demonstrates that the relatively new technology of allowing analyses of genes at the exon level may well lead to discoveries that would have been missed by whole-gene-level analyses (Tian et al. 2011b).

Developmental and Environmental Epigenetics

Epigenetics investigates molecular mechanisms that change gene expression without direct modification of the DNA sequence. *Developmental epigenetics* refers to the processes that regulate cell differentiation, gene activation, gene silencing, and chromosomal instability (Gericke 2006). Research indicates that flawed migration of cells could result as the embryonic and fetal ganglionic eminence develops into the basal ganglia of the fully developed brain. This hypothesis is consistent with TS postmortem study findings of significant reductions of GABA (γ-aminobutyric acid)-ergic parvalbumin-positive cells and fast-spiking GABAergic interneurons in some portions of the basal ganglia and increases of parvalbumin-positive cells in other areas of the basal ganglia (Leckman et al. 2010).

Environmental epigenetics refers to the impact of environmental factors on an organism's development. A number of environmental factors have been implicated as possible contributors to TS, including the mother's prenatal state (severe nausea or vomiting, psychosocial stress) (Burd et al. 1999) and infections, including pediatric autoimmune neuropsychiatric disorders associated with streptococcal infections (PANDAS). A study compared 144 children with TS, OCD, or tic disorders to those without and found that the affected children were more likely to have had a strep infection in the 3 months prior to the onset of their initial tic or obsessive-compulsive behaviors. Moreover, the children who experienced more than one strep infection within 1 year were at a 13-fold greater risk for developing TS (Mell et al. 2005).

Lit et al. (2007) attempted to capture epigenetic changes from blood gene expression measures. Results indicated age-related differences in the expression of interferon responses, viral processing, natural killer genes, and cytotoxic T-lymphocyte cells between children with and without TS.

Neuroanatomical Findings

Imaging studies of the basal ganglia (particularly caudate nucleus and striatum), corpus callosum, prefrontal cortex, limbic-hypothalamic-pituitary-adrenal axis, and sensorimotor area demonstrate differences in brain regions between individuals with TS and individuals without TS. Studies demonstrate that certain areas of the brain activate immediately before tic onset, whereas others activate just after tic presentation. Researchers have speculated that abnormal firing of basal ganglia neurons may initiate a cascade of activation that results in tics as well as premonitory urges. These speculations are substantiated by animal studies in which lesions in this area immediately improve tics (Leckman et al. 2010). The same brain structures that are thought to play a role in habit formation are also thought to be involved with the pathogenesis of tics. In light of these findings, it is interesting to consider the similarity between habits and tics, because both are repeated behaviors that take place without focused consciousness (Leckman et al. 2010).

Neurochemical Findings

A number of neurotransmitters have been implicated in the etiology of TS as the result of position emission tomography, single-photon emission computed tomography, and pharmacological discoveries. Studies indicate more than a 90% increase in the release of putamen and striatum dopamine in individuals with TS compared to those without. The hypothesis that TS is associated with increased dopamine is also supported by the success of dopamine blockers such as haloperidol in reducing tics in most individuals (Leckman et al. 2010).

Research provides clues regarding the role of a number of neurotransmitters in the pathogenesis of TS. Elevated norepinephrine levels were found in the cerebrospinal fluid of adults with TS (Leckman et al. 1995). Additionally, one study found negative associations between the cortisol level of individuals with TS and their subjective feelings of anxiety. Corbett et al. (2008) hypothesized that these results may reflect the anxiolytic aspects of tic expression. An interesting finding is that although selective serotonin reuptake inhibitors (SSRIs) prove effective in treating symptoms of OCD when individuals do not have tics, SSRIs are not as successful in the treatment of tic-related OCD (Scahill et al. 1997). It is known that histamine H_3 receptors are largely localized in the globus pallidus (Martinez-Mir et al. 1990), the region targeted by deep brain stimulation—a treatment that successfully reduces tic severity (Houeto et al. 2005). A recent pilot study found that GABA- and acetylcholine-related genes were correlated with tic severity (Tian et al. 2011a). Finally, a striatal balance between the neurotransmitters acetylcholine and dopamine may be essential for proper striatal functioning. The reduction of acetylcholine, found in some individuals with TS, may contribute to excessive striatal dopamine and result in tics (Threlfell et al. 2010).

Diagnostic Methods

Diagnoses of TS and tic disorders are predominantly based on clinical observation and the gathering of a thorough history. During the initial visit, the clinician documents the patient's age at onset of the first tic as well as the number of motor and phonic tics currently experienced. It is also important to determine if comorbid disorders are present.

It is not uncommon for the family of an individual with TS to recognize some behaviors as tics but to incorrectly conclude that other movements result from various causes. For example, a parent could mistake a sniffing tic for allergies. It is helpful to assist patients and parents in the identification of tics with measures such as the Yale Global Tic Severity Scale (YGTSS). The YGTSS is a structured interview and clinician-rating scale that assists in the determination of the number, frequency, intensity, complexity, and amount of interference of tics (Storch et al. 2005). Questioning about specific tics guided by the YGTSS may temporarily exacerbate a tic the individual currently experiences or reveal a tic that was manifested in the past (Leckman et al. 2010). The consistent use of an instrument such as the YGTSS will assist in tracking the severity and fluctuation of tics over time.

The waxing and waning nature of tics and the tendency of some individuals to suppress tics while in the clinician's office make repeated visits sometimes necessary for diagnosis. A number of visits may be necessary not only to determine an evolving tic profile, but also to reveal the entirety of the disorder, including the presence of undiagnosed comorbid disorders.

Although most tics can be easily identified, there are times that diagnosis takes the thoughtful analysis of an astute clinician. It may help to keep in mind the tic features that differentiate tics from the movements of other disorders. Unique tic characteristics include childhood onset, suggestibility, premonitory urge, temporary suppressibility, waxing and waning nature, occurrence in bouts, coexistence with other tics, and continuation of tics during sleep. For example, when trying to distinguish a TS complex tic from an OCD compulsion, it may be helpful to keep in mind that a tic is often preceded by a premonitory urge, whereas a compulsion is performed to neutralize or prevent anxiety (Robertson 2000). Likewise, ruling out of unrelated illnesses may be necessary for particular tics. For example, sniffing, scratching, and vocal tics may indicate the presence of allergies, skin disorders, and stuttering, respectively.

Once the tic history and current profile are gathered, the information is used to differentiate and diagnose a tic disorder according to the *International Statistical Classification of Diseases and Related Health Problems*, 10th Revision (ICD-10; World Health Organization 2001) or DSM-IV-TR (American Psychiatric Association 2000). Although the two classification systems list slightly different criteria, they are largely comparable (Andrews et al. 1999).

Some research suggests that tics are associated with hyperthyroidism; therefore, levels of thyroid-stimulating hormone can be measured. Additionally, if a patient's history details the sudden onset of tics after pharyngitis or ear infection, the patient should be referred for a throat culture to determine the presence of a β-hemolytic streptococcal infection (Bagheri et al. 1999).

In any case, an accurate differential diagnosis rests on the gathering of a thorough history, keen and careful observation, an awareness of TS, and sometimes the exclusion of other diagnoses. If other diseases are suspected, referral for a neurological examination may be warranted. Selected movement disorders and disease symptoms are described in Table 5–3.

Interventions

Treatment choice is dependent on the intensity of tics, degree of self-harm, level of dysfunction, interpersonal distress, academic challenges, and relationship disruption. It may be necessary to monitor the child for a few months to determine the required intensity of treatment.

In most cases, treatment usually includes a combination of educational and supportive interventions. The objective of TS treatment should emphasize quality of life rather than the suppression or elimination of tics. Just a simple explanation of the condition and prognosis may be appropriate for individuals with transient or mild tics, while more severe cases may require medication and/or behavioral training. Only the most severe cases that result in acute critical injuries (e.g., poking the eyes, resulting in the loss of vision) may require more invasive procedures such as deep brain stimulation. Furthermore, treatment of the comorbid disorders may not require medication. For example, symptoms of OCD are often successfully treated with cognitive-behavioral therapy (Leckman et al. 2010).

Psychopharmacological Interventions

When considering medication, the family and clinician must determine which symptoms are the most disruptive. Many families may identify the

Table 5–3. Differentiating characteristics of other movement disorders

Disease, disorder, or movement symptom	Characteristics
Akathisia, tardive dyskinesia, Parkinson disease, Huntington disease	Involuntary sounds, such as moaning, are infrequently associated
Akathisia as medication/drug side effect or due to Parkinson disease, restless legs syndrome, or other conditions (e.g., attention-deficit/hyperactivity disorder, anxiety)	Purposeful movement to ease feelings of inner restlessness; restless legs syndrome affects lower extremities, increases with inactivity, worsens at night
Blepharospasm and other focal dystonias	Usual onset in adulthood
Chorea	Flow from one muscle to another (dancelike); writhing; unpredictable
Dystonia	Continual twisting; abnormal postures held for sustained periods; usually affects one body region
Myoclonus	Sudden, involuntary twitching of muscle(s); not temporarily suppressible
Obsessive-compulsive disorder	Rituals performed to neutralize or prevent negative consequences
Paroxysmal dyskinesia	Recurrent, brief involuntary movements triggered by sudden voluntary movements; lasts minutes to hours; suppressed by anticonvulsants
Rett syndrome	Usual age at onset before 3 years; fixed pattern of hand wringing
Stereotypies of autism, intellectual disabilities, psychosis	Usual age at onset before 3 years; fixed patterns; frequent involvement of arms, hands, entire body; rhythmic and prolonged; ease when individual is distracted

most distressing symptom to be related to ADHD, OCD, anxiety, depression, or aggression. Furthermore, the advantageous approach might be to initially treat the comorbid symptoms, because simultaneous improvement may occur in tics (Eddy et al. 2011) as well as quality of life.

Psychopharmacological treatment can become complicated when treating both tics and comorbid disorders. Drug interactions and contraindications must be carefully considered. For example, studies of stimulant medications prescribed to treat ADHD in individuals experiencing tics have had conflicting findings; some studies suggest that stimulants exacerbate tics.

α_2-Adrenergic agonists, especially clonidine and guanfacine, are effective not only in the treatment of tics but also for comorbid ADHD symptoms (Leckman et al. 2010). This dual effect may be helpful for individuals whose tics appear to be exacerbated by stimulants. In addition, α_2-adrenergic agonists are frequently considered the first-line psychopharmacological treatment for tics due to their low side-effect profile (Robertson 2000).

Traditional dopamine-related neuroleptics, including haloperidol, pimozide, and fluphenazine, have been used for many years and result in a significant reduction in tics. However, due to their significant side effects, they are not usually the first line of medication to be prescribed (Eddy et al. 2011).

Atypical antipsychotics, such as risperidone, aripiprazole, clozapine, olanzapine, and quetiapine, have fewer side effects and are generally safer than traditional antipsychotics. Not only are these medications successful at tic reduction, but some may successfully target aggressive outbursts associated with some cases of TS (Eddy et al. 2011). Additionally, aripiprazole resulted in a 75% improvement for a 28-year-old patient with coprolalia (Singer 2010).

Aside from traditional and atypical antipsychotic medications, a number of psychopharmacological agents are currently being investigated to determine their efficacy in the treatment of tics. These include benzamides (e.g., sulpiride), tetrabenazine, benzodiazepines (e.g., clonazepam), anticonvulsants (e.g., topiramate), dopamine agonists (e.g., pergolide), anticholinergics (e.g., nicotine patches), and cannabinoids (Eddy et al. 2011).

Among patients with TS who require medication, most need medication for approximately 2 years; only 15% require continued medication beyond that time. When tics appear to be under control for a period of 4–6 months, a gradual dosage decrease should be attempted. Additionally, a patient may be able to discontinue medication temporarily during waning phases of tics (Bagheri et al. 1999).

Behavioral Interventions

Habit reversal training (HRT) is a successful behavioral intervention developed for the treatment of tics. HRT involves increasing the individual's awareness of his or her tics and premonitory urges and then training the person to replace the tics with competing movements. Relatively recently, a novel therapy based on HRT has been developed. Comprehensive behavioral intervention for tics (CBIT) combines elements of HRT with psychoeducation and function-based interventions to replace tics with voluntary behaviors. Over time, both tics and premonitory urges are expected to diminish as a result of therapy. CBIT has proven to be successful, with an effect size comparable to that of antipsychotics (Piacentini et al. 2010);

however, only a limited number of therapists have expertise in implementing this intervention (Kurlan 2010).

Invasive Procedures

Botulinum toxin injected into the tic-affected muscle group prevents acetylcholine release and temporarily reduces muscle activity in the injected muscle. This treatment not only has shown success for motor tics but also has brought relief for phonic tics. Following injection of the toxin into the vocal cords, 94% of subjects demonstrated improvement in phonic tics, with 41% of those individuals becoming tic free. Additionally, relief from the premonitory urge is sometimes experienced (Eddy et al. 2011).

The use of repetitive transcranial magnetic stimulation (rTMS) to emit weak electrical currents directed at the supplementary motor area of the brain is a relatively new technique for the treatment of tics. The theory of rTMS is that low-frequency magnetic stimulation disrupts the neural circuits that perpetuate tics. In some cases, the procedure has resulted in significant tic reduction. Also, a small number of cases show positive findings for the use of electroconvulsive therapy in the treatment of tics (Eddy et al. 2011).

There are rare individuals with TS who have tics that do not respond to medication or to less invasive therapies and that result in severe physical injury or substantial limitation of activities. Deep brain stimulation involves the implantation of electrodes that, when activated, send electrical impulses to targeted areas of the globus pallidus interna or thalamic regions of the brain. Some studies using deep brain stimulation have shown improvement in tics that were otherwise treatment resistant (Leckman et al. 2010).

Alternative Therapies

Some patients with TS have reported improvement in tics from using alternative therapies, such as vitamins, dietary supplements, chiropractic manipulation, and meditation (Mantel et al. 2004). However, robust clinical trials have not been carried out to evaluate the efficacy of these therapies.

Quality of Life

In every case, the clinician should take time to discover and discuss the strengths of the individual with TS or a tic disorder. Often, clinicians focus on the challenges of the disorder and discount the person's strengths. For example, some individuals with tics appear to be remarkably sensitive to others, perhaps due to the development of empathy as a result of their own struggles (Cohen et al. 1992).

The self-esteem and interpersonal relationships of children with TS appear to suffer most during periods of frequent and intense tics when the children are ages 7–12 (Leckman et al. 2006). General awareness of TS may foster understanding and tolerance in others, to the benefit of those with TS. Dooley (2006) advises that tics be referred to as "habits" when talking to young children in the patient's life and that adolescents and adults be informed that TS is a neurobiological disorder. It is essential that patients and parents gain information about TS to educate others. Accurate and up-to-date information is available at the Tourette Syndrome Association Web site (www.tsa-usa.org).

The patient, as well as the family, may benefit from education regarding the clinical course of TS and related issues. Family therapy and/or education might be indicated if it is discovered that the parent punishes the child for tics or feels unduly embarrassed and therefore avoids social outings with the child. Additionally, parents and patients may feel increased levels of stress when tics are severe and disruptive (Dooley 2006).

Research reports that were gathered 20 years apart suggest strikingly similar strategies as helpful for children and adolescents with TS in the academic environment. Extended time can be provided for tests, classwork, and homework to accommodate for the decreased attention due to tics or possible handwriting deficits. Permitting the individual to leave the room and go to a safe location during intense periods of tics, as well as allowing preferential seating so that the individual is able to leave the room without drawing unnecessary attention, appears to be helpful. Finally, offering education and support regarding TS to the child, teachers, and peers allows the child to be more comfortable and provides the opportunity for the child to build resilience (Packer 2005). Children with TS whose educational performance is disrupted by their condition are entitled to such educational accommodations under the Individuals With Disabilities Education Act (IDEA), the federal law that guarantees special educational accommodations and support for children with health impairments as well as other types of educational impairments, and through Section 504 of the Rehabilitation Act. Families in need of such services should contact the office of special education in their local school district.

New Research Directions

The diagnoses of TS and the related tic and comorbid disorders are currently based on criteria from DSM-IV-TR or ICD-10, which are generally compatible manuals (Andrews et al. 1999). DSM-5 is scheduled to be published in 2013, with a similar update of ICD-10 following soon thereafter.

A number of changes proposed for DSM-5 are meant to address short-comings in the tic disorder criteria in the current edition. Recommended changes include reclassification, more precise definitions, and unified criteria across tic disorders. More precisely defined disorders are expected to simplify diagnosis, improve communication between clinicians and researchers, eluci-date the influence of comorbid disorders, and help to more accurately deter-mine prevalence estimates (Roessner et al. 2011). Current findings are complicated by overlapping phenotypes and sometimes by the presence of undetected comorbid disorders (Dooley 2006). Carefully defined study pop-ulations that separate discrete groups, such as those with TS alone, those with TS along with comorbidity, and those who exhibit explosive outbursts, will al-low more concentrated research and help define targeted treatments.

Recent advances in the fields of genetics, epigenetics, and biology provide exciting opportunities to improve diagnoses, specify the impact of comorbid disorders, design effective interventions, confirm existing findings, and make novel discoveries regarding etiology and disease progression. For example, the ability to analyze genes at the exon level provides denser genetic information in the form of number of probes and allows for discovery of alternative splic-ing. The breadth and depth of these analyses may eventually permit measure-ment of gene expression specific to etiology, severity, and clinical course and help determine which genes are contributors to disease onset, which contrib-ute to disease progression, and which are associated with comorbidities.

The use of imaging technology to measure biochemical information will allow the targeting of specific brain areas and specific neurochemical processes for rigorous study. Not only will these studies provide clues to the etiology and course of tics and related disorders; they also may enable tracking of the biological and metabolic changes in response to medication and behavioral treatment. A relatively recent study demonstrated the im-portance of accounting for the effect of medication on the alteration of neurotransmitters and on the modulation of tics (Liao and Sharp 2010).

Studies are needed to determine and design successful peer interven-tions and academic strategies. High-quality, well-designed studies are needed to replicate findings of possible therapeutic agents such as vitamins and nutritional supplements. Additionally, although behavioral therapies have been proven successful in the treatment of tics, the limited number of HRT- and CBIT-trained therapists makes it challenging to provide these therapies to a broad population; therefore, research is needed to determine the efficacy of providing long-distance therapy through technologies such as telemedicine (Kurlan 2010).

Finally, although past studies have offered exciting discoveries relating to TS, studies with larger sample sizes are needed to replicate or refute cur-rent findings.

Key Points

- Approximately 80% of individuals with Tourette syndrome (TS) also have at least one other comorbid disorder. Evaluation for comorbid disorders is essential for complete diagnoses. Comorbid disorders include but are not limited to attention-deficit/hyperactivity disorder, obsessive-compulsive disorder, depression, and anxiety disorders.

- The most problematic symptom may not be the tics. Clinicians should discuss what symptom the patient and parents find most disruptive or worrisome and consider that symptom for initial treatment focus.

- Because of the waxing and waning nature of tics, the presence of comorbidities, and the challenge of differentiating tics from the movements found in other disorders or diseases, accurate diagnosis may take more than one visit.

- The parents and patient should be educated (when appropriate) regarding the typical clinical course of TS, including the possibility of comorbidities. Additionally, they should be provided with information regarding the symptoms of common comorbid disorders.

- The family should be encouraged to consider sharing their newfound knowledge with people with whom the child has regular contact and to seek educational supports and accommodations if needed through their school district.

Recommended Readings

Bloch MH, Leckman JF: Clinical course of Tourette syndrome. J Psychosom Res 67:497–501, 2009

Eddy CM, Rickards HE, Cavanna AE: Treatment strategies for tics in Tourette syndrome. Ther Adv Neurol Disord 4:25–45, 2011

Jankovic J, Kurlan R: Tourette syndrome: evolving concepts. Mov Disord 26:1149–1156, 2011

Leckman JF, Bloch MH, Scahill L, et al: Tourette syndrome: the self under siege. J Child Neurol 21:642–649, 2006

Müller N: Tourette's syndrome: clinical features, pathophysiology, and therapeutic approaches. Dialogues Clin Neurosci 9:161–171, 2007

Robertson MM: Tourette syndrome, associated conditions and the complexities of treatment. Brain 123:425–462, 2000

References

American Psychiatric Association: Diagnostic and Statistical Manual of Mental Disorders, 4th Edition, Text Revision. Washington, DC, American Psychiatric Association, 2000

Andrews G, Slade T, Peters L: Classification in psychiatry: ICD-10 versus DSM-IV. Br J Psychiatry 174:3–5, 1999

Bagheri MM, Kerbeshian J, Burd L: Recognition and management of Tourette's syndrome and tic disorders. Am Fam Physician 59:2263–2272, 2274, 1999

Bloch MH, Leckman JF: Clinical course of Tourette syndrome. J Psychosom Res 67:497–501, 2009

Brooks M: Anxiety exacts a toll in adults with Tourette's syndrome. Medscape News. 2010. Available at: http://www.medscape.com/viewarticle/724053. Accessed April 16, 2012.

Burd L, Severud R, Klug MG, et al: Prenatal and perinatal risk factors for Tourette disorder. J Perinat Med 27:295–302, 1999

Burd L, Freeman RD, Klug MG, et al: Tourette syndrome and learning disabilities. BMC Pediatr 5:34, 2005

Cáceres JF, Kornblihtt AR: Alternative splicing: multiple control mechanisms and involvement in human disease. Trends Genet 18:186–193, 2002

Centers for Disease Control and Prevention: Prevalence of diagnosed Tourette syndrome in persons aged 6–17 years—United States, 2007. MMWR Morb Mortal Wkly Rep 58:581–585, 2009

Cheung MY, Shahed J, Jankovic J: Malignant Tourette syndrome. Mov Disord 22:1743–1750, 2007

Cohen DJ, Friedhoff AJ, Leckman JF, et al: Tourette syndrome: extending basic research to clinical care. Adv Neurol 58:341–362, 1992

Cohrs S, Rasch T, Altmeyer S, et al: Decreased sleep quality and increased sleep related movements in patients with Tourette's syndrome. J Neurol Neurosurg Psychiatry 70:192–197, 2001

Conelea CA, Woods DC: Examining the impact of distraction on tic suppression in children and adolescents with Tourette syndrome. Behav Res Ther 46:1193–1200, 2008

Corbett BA, Mendoza SP, Baym CL, et al: Examining cortisol rhythmicity and responsivity to stress in children with Tourette syndrome. Psychoneuroendocrinology 33:810–820, 2008

Díaz-Anzaldúa A, Joober R, Rivière JB, et al: Tourette syndrome and dopaminergic genes: a family-based association study in the French Canadian founder population. Mol Psychiatry 9:272–277, 2004

Dooley JM: Tic disorders in childhood. Semin Pediatr Neurol 13:231–242, 2006

Du JC, Chiu TF, Lee KM, et al: Tourette syndrome in children: an updated review. Pediatr Neonatol 51:255–264, 2010

Eddy CM, Rickards HE, Cavanna AE: Treatment strategies for tics in Tourette syndrome. Ther Adv Neurol Disord 4:25–45, 2011

Freeman RD, Zinner SH, Müller-Vahl KR, et al: Coprophenomena in Tourette syndrome. Dev Med Child Neurol 51:218–227, 2009

Gericke GS: Chromosomal fragility, structural rearrangements and mobile element activity may reflect dynamic epigenetic mechanisms of importance in neurobehavioural genetics. Med Hypotheses 66:276–285, 2006

Gorman DA, Thompson N, Plessen KJ, et al: Psychosocial outcome and psychiatric comorbidity in older adolescents with Tourette syndrome: controlled study. Br J Psychiatry 197:36–44, 2010

Hoekstra PJ, Steenhuis MP, Troost PW, et al: Relative contribution of attention-deficit hyperactivity disorder, obsessive-compulsive disorder, and tic severity to social and behavioral problems in tic disorders. J Dev Behav Pediatr 25:272–279, 2004

Houeto JL, Karachi C, Mallet L, et al: Tourette's syndrome and deep brain stimulation. J Neurol Neurosurg Psychiatry 76:992–995, 2005

Jankovic J, Kurlan R: Tourette syndrome: evolving concepts. Mov Disord 26:1149–1156, 2011

Kessler RC, Chiu WT, Demler O, et al: Prevalence, severity, and comorbidity of 12-month DSM-IV disorders in the National Comorbidity Survey Replication. Arch Gen Psychiatry 62:617–627, 2005

Kurlan R: Clinical practice: Tourette's syndrome. N Engl J Med 363:2332–2338, 2010

Kurlan R, Daragjati C, Como PG, et al: Non-obscene complex socially inappropriate behavior in Tourette's syndrome. J Neuropsychiatry Clin Neurosci 8:311–317, 1996

Kwak C, Dat Vuong K, Jankovic J: Premonitory sensory phenomenon in Tourette's syndrome. Mov Disord 18:1530–1533, 2003

Lawson CA, Donaldson IJ, Bowman SJ, et al: Analysis of the insertion/deletion related polymorphism within T cell antigen receptor beta variable genes in primary Sjögren's syndrome. Ann Rheum Dis 64:468–470, 2005

Leckman JF, Goodman WK, Anderson GM, et al: Cerebrospinal fluid biogenic amines in obsessive compulsive disorder, Tourette's syndrome, and healthy controls. Neuropsychopharmacology 12:73–86, 1995

Leckman JF, Bloch MH, Scahill L, et al: Tourette syndrome: the self under siege. J Child Neurol 21:642–649, 2006

Leckman JF, Bloch MH, Smith ME, et al: Neurobiological substrates of Tourette's disorder. J Child Adolesc Psychopharmacol 20:237–247, 2010

Liao IH, Sharp FR: Tourette syndrome: gene expression as a tool to discover drug targets. Neurotherapeutics 7:302–306, 2010

Lit L, Gilbert DL, Walker W, et al: A subgroup of Tourette's patients overexpress specific natural killer cell genes in blood: a preliminary report. Am J Med Genet B Neuropsychiatr Genet 144B:958–963, 2007

Mantel BJ, Meyers A, Tran QY, et al: Nutritional supplements and complementary/alternative medicine in Tourette syndrome. J Child Adolesc Psychopharmacol 14:582–589, 2004

Martinez-Mir MI, Pollard H, Moreau J, et al: Three histamine receptors (H1, H2 and H3) visualized in the brain of human and non-human primates. Brain Res 526:322–327, 1990

Mathews CA, Reus VI, Bejarano J, et al: Genetic studies of neuropsychiatric disorders in Costa Rica: a model for the use of isolated populations. Psychiatr Genet 14:13–23, 2004a

Mathews CA, Waller J, Glidden D, et al: Self injurious behaviour in Tourette syndrome: correlates with impulsivity and impulse control. J Neurol Neurosurg Psychiatry 75:1149–1155, 2004b

Mejia NI, Jankovic J: Secondary tics and tourettism. Rev Bras Psiquiatr 27:11–17, 2005

Mell LK, Davis RL, Owens D: Association between streptococcal infection and obsessive-compulsive disorder, Tourette's syndrome, and tic disorder. Pediatrics 116:56–60, 2005

Müller N: Tourette's syndrome: clinical features, pathophysiology, and therapeutic approaches. Dialogues Clin Neurosci 9:161–171, 2007

National Institute of Neurological Disorders and Stroke: Sensory sensitivity in Tourette syndrome. March 9, 2010. Available at: http://www.ninds.nih.gov/jobs_and_training/summer/2009_students/Veronica-Watters-Abstract.htm?css=print. Accessed April 16, 2012.

O'Rourke JA, Scharf JM, Yu D, et al: The genetics of Tourette syndrome: a review. J Psychosom Res 67:533–545, 2009

Packer LE: Tic-related school problems: impact on functioning, accommodations, and interventions. Behav Modif 29:876–899, 2005

Packer LE: Tourette Syndrome "Plus": Overview of "rage attacks." February 2009. Available at: http://www.tourettesyndrome.net/disorders/rage-attacks-or-storms/overview-of-rage-attacks. Accessed April 16, 2012.

Pastor PN, Reuben CA: Diagnosed attention deficit hyperactivity disorder and learning disability: United States, 2004–2006. Vital Health Stat 10 (237):1–14, 2008

Piacentini J, Woods DW, Scahill L, et al: Behavior therapy for children with Tourette disorder: a randomized controlled trial. JAMA 303:1929–1937, 2010

Robertson MM: Tourette syndrome, associated conditions and the complexities of treatment. Brain 123:425–462, 2000

Roessner V, Hoekstra PJ, Rothenberger A: Tourette's disorder and other tic disorders in DSM-5: a comment. Eur Child Adolesc Psychiatry 20:71–74, 2011

Scahill L, Riddle MA, King RA, et al: Fluoxetine has no marked effect on tic symptoms in patients with Tourette's syndrome: a double-blind placebo-controlled study. J Child Adolesc Psychopharmacol 7:75–85, 1997

Schmidt RE, Harvey AG, Van der Linden M: Cognitive and affective control in insomnia. Front Psychol 2:349, 2011

Simonic I, Gericke GS, Ott J, et al: Identification of genetic markers associated with Gilles de la Tourette syndrome in an Afrikaner population. Am J Hum Genet 63:839–846, 1998

Singer HS: Treatment of tics and Tourette syndrome. Curr Treat Options Neurol 12:539–561, 2010

Stefanoff P, Wolanczyk T, Gawrys A, et al: Prevalence of tic disorders among schoolchildren in Warsaw, Poland. Eur Child Adolesc Psychiatry 17:171–178, 2008

Storch EA, Murphy TK, Geffken GR, et al: Reliability and validity of the Yale Global Tic Severity Scale. Psychol Assess 17:486–491, 2005

Threlfell S, Clements MA, Khodai T, et al: Striatal muscarinic receptors promote activity dependence of dopamine transmission via distinct receptor subtypes on cholinergic interneurons in ventral versus dorsal striatum. J Neurosci 30:3398–3408, 2010

Tian Y, Gunther JR, Liao IH, et al: GABA- and acetylcholine-related gene expression in blood correlate with tic severity and microarray evidence for alternative splicing in Tourette syndrome: a pilot study. Brain Res 1381: 228–236, 2011a

Tian Y, Liao IH, Zhan X, et al: Exon expression and alternatively spliced genes in Tourette syndrome. Am J Med Genet B Neuropsychiatr Genet 156B:72–78, 2011b

Walusinski O, Bogousslavsky J: Georges Gilles de la Tourette (1857–1904). J Neurol 258:166–167, 2011

World Health Organization: International Statistical Classification of Diseases and Related Health Problems, 10th Revision. Geneva, World Health Organization, 2001

CHAPTER 6

DOWN SYNDROME

Liga Bivina, M.S., C.G.C.
Billur Moghaddam, M.D.
Terry D. Wardinsky, M.D.

Down syndrome (DS) has long been recognized as a leading cause of intellectual disability, and individuals with DS and their families have played a major role in changing attitudes, legislation, public policy, and expectations for care and inclusion of all individuals with intellectual and other disabilities. The syndrome was named for John Langdon Haydon Down, an Edinburgh physician and superintendent of the Earlswood Asylum in England, who first described the physical and behavioral characteristics that are typically found in this syndrome.

In 1959, Jerome Lejeune and Patricia Jacobs, working independently, discovered that tissue cultures from individuals with DS had 47 chromosomes, with three copies of chromosome 21 (Jacobs et al. 1959; Lejeune et al. 1959). By the mid-1960s, the syndrome hallmarks were well described, the cytogenetic causes identified, and the most significant risk factor of advanced maternal age recognized. Advances in understanding the health risks and behavioral and learning profiles, improved community living opportunities, and continued scientific breakthroughs are allowing children and adults with DS to live increasingly independent and productive lives.

Epidemiology

DS is the most commonly identified genetic cause of intellectual disability. DS has an estimated occurrence of 1 in 691 live-born infants in the United States (Parker et al. 2010). The estimated rate of spontaneous loss of fetuses with trisomy 21 is 32% between the time of chorionic villus sampling at

10 weeks' gestation and term and 25% between the time of amniocentesis at 16 weeks' gestation and term (Savva et al. 2006). It is estimated that larger percentages are spontaneously aborted in early pregnancy.

DS occurs in all ethnic groups and among all economic classes, with analogous effects found in other species, such as chimpanzees and mice. Maternal age influences the chances of conceiving a baby with DS. At a maternal age of 20, the probability of having a live-born child with DS is 1 in 1,441; at age 30, the probability is 1 in 959; at age 35, the probability is 1 in 338; and at age 40, the probability is 1 in 84 (Morris et al. 2002). Although the probability increases with maternal age, 61% of children with DS are born to women under age 35 (Egan et al. 2011), reflecting the overall fertility and higher delivery rate of that group.

Etiology

DS is caused by a triple copy of genes on chromosome 21. The most common etiology is an extra freestanding copy of chromosome 21 due to the mechanism of nondisjunction. This nondisjunction variation of DS, also called trisomy 21, accounts for 95% of cases. Individuals with trisomy 21 have a total of 47 chromosomes. Advanced maternal age is the single most important determinant of nondisjunction trisomy 21. Approximately 85%–90% of cases of trisomy 21 result from maternal nondisjunction, 5%–10% result from paternal nondisjunction, and 5% result from postzygotic mitotic nondisjunction.

Robertsonian translocation, caused by unbalanced structural rearrangements involving chromosome 21 and another acrocentric chromosome (13, 14, 15, 21, or 22), is the etiology in 3%–4% of cases. In approximately one-third of these cases, the translocation is inherited from a parent carrying a balanced form of the translocation. Individuals with translocation DS have a total of 46 chromosomes. The parents of children with translocation DS should undergo karyotype analysis for the purpose of genetic counseling and recurrence risk estimates.

Mosaic DS accounts for 1%–2% of cases. Mosaicism may arise by postzygotic (mitotic) nondisjunction of a normal zygote or the postzygotic loss of a chromosome 21 from a trisomic zygote (partial trisomy rescue).

The recurrence risk of DS in subsequent children varies with the age of the mother at the time the child with DS was born, as well as the etiology of DS in the child. Mothers who have had a child with nondisjunction DS and are of advanced maternal age (≥35 years) have a recurrence risk of 1.7 times their current age-related risk. Mothers who have children with nondisjunction DS and who are younger (<35 years) have a recurrence risk of 3.5 times their current age-related risk (Sheets et al. 2011). The basis of the increased risk remains unknown.

The risk is different for parents of children with translocation DS because of the possibility that one parent may be a balanced translocation carrier. Parental chromosome analysis and genetic counseling is recommended for these families. The parents of a child with a de novo translocation are not at significantly increased risk for recurrence. A male carrier of a balanced Robertsonian translocation has an estimated <0.5%–1.0% risk for recurrence, whereas a female carrier of a balanced translocation has as much as a 15% risk for recurrence of translocation DS in future children (Gardner and Sutherland 2004). The exact risks of recurrence vary by the specific translocation of the carrier. It is important to note that if a parent is a carrier of a Robertsonian translocation between two copies of chromosome 21, the risk of having a child with DS is 100%. Prenatal diagnosis is available via chorionic villus sampling and amniocentesis.

Trisomy 21 is the result of a random event during gametogenesis or shortly after in the postzygotic period, as in cases of mosaic DS. Research shows that there is no association between the maternal age–adjusted incidence rates of DS and paternal age, birth order, ancestral origin, country of birth, maternal education level, maternal ABO and Rh blood groups, pregnancy interval, and paternal consanguinity (Carothers et al. 2001).

Signs and Symptoms

Physical Features

Individuals with DS have characteristic facial and physical features (Figures 6–1 through 6–5) and, across ethnic lines, appear more related to each other than to their biological brothers or sisters. Recognizing facial characteristics may be challenging in the case of infants who are premature or who have certain ethnic characteristics (i.e., individuals of Asian or Hispanic ancestry), or those who may have significant mosaicism. Physical findings that suggest a clinical diagnosis of DS include a rounded facies that becomes more oval in shape with age; relative microcephaly and brachycephaly with large fontanelles, often including a third fontanelle in the midline between the anterior and posterior fontanelles; and midface hypoplasia with frequent tongue protrusion because the oral cavity and nasal pharyngeal spaces are smaller secondary to midface hypoplasia. As the midface grows, the tongue protrusion recedes and noisy respiration tends to improve. Generalized hypotonia and laxity of the joints with unusual ability to flex and extend extremities are often striking and, in the newborn period, may be significant clues to the diagnosis. Other features include upslanting palpebral fissures, epicanthal folds, strabismus, nystagmus, Brushfield spots of the iris (especially in blue-eyed babies), nuchal neck skin folds or appearance of a thick neck skin, transverse palmar creases (single palmar creases) with shorter digits (brachydactyly), fifth finger incurving (clinodactyly), and wide gaps between great and second toes. Frequently the skin is mottled (cutis marmorata), often a persistent finding. Occasional subluxation of hips and later of the patellae is found.

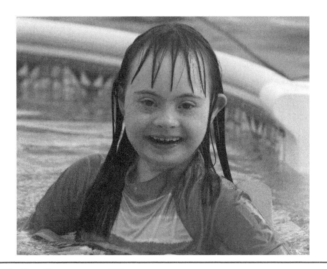

FIGURE 6–1. Emma, age 10.

Source.   Courtesy of National Down Syndrome Society. Used with permission.

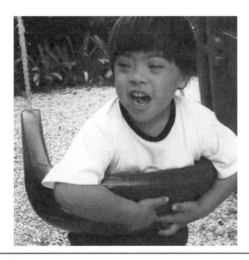

FIGURE 6–2. Ricardo, age 4.

Source.   Courtesy of National Down Syndrome Society. Used with permission.

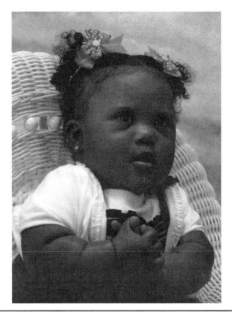

FIGURE 6–3. Lensey, age 1.

Source. Courtesy of National Down Syndrome Society. Used with permission.

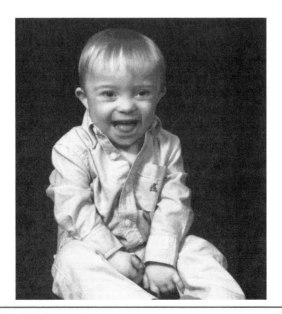

FIGURE 6–4. Caleb, age 3.

Source. Courtesy of National Down Syndrome Society. Used with permission.

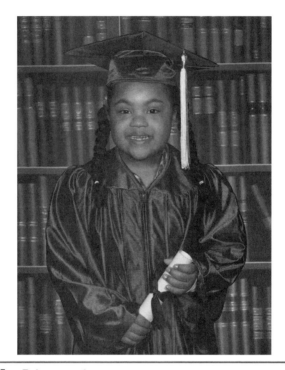

FIGURE 6–5.   Priya, age 6.

Source.   Courtesy of National Down Syndrome Society. Used with permission.

Congenital heart defects are found in 44% of patients with DS (Freeman et al. 2008), with atrioventricular septal defects (39%), ventricular septal defects (43%), and secundum atrial septal defects (42%) being the most common. Congenital heart defects in newborns with DS may be asymptomatic; therefore, echocardiograms are routinely indicated in the newborn period regardless of whether a fetal echocardiogram was performed (Bull 2011).

Hearing and vision impairments are both common in DS and require routine assessment in the newborn period and regularly thereafter to identify impairments that can be treated before they affect early development, learning, and adaptive function (Bull 2011). Two-thirds of adults with DS will have hearing problems by age 50, with increasing rates thereafter, and visual problems occur with similar frequencies across studies (Steingass et al. 2011).

Many factors contribute to an increased risk for obstructive sleep apnea, including facial structure, small upper airway, hypotonia, and obesity; up to 50% of 3-year-olds have abnormal sleep studies, although most parents report no sleep problems (Shott 2006). Sleep disorders may present as fatigue, problems with concentration, poor work performance, depression, and mood disturbance. Findings suggestive of sleep apnea include noisy breathing with snoring, long pauses (20–30 seconds) between breaths, startling awake with air hunger, sweating during sleep, and being tired, with reports of sleeping in school. Routine sleep studies should be done by age 4 in all children with DS, and when indicated thereafter based on clinical symptoms.

Managing diet and exercise to prevent obesity is important. Individuals with DS have a lower resting metabolic rate, and almost 90% of adults with DS are obese (Steingass et al. 2011). Individuals with DS have a 20-fold higher risk of leukemia, and this is particularly the case for those with transient myeloproliferative disease in infancy, which occurs in 4%–10% of newborns with DS (Alford et al. 2011; Malinge et al. 2009). Of these infants, 20% will develop acute megakaryocytic leukemia within 4 years.

About 10.8% of children with DS have medically treated thyroid disease (Carroll et al. 2008), a significantly greater percentage than in the general population. Thyroid abnormalities increase with age and are often not recognized without routine screening or until significant secondary health problems occur. After the newborn period, monitoring is recommended at 6 months, at 12 months, and yearly thereafter (Bull 2011).

Celiac disease is much more common in individuals with DS than previously recognized, and it may present with gastrointestinal symptoms, poor growth, and weight loss. Any of these symptoms should prompt screening assessment with transglutaminase immunoglobulin A (IgA) and quantitative IgA (Bull 2011).

Because of joint and ligament laxity, atlantoaxial joint instability is a concern for spinal cord compression. Routine cervical spine X rays are not helpful, but prompt assessments and referrals to neurology and/or orthopedic surgery should be made if *any* signs of neurological impairment occur, such as loss of motor skills, stiff neck, or change in bowel or bladder function.

Development

In children with DS, the early developmental profile, particularly of motor skills, is slow due to low muscle tone and joint laxity. Social and self-help skills are often the best early developmental abilities. Compared with children without DS, infants with DS begin to develop language similarly, but around age 17 months, their language acquisition slows. Young children with DS appear to have significant language sensory processing problems, with much better receptive than expressive skills. For these reasons, multimedia language supports have been used, such as language therapy, signing, picture boarding, and other augmentative techniques. Computers have been used to enhance language processing and ultimate expression.

Cognitive Function

In longitudinal cohort studies (Carr 1988; Cuckle et al. 2008), IQ of individuals with DS declined from an average of 80 at age 6 months to scores in the 40s from age 4 years up to 42 years. At 30 years, the mean mental age in this sample was 5 years 6 months on the Leiter International Performance Scale—Revised, a test of nonverbal intelligence. Reading, writing, and math skills in another cohort were found to be at a 5-year level for most, with skills up to 11 years in 25% (Turner and Alborz 2003). IQ measures may be a poor representation of the spectrum of abilities in individuals with DS, who have better adaptive function than do individuals with similar IQ levels from other etiologies (Esbensen et al. 2008).

Adaptive function generally shows improvement into young adulthood, followed by a period of stability and then decline beginning in the mid-40s (Hawkins et al. 2003). Carr (2005) found that declines in IQ in individuals with DS generally began 10 years earlier than in the general population, with verbal abilities declining more significantly than performance. The overall prevalence of Alzheimer dementia in individuals with DS is 16.8%. The prevalence is 8.9% until age 49 years, 17.7% for ages 50–54 years, and 32.1% for ages 55–59 (Coppus et al. 2006). When cognitive or adaptive function declines are recognized, it is important to assess carefully for other contributing factors, such as hypothyroidism, visual or hearing impairments, stressful life events, and depression.

Behavioral and Psychiatric Disorders

Children with DS are often described as affectionate and easy in temperament; however, research indicates that temperament profiles in children with DS are not uniform and that these children demonstrate a wide range of behaviors and considerable individual differences. Children with DS may develop behavior issues that interfere with ideal learning practices; for example, children with DS may exhibit avoidance strategies when faced with challenges, as well as less efficient use of problem-solving skills, failure to consolidate newly acquired cognitive skills, and reluctance to take initiative in learning.

Psychiatric disorders need to be recognized in individuals with DS who are having behavioral changes; such changes should not be ignored as being "part of DS." Childhood psychiatric disorders, along with less adaptive function and greater severity of intellectual disability, are predictive of be-havior problems in adults with DS (Esbensen et al. 2008; McCarthy 2008).

Autism spectrum disorders (ASDs) are estimated to occur in approximately 10% of individuals with DS (Dykens 2007), and overall function in individuals with both DS and ASD is significantly lower (Molloy et al. 2009). Regression of language, when observed in children with DS and ASD, generally tends to occur later than in children with ASD. A 2008 study (Castillo et al. 2008) reported that the average age at occurrence of language regression in children with DS and ASD was 46.2 months, compared to 19.5 months in children with ASD without DS. Attention-deficit/hyperactivity disorder is estimated to occur in about 6%–8% of individuals with DS, and oppositional defiant disorder/conduct disorder in 10%–15% (Dykens 2007).

Differential Diagnosis

DS is a common condition and not often confused with other syndromes. Because mosaic DS can be associated with a milder phenotype and more subtle facial features, recognition of the syndrome can be more difficult.

The physical characteristics seen in DS overlap with those seen in other syndromes. Macroglossia also occurs in individuals with Beckwith-Wiedemann syndrome. Smith-Magenis syndrome and DS share overlapping facial features, such as brachycephaly, upslanting palpebral fissures, midface hypoplasia, and a small, wide nose. Zellweger syndrome and DS have in common hypotonia, large fontanelles, flat occiput and face, anteverted nares, epicanthal folds, Brushfield spots, cataracts, and cardiac septal defects (Cassidy and Allanson 2010).

Management and Intervention

The birth of a child with DS may come as a surprise to some families, whereas families who have chosen prenatal diagnostic assessments may have been made aware and had time for preparation. Early bereavement support is very important, as is the way that professionals present the news of a clinical diagnosis of DS to the parents. Professionals should meet with the parents and family members in a private area, reveal the diagnostic impression as early as possible, have the infant present to identify what findings suggest the diagnosis, give value to the newborn with the diagnosis of DS, and avoid providing too much initial overwhelming information. A congenital birth defect, such as a congenital heart defect or gastrointestinal malformation, can add another level of concern to the scenario. Additional worries and unknowns for surgical outcomes must be recognized and supported, especially if the family will be traveling to an outside location and working with new health care providers. Professional bereavement counseling by a trained child psychologist, if desired, can be very helpful for "resetting" the family's dream for a new child. In general, several researchers report that families of children with DS cope better, have less family conflict, and report less burden and stress when compared to parents of children and adults with other disabilities (Hodapp 2007; Seltzer et al. 1993).

Medical Management

New guidelines for the primary management of individuals with DS were recently published by the Committee on Genetics of the American Academy of Pediatrics (Bull 2011) and are recommended as a reference to all health care professionals caring for individuals with DS to optimally manage and/or prevent the multiple health risks common in DS. In general, routine assessments in the newborn period, after the diagnosis of DS has been made, include the following: echocardiogram, hearing screen, ophthalmological examination to look for cataracts, and complete blood test with differential to assess for transient myeloproliferative disease or polycythemia. Hearing should be screened again at 6 months and every year thereafter. Ophthalmological examinations should be performed annually for the first 5 years, every 2 years until age 13, and then every 3 years. Thyroid function should be assessed in the newborn screen, again at 6 and 12 months, and annually thereafter.

Symptomatic monitoring should be done at each visit for atlantoaxial subluxation, celiac disease, feeding and swallowing difficulties, and obstructive sleep apnea. Parents, caregivers, and individuals with DS need to know the symptoms of atlantoaxial subluxation, including complaints of neck pain (holding the back of one's neck); developing torticollis or head tilt as a protective mechanism; complaints of sensations of pain, tingling, or paresthesias radiating down the arms, back, or back of legs, with hypertonicity of calf muscles; weakness of the arms or legs; walking on toes; and loss of bowel or bladder function after normal acquisition of training. If the individual with DS has any of the above complaints, X ray of the spine and/ or magnetic resonance imaging as soon as possible is recommended for measurements to rule out compression of cervical vertebra 1 or 2. Routine X rays of the neck are no longer recommended, although organizations that sponsor equestrian therapy and Special Olympics may require screening neck X rays and exams prior to participation.

Every child should undergo a sleep study or polysomnography by age 4 years, regardless of symptoms, or whenever symptoms are reported. Treatments for sleep problems include weight reduction, supplemental oxygen, tonsillectomy, mouthpieces, and continuous positive airway pressure. Swallowing assessment should be done when a child experiences failure to thrive, slow feeding, choking, or recurrent or persistent respiratory problems.

Increased vigilance is recommended for other medical problems for which individuals with DS are at somewhat increased risk, including arthritis, diabetes, gastrointestinal and renal malformations, and seizures (Bull 2011). Attention to growth and dental hygiene is important to prevent obesity, gingivitis, and caries.

Discussing issues related to self-care, bodily functions, and sexuality with individuals with DS is important, beginning at an early age. Several excellent resources are available to help support these discussions, in conjunction with school and community agency personnel (see "Recommended Resources" section at end of chapter). *Teaching Children With Down Syndrome About Their Bodies, Boundaries, and Sexuality: A Guide for Parents and Professionals* (Couwenhoven 2007) is a particularly important publication that teaches individuals with DS and their caretakers to participate safely in extracurricular activities in the community with peers and other adults.

Usually adults with DS should be transitioned to receive health care from an adult physician (i.e., an internist or family physician) because pediatricians are not generally trained to support adult diseases such as hypertension or type 2 diabetes mellitus or to do cancer screening. Because of a higher frequency of testicular cancer in males with DS, it is important that they have routine testicular exams as well as perform self-examinations. Compared with typical-population adults, adults with DS are more prone to mental health disorders (i.e., dual diagnosis), including anxiety, depression, obsessive-compulsive disorder, and conduct disorder, and should be monitored because these disorders are treatable with behavioral modifications and medications.

Educational Interventions

Early intervention is important for both infants with DS and their families. For some families, parent support groups are also very important. Because children and adolescents with DS are frequently visual learners, approaches that might enhance their learning abilities include using a schedule of pictures to break down a task or an activity into a series of steps and preparing for a transition by presenting a calendar marked with the timing of the transition event.

Behavioral Interventions

Significant behavioral changes can occur due to medical or psychosocial stressors, as well as due to onset of psychiatric disorders common in individuals with DS. Because these individuals often have difficulties communicating their feelings, discovering the exact cause of behavioral changes can be difficult and may require comprehensive investigations. For instance, medical causes, such as pain from dental caries, sinus infection, reflux esophagitis, thyroid problems, celiac disease, or sleep apnea, need to be ruled out. A workup should include blood analysis to rule out renal and liver function abnormalities, anemia (complete blood count and iron level), B_{12} and folic acid deficiencies, and thyroid dysfunction. Vision and hearing evaluations should also be performed. Other etiologies of behavioral changes can be life stressors, including employment problems, threats and teasing, and sexual and physical abuse. Self-talk and imaginary friends are common and usually developmentally appropriate, rather than representing psychotic behaviors (which are rare in DS). Obsessions and compulsive behaviors are not uncommon, particularly in individuals with underlying anxiety. Any persistent behavioral disturbances or decline in functioning occurring within months of a parent's or close family member's death should be considered a grief reaction. Symptoms of major depression include at least 2 weeks of sad or agitated mood, sleep disturbance, appetite disturbance, crying spells, loss of enjoyment of previously pleasurable activities, and withdrawal. Depression shows an up-and-down pattern, with improvement and eventual return to baseline, whereas onset of Alzheimer dementia shows a persistent decline in function.

Psychopharmacological Interventions

Medication should not be used as a substitute for appropriate supportive therapy, and the decision to medicate should be periodically reexamined. If a decision to treat with medication is made, care providers need to be properly educated about the medications and side effects, as well as how to properly dispense them. When medication is being prescribed, the best interests of the patient, rather than those of the caretaker, should be kept in mind. Medication use and dosing should be predicated on results from adequate clinical trials whenever possible.

A comprehensive list of medications, as well as their uses, chemistry, and side effects, can be found in *Mental Wellness in Adults With Down Syndrome: A Guide to Emotional and Behavioral Strengths and Challenges*, by McGuire and Chicoine (2006). Table 6–1 includes a modified list of medications and their intended indications.

Table 6–1. Medications for management of Down syndrome

Medication class	Examples	Symptoms targeted
Acetylcholine receptor inhibitors	Benztropine mesylate (Cogentin)	Extrapyramidal side effects to psychotropic medications
α-Adrenergic antihypertensives	Clonidine (Catapres), guanfacine (Tenex)	Anxiety and ADHD
Antianxiety agents	Benzodiazepines (both long and short acting)	Anxiety and insomnia
Antidepressant agents	Bupropion (Wellbutrin), fluoxetine (Prozac), sertraline (Zoloft), clomipramine (Anafranil), amitriptyline (Elavil)	Depression, obsessive-compulsive disorder, anxiety, and aggressive behaviors
Antihistamines	Hydroxyzine (Atarax)	Anxiety, sedation, and insomnia
Antiseizure medications	Valproic acid (Depakote), carbamazepine (Tegretol)	Seizures and off-label use for mood, aggressive behaviors, and impulse control
Antithyroid agents	Methimazole (Tapazole), propylthiouracil	Hyperthyroidism
Thyroid supplements	Desiccated thyroid, levothyroxine (Synthroid)	Hypothyroidism
ADHD medications	Atomoxetine (Strattera), amphetamine and dextroamphetamine (Adderall), dextroamphetamine (Dexedrine)	ADHD
β-Blockers	Atenolol (Tenormin)	Anxiety, impulse control, and aggressive behaviors
Cholinesterase inhibitors	Donepezil (Aricept), rivastigmine (Exelon)	Alzheimer dementia
Contraceptives	Ortho-Novum, Tri-Norinyl, Depo-Provera	For contraception; also, dysmenorrhea
Lithium	Eskalith, Lithobid	Mania and bipolar disorder
Sleep agents	Melatonin, zolpidem (Ambien), eszopiclone (Lunesta), trazodone (Desyrel), antihistamines	Insomnia

Table 6–1.   Medications for management of Down syndrome *(continued)*

Medication class	Examples	Symptoms targeted
NMDA receptor antagonists	Memantine (Namenda)	Alzheimer's dementia
Nonsteroidal anti-inflammatory agents	Naproxen (Aleve), ibuprofen (Advil)	Pain, arthritis, dysmenorrhea, and gout
Opioid antagonists	Naltrexone (Revia)	Self-injurious behavior

Note.   ADHD=attention-deficit/hyperactivity disorder; NMDA=*N*-methyl-D-aspartate.
Source.   Based on data from McGuire and Chicoine 2006.

Over the years, many alternative and testimonial therapies have been proposed for DS. It is important that clinicians help parents understand information regarding the many alternative therapies. It is also important to review the evidence-based research outcomes and side effects in order to be able to explain whether sufficient support exists for the use of a therapy. Some of the alternative therapies that have not been found to benefit people with DS include sicca cell injection therapy, nutritional supplements, megavitamins, and piracetam. In their attempts to help their child, parents may be vulnerable to these unusual treatments.

Outcomes

In 1936, the life expectancy for individuals with DS was 20 years; in contrast, the current life expectancy is greater than 60 years. A cohort study in Western Australia found that the life expectancy of people with DS was 58.6 years; 25% of participants lived to age 62.9 (Glasson et al. 2002). Among individuals with DS, males have an increased average survival of 3.3 years (Glasson et al. 2003) compared with females.

Even though the word *syndrome* implies "features that run together," and people with DS indeed have similar appearances, the assumption that all people with DS have the same characteristics and abilities reinforces the stereotype that all persons with DS are the same. Even though we have described the typical health, learning, and behavioral profiles of individuals with DS, we emphasize that each person has his or her own unique strengths, capabilities, and talents, just as do individuals without DS.

The majority of individuals with DS have mild to moderate intellectual disability, but there can be a high degree of variability in their abilities. Predictors of adaptive function and employment of individuals with DS include higher cognitive ability, social supports, emotional and physical health, and vocational training or assistance (McDermott et al. 1999; McGuire and Chicoine 2006; Moore et al. 2004).

Parent groups and national support organizations (see "Recommended Resources" section) have had major roles in advocacy, social attitudes, education, and community networking. The annual convention of the DS national support group, the National Down Syndrome Congress, demonstrates the amazing progress that has been made. Transitions are always difficult for individuals with neurodevelopmental disabilities and their parents. Planning and reassessment should be done as individuals transition from early intervention services to preschool; then to grade school, middle school, high school, and further secondary education such as a community college or vocational training; and ultimately to community residential living and employment. It is important for parents to understand the importance of planning ahead for these transitions, rather than be thrust suddenly into decision making when their son or daughter becomes an adolescent or adult. Programs that assist parents in planning for these transitions include Making Action Plans (MAPS; www.inclusion.com/maps.html), Planning Alternative Tomorrows with Hope (PATH; www.ont-autism.uoguelph.ca), and Personal Futures Planning (PFP; www.ilr.cornell.edu/edi/PCP/course05d.html). Information about these programs is available online and at local resource centers.

Decisions about conservatorship, guardianship, or alternatives such as power of attorney for finances or health care matters are important but often difficult, and the person with DS must be included in determining the best alternative. Laws vary by state, and information is available through State Councils on Developmental Disabilities in each state.

New Research Directions

Studies indicate that individuals with DS have cholinergic dysfunction (Beccaria et al. 1998), which may be due to lifelong overexpression of the gene *APP* located on chromosome 21. *APP* encodes the amyloid-β (A4) precursor protein involved in the production of β-amyloid. In recent years, there has been growing interest in treatment with cholinesterase inhibitors (ChEIs). These inhibitors increase the availability of acetylcholine to postsynaptic receptors by limiting its breakdown in the synapse. Increased concentrations of acetylcholine in the brain lead to increased communication between nerve cells. Initial pharmacological studies with donepezil hydrochloride, a ChEI approved for the treatment of Alzheimer disease in the general population, in small groups of individuals with DS seemed to support this theory. Treatment was demonstrated in a 12-week randomized double-blind placebo-controlled study with a 12-week open-label extension phase that enrolled 123 individuals, ages 18–35, with DS but without Alzheimer disease (Kishnani et al. 2009). Efficacy (measured using the Severe Impairment Battery) was shown in some subjects but not others. A 10-week randomized double-blind placebo-controlled multicenter study that enrolled 129 individuals, ages 10–17, with DS failed to demonstrate any benefit for donepezil versus placebo (Kishnani et al. 2010). However, a 24-week trial with 21 older adults, ages 32–58, who were severely impaired with DS showed positive effect of donepezil over placebo (Kondoh et al. 2011).

Memantine hydrochloride, another approved treatment for Alzheimer disease in the general population, is an N-methyl-D-aspartate (NMDA) receptor antagonist. The mechanism and its association with DS are not well understood. One hypothesis is that individuals with DS may have hyperactivity of the NMDA receptor. In a 52-week randomized double-blind trial that enrolled adults with DS over age 40, memantine was not found to be effective in decreasing the rate of decline in cognition and function (Hanney et al. 2012). At the time of this publication, recruitment for additional studies to build on previous findings was taking place.

Key Points

- Down syndrome has long been recognized as a leading cause of intellectual disability. People with DS and their families have played a major role in changing attitudes, legislation, public policy, and expectations for care and inclusion of all individuals with intellectual and other disabilities.

- Clinicians should always obtain a karyotype on each child with DS to differentiate between nondysjunctive type (95% of cases) and Robertsonian translocation type. The latter type may carry a much higher recurrence risk if one of the parents has a balanced translocation.

- Early physical recognition features of Down syndrome that suggest a clinical diagnosis include rounded facies, relative microcephaly/brachycephaly, large fontanelles (often with a midline third fontanelle), neck folds, tongue protrusion, and generalized and striking hypotonia and laxity.

- Behavioral and psychiatric disorders, especially in adolescents and adults with DS, are not uncommon. Because these individuals often have difficulty communicating their feelings, discovering the exact cause of behavioral changes can be difficult and requires comprehensive investigation. For example, medical causes such as pain, dental caries, sinus infection, reflux esophagitis, thyroid problems, celiac disease, or sleep apnea need to be ruled out. In addition, other etiologies such as life stressors should be considered; these may include employment problems, threats and teasing, sexual or physical abuse, or depression.

- Transitions are always difficult for individuals with neurodevelopmental disabilities and for their parents. Planning and assessment should always be considered from early childhood to adolescent and adult life. Programs that assist parents, described in the Outcomes section of this chapter, include MAPS, PATH, and PFP.

- A road map to medical monitoring that is unique to people with DS has been established. It calls for periodic monitoring of vision, hearing, thyroid function, atlantoaxial subluxation, celiac diseases, sleep apnea, and other conditions.

Recommended Readings

Couwenhoven T: Teaching Children With Down Syndrome About Their Bodies, Boundaries and Sexuality. Bethesda, MD, Woodbine House, 2007

Chicoine B, McGuire D: The Guide to Good Health for Teens and Adults With Down Syndrome. Bethesda, MD, Woodbine House, 2010

McGuire D, Chicoine B: Mental Wellness in Adults With Down Syndrome: A Guide to Emotional and Behavioral Strengths and Challenges. Bethesda, MD, Woodbine House, 2006

Pueschel S, Sustrova M: Adolescents With Down Syndrome: Toward a More Fulfilling Life. Baltimore, MD, Brookes, 1997

Recommended Resources

Information for Health Care Providers

National Center for Biotechnology Information—Resources for Down syndrome
http://www.ncbi.nlm.nih.gov/sites/ga?disorder=Down%20Syndrome

Online Mendelian Inheritance in Man—Down syndrome
http://omim.org/entry/190685

Information for Families and Health Care Providers

Association for Children with Down Syndrome
http://www.acds.org

International Mosaic Down Syndrome Association
http://www.imdsa.org

National Down Syndrome Congress
http://www.ndsccenter.org

National Down Syndrome Society
http://www.ndss.org

References

Alford KA, Reinhardt K, Garnett C, et al: Analysis of GATA1 mutations in Down syndrome transient myeloproliferative disorder and myeloid leukemia. Blood 118:2222–2238, 2011

Beccaria L, Marziani E, Manzoni P, et al: Further evidence of cholinergic impairment of the neuroendocrine control of the GH secretion in Down's syndrome. Dement Geriatr Cogn Disord 9:78–81, 1998

Bull MJ; Committee on Genetics: Health supervision for children with Down syndrome. Pediatrics 128:393–406, 2011

Carothers AD, Castilla EE, Dutra MG, et al: Search for ethnic, geographic, and other factors in the epidemiology of Down syndrome in South America: analysis of data from the ECLAMC project, 1967–1997. Am J Med Genet 103:149–156, 2001

Carr J: Six weeks to twenty-one years old: a longitudinal study of children with Down's syndrome and their families. Third Jack Tizard Memorial Lecture. J Child Psychol Psychiatry 29:407–431, 1988

Carr J: Stability and change in cognitive ability over the life span: a comparison of populations with and without Down's syndrome. J Intellect Disabil Res 49:915–928, 2005

Carroll KN, Arbogast PG, Dudley JA, et al: Increase in incidence of medically treated thyroid disease in children with Down syndrome after rerelease of American Academy of Pediatrics Health Supervision guidelines. Pediatrics 122: E493–E498, 2008

Cassidy SB, Allanson JE: Management of Genetic Syndromes, 3rd Edition. Hoboken, NJ, Wiley-Blackwell, 2010

Castillo H, Patterson B, Hickey F, et al: Difference in age at regression in children with autism with and without Down syndrome. J Dev Behav Pediatr 29:89–93, 2008

Coppus A, Evenhuis H, Verberne GJ, et al: Dementia and mortality in persons with Down's syndrome. J Intellect Disabil Res 50:768–777, 2006

Couwenhoven T: Teaching Children With Down Syndrome About Their Bodies, Boundaries, and Sexuality: A Guide for Parents and Professionals. Bethesda, MD, Woodbine House, 2007

Cuckle HS, Malone FD, Wright D, et al: Contingent screening for Down syndrome: results from the FaSTER trial. Prenat Diagn 28:89–94, 2008

Dykens EM: Psychiatric and behavioral disorders in persons with Down syndrome. Ment Retard Dev Disabil Res Rev 13:272–278, 2007

Egan JF, Smith K, Timms D, et al: Demographic differences in Down syndrome livebirths in the U.S. from 1989 to 2006. Prenat Diagn 31:389–394, 2011

Esbensen AJ, Seltzer MM, Krauss MW: Stability and change in health, functional abilities, and behavior problems among adults with and without Down syndrome. Am J Ment Retard 113:263–277, 2008

Freeman SB, Bean LH, Allen EG, et al: Ethnicity, sex, and the incidence of congenital heart defects: a report from the National Down Syndrome Project. Genet Med 10:173–180, 2008

Gardner RJM, Sutherland GR: Chromosome Abnormalities and Genetic Counseling, 3rd Edition (Oxford Monographs on Medical Genetics, no. 46). New York, Oxford University Press, 2004

Glasson EJ, Sullivan SG, Hussain R, et al: The changing survival profile of people with Down's syndrome: implications for genetic counselling. Clin Genet 62:390–393, 2002

Glasson EJ, Sullivan SG, Hussain R, et al: Comparative survival advantage of males with Down syndrome. Am J Hum Biol 15:192–195, 2003

Hanney M, Prasher V, Williams N, et al: Memantine for dementia in adults older than 40 years with Down's syndrome (MEADOWS): a randomised, double-blind, placebo-controlled trial. Lancet 379:528–536, 2012

Hawkins BA, Eklund SJ, James DR, et al: Adaptive behavior and cognitive function of adults with Down syndrome: modeling change with age. Ment Retard 41:7–28, 2003

Hodapp RM: Families of persons with Down syndrome: new perspectives, findings, and research and service needs. Ment Retard Dev Disabil Res Rev 13:279–287, 2007

Jacobs PA, Baikie AG, Court Brown WM, et al: The somatic chromosomes in mongolism. Lancet 1:710, 1959

Kishnani PS, Sommer BR, Handen BL, et al: The efficacy, safety, and tolerability of donepezil for the treatment of young adults with Down syndrome. Am J Med Genet A 149A:1641–1654, 2009

Kishnani PS, Heller JH, Spiridigliozzi GA, et al: Donepezil for treatment of cognitive dysfunction in children with Down syndrome aged 10–17. Am J Med Genet A 152A:3028–3035, 2010

Kondoh T, Kanno A, Itoh H, et al: Donepezil significantly improves abilities in daily lives of female Down syndrome patients with severe cognitive impairment: a 24-week randomized, double-blind, placebo-controlled trial. Int J Psychiatry Med 41:71–89, 2011

Lejeune J, Gauthier M, Turpin R: Human chromosomes in tissue cultures [in French]. CR Hebd Seances Acad Sci 248:602–603, 1959

Malinge S, Izraeli S, Crispino JD: Insights into the manifestations, outcomes, and mechanisms of leukemogenesis in Down syndrome. Blood 113:2619–2628, 2009

McCarthy J: Behaviour problems and adults with Down syndrome: childhood risk factors. J Intellect Disabil Res 52:877–882, 2008

McDermott S, Martin M, Butkus S: What individual, provider, and community characteristics predict employment of individuals with mental retardation? Am J Ment Retard 104:346–355, 1999

McGuire DE, Chicoine B: Mental Wellness in Adults With Down Syndrome: A Guide to Emotional and Behavioral Strengths and Challenges. Bethesda, MD, Woodbine House, 2006

Molloy CA, Murray DS, Kinsman A, et al: Differences in the clinical presentation of Trisomy 21 with and without autism. J Intellect Disabil Res 53:143–151, 2009

Moore CL, Harley DA, Gamble D: Ex-post-facto analysis of competitive employment outcomes for individuals with mental retardation: national perspective. Ment Retard 42:253–262, 2004

Morris JK, Mutton DE, Alberman E: Revised estimates of the maternal age specific live birth prevalence of Down's syndrome. J Med Screen 9:2–6, 2002

Parker SE, Mai CT, Canfield MA, et al: Updated National Birth Prevalence estimates for selected birth defects in the United States, 2004–2006. Birth Defects Res A Clin Mol Teratol 88:1008–1016, 2010

Savva GM, Morris JK, Mutton DE: Maternal age-specific fetal loss rates in Down syndrome pregnancies. Prenat Diagn 26:499–504, 2006

Seltzer MM, Krauss MW, Tsunematsu N: Adults with Down syndrome and their aging mothers: diagnostic group differences. Am J Ment Retard 97:496–508, 1993

Sheets KB, Crissman BG, Feist CD, et al: Practice guidelines for communicating a prenatal or postnatal diagnosis of Down syndrome: recommendations of the National Society of Genetic Counselors. J Genet Couns 20:432–441, 2011

Shott SR: Down syndrome: common otolaryngologic manifestations. Am J Med Genet C Semin Med Genet 142C:131–140, 2006

Steingass KJ, Chicoine B, McGuire D, et al: Developmental disabilities grown up: Down syndrome. J Dev Behav Pediatr 32:548–558, 2011

Turner S, Alborz A: Academic attainments of children with Down's syndrome: a longitudinal study. Br J Educ Psychol 73:563–583, 2003

ANGELMAN AND PRADER-WILLI SYNDROMES

Molly McGinniss, M.S., L.C.G.C.
Billur Moghaddam, M.D.

Angelman syndrome (AS) and Prader-Willi syndrome (PWS) are clinically distinct neurodevelopmental disorders caused by deletions or abnormal imprinting of the Angelman syndrome/Prader-Willi syndrome (AS/PWS) region at 15q11.2–q13. AS is caused by loss of function of the maternally contributed AS/PWS region; PWS is caused by loss of the paternally derived AS/PWS region.

PWS and AS are the first known examples of human disease involving imprinted genes, and research surrounding the underlying genetic mechanisms of both conditions has led to a much greater understanding of imprinting. *Imprinting* is defined as "the process by which maternally and paternally derived chromosomes are uniquely chemically modified leading to different expression of a certain gene or genes on those chromosomes depending on their parental origin" (Pagon et al. 1993).

Angelman Syndrome

AS is a severe neurodevelopmental genetic disorder that was first described in 1965 (Angelman 1965). The syndrome is characterized by severe global developmental delay, ataxic gait, seizures, and a unique behavioral phenotype associated with happy demeanor coupled with bursts of laughter and excitability.

147

Epidemiology

The incidence of AS is estimated to be between 1 in 10,000 and 1 in 20,000 in the general population (Williams 2005).

Etiologies

AS is caused by deficient expression or function of the maternally inherited ubiquitin-protein ligase E3A allele (*UBE*3A*) located within the 15q11.2–q13 AS/PWS region. *UBE*3A* is involved in the ubiquitination pathway, which targets selected proteins for degradation. Although *UBE*3A* demonstrates normal biallellic expression in most tissues, preferential expression of the maternal allele in the brain of humans and mice has been well documented (Horsthemke and Wagstaff 2008). The majority of individuals with AS (~70%) have a common 5- to 7-megabase (Mb) deletion at 15q11.2–q13 on the maternal allele. Paternal uniparental disomy (UPD), in which the father contributes both copies of chromosome 15, accounts for approximately 7% of cases, whereas *UBE*3A* sequence alterations are detected in 11% of cases, and imprinting center defects account for approximately 3% of cases (Dagli and Williams 2011). In approximately 10%–15% of cases, clinical features of AS are present although an AS-causing genetic mechanism cannot be identified, indicating the possibility of additional mechanisms or genes being involved in *UBE*3A* function (Dagli and Williams 2011). A very small number of patients (1%) have a deletion as the result of a cytogenetically visible chromosomal rearrangement (i.e., translocation or inversion) involving the AS/PWS region.

Initial testing strategies to establish a diagnosis of AS include methylation analysis and *UBE*3A* sequence analysis, which together can detect abnormalities in approximately 89% of cases. Among these, parent-specific DNA methylation analysis will be abnormal in 78% of cases, and *UBE*3A* sequencing will detect another 11% of cases expected to have a molecular diagnosis (Dagli and Williams 2011). Methylation analysis will not distinguish among duplications, paternal UPD, or AS imprinting center defects; therefore, further molecular testing is important to establish the exact molecular etiology so that accurate genetic counseling can be provided.

Recurrence risks for AS depend on the genetic mechanism leading to the loss of *UBE*3A* function. The risk to siblings of an individual with AS is typically less than 1% for probands with a deletion of paternal UPD and as high as 50% for probands with an imprinting center defect or *UBE*3A* sequence alteration. While uncommon, the risk to siblings can approach 100% if the father of the proband has a 15;15 Robertsonian translocation. Only one case has been reported of an individual with AS reproducing (Lossie and Driscoll 1999). The risk to offspring of individuals with AS would depend on the AS-causing genetic mechanism and the sex of the individual with AS.

Even though all possible genetic mechanisms lead to severe to profound levels of intellectual disability, movement disorder, characteristic behaviors, and speech limitations, some genotype-phenotype correlations have been reported (Fridman et al. 2000; Lossie et al. 2001; Smith et al. 1997; Varela et al. 2004). In summary, the 5- to 7-Mb deletion leads to the most severe phenotype; patients with UPD have better physical growth, less severe movement disorder, and a lower prevalence of seizures. Individuals with imprinting center defects or UPD or *UBE*3A* mutations often have less motor milestone delay and higher communication ability than do individuals with AS due to the 5- to 7-Mb deletion, who typically have absent speech. Individuals with a maternal deletion of the AS/PWS region encompassing the oculocutaneous albinism II gene *OCA2* may have hypopigmentation of the hair, eyes, and skin. Homozygous loss of *OCA2* results in tyrosine-positive oculocutaneous albinism.

Signs and Symptoms

Newborns with AS typically have a normal physical phenotype, and developmental delay is typically noted around age 6 months. Other characteristic manifestations of this disorder emerge gradually and become quite evident after age 1 year, but the classic presentation may not manifest until several years later. The Scientific Advisory Committee of the U.S. Angelman Syndrome Foundation has developed consensus criteria for the clinical diagnosis of this entity (Williams et al. 2006). The typical manifestations and findings that are present in all individuals with AS include a normal prenatal, birth, and neonatal history; no major birth defects; and normal hematological, biochemical, and metabolic profiles. Magnetic resonance imaging (MRI) shows that the brain is structurally normal, except that mild cortical atrophy and dysmyelinization occur in some cases. Development is delayed, but there is no developmental regression. The developmental delay is usually severe and evident by age 6–12 months. Patients' receptive language abilities far exceed their expressive language abilities, which remain strikingly limited. Extremity movements are tremulous and ataxic; as gait is acquired, the ataxia becomes more noticeable. Individuals with AS are often described as hypermotoric, and they have short attention spans. Their ataxic gait and unique behavior patterns, with frequent laughing and smiling for no apparent reason, have led to the descriptive term "happy puppet syndrome" (Angelman 1965).

The majority of individuals with AS (more than 80%) have absolute or relative microcephaly by age 2 years, and electroencephalography (EEG) may show abnormal results, including characteristic large-amplitude and slow-spike waves. Most have some facial dysmorphism, such as protruding tongue, midface hypoplasia, flat occiput, prognathia, tongue thrusting, suck and swallowing problems, a wide mouth, and wide-spaced teeth (see Figure 7–1). Tongue thrusting and oral-motor dysfunction lead to drooling and feeding difficulties. Patients may also have strabismus. As previously mentioned, individuals with deletions encompassing *OCA2* may have hypopigmentation of the skin, hair, and eyes. Other clinical features include increased heat sensitivity, abnormal sleep-wake cycles, fascination with water, obesity, scoliosis, and constipation.

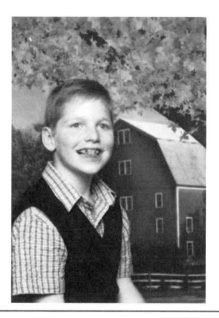

FIGURE 7–1.   A young male with Angelman syndrome. Note the midface hypoplasia, prognathia, and wide mouth.

Source.   Image used with parental permission.

AS should be suspected when a child has global developmental delay, particularly in expressive language skills, combined with other neurological findings such as muscular hypotonia, tremulousness, ataxia, and seizures, which typically emerge over time. The seizures are quite variable and may be generalized or focal (Fiumara et al. 2010; Thibert et al. 2009). The average child with AS begins walking between ages 2.5 and 6 years, and the gait is quite stiff and robotlike with uplifted, flexed, and pronated arms (Lossie et al. 2001). The language impediment is typically so severe that it is very unusual for a child with AS to have more than one or two understandable words. Effective use of sign language is not common; however, individuals with AS can benefit from the use of communication boards or electronic devices. They generally have good physical health through adulthood, and fertility and onset of puberty are typically not affected. Life span is nearly normal; however, due to the severity of cognitive delays, independent living is rarely possible for adults with AS.

Differential Diagnosis

Because patients with AS typically present initially with nonspecific developmental delay and/or seizure disorder, the differential diagnosis can be quite extensive and may include cytogenetic abnormalities (such as 22q13.3 deletion), mitochondrial disorders, cerebral palsy, and nonspecific encephalopathies. Several rare syndromes, such as Mowat-Wilson syndrome, Pitt-Hopkins syndrome, and Christianson syndrome, may have some clinical overlap, although these syndromes are typically distinguishable by the distinct facial or electroencephalographic phenotypes. Females with developmental delay, seizure disorder, speech impairment, and acquired microcephaly can resemble girls with Rett syndrome, a progressive neurodevelopmental disorder due to mutations within the methyl CpG binding protein 2 gene (*MECP2*). *MECP2* analysis should be considered in this patient population. Additionally, *MECP2* duplication in males may be characterized by developmental delay, seizures, absent speech, and ataxic gait with spastic paraparesis (Lugtenberg et al. 2009). Rare metabolic disorders such as disorders of glycosylation and adenylosuccinate lyase deficiency can cause autistic traits, seizures, and hypotonia.

For diagnostic purposes, the ideal testing strategy begins with a DNA methylation analysis, which covers the microdeletions as well as UPD cases and AS imprinting center defects. If results of this test are abnormal, the next step would be to obtain fluorescence in situ hybridization (FISH) analysis for the detection of microdeletions. This test may be important in family counseling. If the methylation study results are normal and there is sufficient clinical suspicion, *UBE*3A* sequencing would pick up an additional 11% of patients. Regardless, genetic counseling is strongly recommended for families of individuals with AS.

Management

Once the diagnosis of AS is established, the following studies are recommended as baseline evaluations:

- Baseline brain MRI and EEG
- Musculoskeletal evaluation for scoliosis and gait abnormalities

- Ophthalmological evaluation
- Developmental evaluation and initiation of intervention services
- Feeding and nutritional evaluation for children with feeding and growth problems
- Evaluation for reflux, if indicated

After the results are available, patients can be provided with individualized help. Feeding aids may include special nipples and formulas to provide more caloric intake. Seizures are treated with antiepileptic medications and pediatric neurology management. Behavioral therapies to address hypermotoric behaviors and short attention span may be helpful. Physical, occupational, and speech therapy focusing on nonverbal communication are essential parts of the management protocol. The management generally requires multidisciplinary involvement.

Many families benefit from involvement in AS support groups, which exist in most developed countries and have proven instrumental in bringing together both parents and medical professionals interested in the management and treatment of AS. These groups include the Angelman Syndrome Foundation (ASF; www.angelman.org) and the Angelman Syndrome Support Education and Research Trust (ASSERT; www.angelmanuk.org).

Prader-Willi Syndrome

PWS is a multisystem disorder first described clinically in 1956. PWS was the first microdeletion syndrome identified after high-resolution chromosome studies became available and was the first recognized human genetic imprinting disorder (Ledbetter et al. 1981; Nicholls et al. 1989). PWS is characterized by severe infantile hypotonia and feeding difficulties, followed by excessive eating behaviors in childhood, which gradually result in morbid obesity unless eating is externally controlled.

Epidemiology

A wide range of prevalence rates have been reported for PWS, with previous estimates ranging from 1 in 8,000 to 1 in 20,000 in the United States; however, recent epidemiological surveys in Europe and Australia have estimated a lower birth incidence of approximately 1 in 30,000 (Jin 2011).

Etiologies

PWS is caused by absent or deficient expression of the paternally derived AS/PWS region at 15q11.2–q13. Several genes in the AS/PWS deleted region (*SNURF-SNRPN, MKRN, MAGEL2*, and *NDN*) are subject to genomic imprinting and are therefore normally active only from the paternally contributed chromosome 15. The absence of one or more of the paternally inherited genes must contribute to the phenotype of PWS; however, the precise cause of PWS is still unknown. Unlike AS, for which the causative factor is deficient expression or function of one gene (*UBE*3A*), PWS is thought to be a contiguous gene disorder, because studies thus far have indicated that the complete phenotype is due to the loss of expression of multiple genes (Cassidy et al. 2012). Despite the lingering ambiguity of the causative molecular mechanism for PWS, *SNORD116* (snoRNA gene cluster previously named *HBII-85*) has recently proven to be of significant interest to researchers. Three individuals have been reported with overlapping microdeletions (175–236 kilobase) that all encompass the *SNORD116* gene cluster (de Smith et al. 2009; Duker et al. 2010; Sahoo et al. 2008). Although all three individuals have had multiple clinical features suggestive of PWS, they also have other features not associated with classic PWS, including tall stature as a child, large head circumference, absence of typical PWS facial features, and atypical hand features. Although formal neurodevelopmental studies have not been performed to determine whether classical PWS behaviors are present, these reports emphasize the importance of the paternally derived *SNORD116* gene cluster in determining a PWS phenotype.

Absence of the paternally derived AS/PWS region at 15q11.2–q13 can be caused by a paternal deletion, maternal UPD, or an imprinting center defect. The majority of individuals (70%) have a deletion at 15q11.2–q13 on the paternal allele. There are two common deletion sizes, both of which can be detected by FISH testing. Maternal UPD, in which the mother contributes both copies of chromosome 15, accounts for approximately 25%–29% of cases, whereas imprinting center defects are suspected in less than 1% of cases. Approximately 1% of individuals with PWS have a detectable chromosomal rearrangement resulting in deletion of the AS/PWS region, whereas less than 1% of individuals have a balanced chromosomal rearrangement breaking within the 15q11.2–q13 region (Cassidy and Schwartz 2009).

Methylation analyses will correctly diagnosis PWS in more than 99% of cases. Although methylation analysis is the only technique that will diagnosis PWS in all three molecular classes (deletion, UPD, imprinting center defect), it does not distinguish between molecular classes. Further studies to determine the underlying molecular mechanism would be necessary so that accurate genetic counseling can be provided. An imprinting defect is presumed to be present in individuals with an abnormality of the parent-specific methylation imprint without evidence of a deletion or UPD

(Ohta et al. 1999). Most imprinting defects are epimutations; however, approximately 15% of individuals are found to have a small deletion in the PWS imprinting center region located at the 5´ end of the SNRPN gene and promoter (Ohta et al. 1999).

Recurrence risks for PWS depend on the genetic mechanism leading to the absence of the paternally derived AS/PWS region. The risk to siblings of an individual with PWS is typically less than 1% if the proband has a deletion or maternal UPD, and as high as 50% for probands with an imprinting center defect. The theoretical recurrence risk is 25%–50% if the father of the proband has a balanced rearrangement, and the risk approaches 100% if the mother of the proband is found to have a 15;15 Robertsonian translocation (Cassidy et al. 2012). Very few individuals with PWS have been reported to reproduce (Cassidy et al. 2012). The risk to offspring of individuals with PWS would depend on the PWS-causing genetic mechanism and the sex of the individual with PWS.

Some clinical differences exist between individuals with PWS who have a paternal deletion and those who have maternal UPD. The individuals with maternal UPD are less likely to have the classic facial features, hypopigmentation, or skill with jigsaw puzzles often noted in PWS (Dykens 2002). They also have higher IQs and fewer behavior problems (Hartley et al. 2005). Individuals with maternal UPD are more likely to have autism spectrum disorders and psychosis (Veltman et al. 2005). Hypopigmentation of the hair, eyes, and skin is common in individuals with a deletion of the AS/PWS region due to the concomitant loss of one copy of the gene *OCA2*; homozygous loss of *OCA2* results in tyrosine-positive oculocutaneous albinism (Cassidy et al. 2012).

Signs and Symptoms

The initial presentation of PWS in the infantile period involves typically significant hypotonia and feeding difficulties resulting from a weak suck and decreased arousal. Fetal size is generally normal, but infants are often diagnosed with failure to thrive because of their feeding difficulties. PWS should always be considered in the differential diagnosis of early infantile hypotonia. Electrophysiological and muscle histological studies generally show nonspecific changes, and hypotonia tends to improve gradually (Cassidy et al. 2012).

Dysmorphic features of PWS can be quite subtle but nonetheless present even in early infancy; these include face and head with narrow bifrontal diameter, almond-shaped palpebral fissures, a narrow nasal bridge, a thin upper lip, and downturned corners of the mouth. The features may become more pronounced with age. The hands are small with tapering fingers, and the feet are short and broad. Hypogonadism may manifest as a micropenis and/or cryptorchidism in males in the neonatal period and may be more subtle or not notable in female infants. Individuals with PWS also have sloping shoulders, truncal obesity, and genu valgum. Strabismus, scoliosis, and kyphosis are common. Short stature is characteristic, with lack of a pubertal growth spurt. The average height is 155 cm for males and 148 cm for females (Cassidy et al. 2012).

Global developmental delays are common in individuals with PWS. Motor delays relate, at least in part, to the underlying hypotonia. Average age for sitting is 12 months and for walking is 24 months (Cassidy et al. 2012). Even though the hypotonia improves with age, adults remain mildly hypotonic with decreased muscle bulk and tone. Language development is also delayed. Speech is usually poorly articulated with a nasal or slurred character. Cognitive abnormalities are common, with a characteristic profile of strengths and weaknesses. Approximately 40% of individuals with PWS are in the borderline to mild intellectual disability range, and another 20% are in the moderate range (Whittington et al. 2004a, 2004b). Individuals with PWS have relative strengths in reading, visuospatial skills, and long-term memory, with weaknesses in mathematics and short-term memory (Dykens et al. 1999). Their visuospatial skills help them excel in solving jigsaw puzzles (Dykens 2002).

As previously mentioned in the sections on etiologies for both PWS and AS, individuals with a paternal deletion of the AS/PWS region encompassing the gene *OCA2* may have hypopigmentation of the hair, eyes, and skin.

Hypogonadism is observed in both sexes and may present at birth with hypoplastic genitalia; later in life, it manifests as abnormal pubertal development. Males may have cryptorchidism, small testes, and scrotal hypoplasia, whereas females may have labial hypoplasia, small clitorises, and primary amenorrhea (Akefeldt et al. 1999).

Hyperphagia is not evident at birth and emerges later, usually between ages 2 and 4 years (range: 1–6 years). It is recognized later due to lack of satiety related to hypothalamic dysfunction (Butler and Bittel 2007) as well as a high threshold for emesis. Extreme food-seeking behaviors, including the eating of garbage, pet food, and frozen foods, are common and difficult to manage. Central obesity develops due to excessive eating coupled with low metabolic rate and decreased activity. There is relative sparing of obesity in the lower extremities.

Obesity and its complications, including cardiopulmonary complications, sleep apnea, hypertension, thrombophlebitis, and type II diabetes, are the major causes of morbidity and mortality in individuals with PWS. Non-insulin-dependent diabetes emerges in about 25% of adults with PWS (Butler et al. 2002).

Individuals with PWS demonstrate a unique behavioral profile, which can include temper tantrums, controlling and manipulative behavior, stubbornness, obsessive-compulsive characteristics, and difficulty with changes in routine. Lying, stealing, and aggression are common, particularly related to food seeking. Attention-deficit and hyperactivity disorders are also common (Wigren and Hansen 2005). Recent studies have reported psychosis in up to 20% of individuals with PWS (Joshi et al. 2010). Although PWS has been associated with an increased risk for autism spectrum disorders, few studies have assessed the exact risk. Estimates are that approximately 40% of those with PWS due to maternal UPD and 15%–18% of those with PWS due to a 15q11.2–q13 deletion will have an autism spectrum disorder (Descheemaeker et al. 2006; Dykens et al. 2011; Veltman et al. 2005).

Individuals with PWS experience sleep disturbances. These include central and obstructive sleep apnea, abnormal circadian rhythms in rapid eye movement sleep, and excessive daytime sleepiness (Dykens et al. 2011; Festen et al. 2006; Nixon and Brouillette 2002; Priano et al. 2006).

Clinical diagnostic criteria were developed in 1993 and reviewed for accuracy in 2001 (Gunay-Aygun et al. 2001; Holm et al. 1993). The major criteria are weighted 1 point each and the minor criteria are ½ point each (Table 7–1). Supportive criteria serve to increase or decrease the suspicion for the diagnosis but do not add any points. For children under age 3 years, 5 points are required for diagnosis, 4 of which must be major criteria. For individuals age 3 years and older, a total of 8 points is required for diagnosis, with at least 5 points coming from the major group. Despite the accuracy of molecular genetic testing, clinical diagnostic criteria remain a crucial tool in raising diagnostic suspicion prior to genetic testing.

Differential Diagnosis

Many disorders have features similar to those of the PWS phenotype. Craniopharyngiomas, particularly if they occur at a young age, share many common findings with PWS because of the damage to the hypothalamus. In addition, hyperphagic short stature, an acquired condition that develops because of psychosocial stressors, is associated with growth hormone deficiency, hyperphagia, and mild learning disabilities (Gilmour et al. 2001). Methylation analysis will distinguish craniopharyngiomas and hyperphagic short stature from PWS. One of the most prevalent features of PWS is neonatal hypotonia, which can also be noted in many other conditions. The differential diagnosis of neonatal hypotonia is quite extensive and includes the following disorders: congenital myotonic dystrophy type 1, neonatal sepsis, central nervous system depression, and several myopathies and neuropathies, such as spinal muscular atrophy.

TABLE 7–1. Consensus diagnostic criteria for Prader-Willi syndrome

Major criteria (1 point each)	Minor criteria (½ point each)	Supportive findings
Neonatal/infantile hypotonia with poor suck	Decreased fetal movement and infantile lethargy	High pain threshold
		Decreased vomiting
Feeding problems and failure to thrive in infancy	Characteristic behavior issues	Scoliosis; kyphosis
	Sleep disturbances; sleep apnea	Early adrenarche
Weight gain at 1–6 years causing obesity	Short stature for family by age 15 years	Osteoporosis
		Unusual skill with jigsaw puzzles
Hyperphagia	Hypopigmentation	Normal results on neuromuscular studies (i.e., muscle biopsy, EMG, NCV)
Characteristic facial features	Small hands and feet for height	
Hypogonadism manifesting as genital hypoplasia, pubertal delay/insufficiency, and infertility	Narrow hands; straight ulnar border	
	Esotropia; myopia	
	Thick, viscous saliva	
Developmental delay/ intellectual disability	Speech articulation defects	
	Skin picking	

Note. EMG=electromyography; NCV=nerve conduction velocity.
Source. Based on criteria from Gunay-Aygun et al. 2001; Holm et al. 1993.

Disorders causing autism spectrum disorder and developmental delay, such as fragile X syndrome, should also be included in the differential diagnosis of PWS (Nowicki et al. 2007).

Additionally, differential diagnosis is necessary because developmental delay and obesity with or without hypogonadism can also be seen in the following disorders: AS, Albright hereditary osteodystrophy, Bardet-Biedl syndrome, Cohen syndrome, Börjeson-Forssman-Lehmann syndrome, and Alström syndrome.

Management

Intervention and management of PWS patients can have a significant impact on their health, longevity, and ability to achieve maximum neurodevelopmental potential. A multidisciplinary team approach is extremely important in the care of individuals with PWS. The family and the health care professionals (geneticist, developmental pediatrician, psychotherapist, psychiatrist, dietitian, endocrinologist, ophthalmologist) should work together to help the patient achieve his or her maximum health and functional potential.

Infantile hypotonia and related feeding difficulties and failure to thrive usually pose the initial challenge in the management of individuals with PWS. Breast-feeding is usually not possible, and feeding methodologies such as gavage feeding and even gastrostomy tubes may be necessary to deliver adequate nutrition to the patients. During this period, high-calorie formulas may be used. This period may last from weeks to months. As muscle tone improves, there is a period of adequate feeding, which is typically followed by the characteristic hyperphagia.

Avoidance of obesity is one of the most difficult challenges in the management of patients with PWS. As a consequence of hypotonia, patients have decreased lean muscle mass, and therefore their caloric requirement is decreased. Individuals with PWS want to eat excessively and persistently seek food. A supportive environment and parental education are crucial. Monitoring of caloric intake, close supervision to minimize food-stealing behavior, prevention of unsupervised access to food, and regular exercise regimens are essential. Intake should typically not be above 1,000–1,200 calories/day. Many families have to resort to locking refrigerators and cabinets. Another strategy parents commonly use to prevent food access is avoidance of social gatherings; this can be isolating for the entire family unless other social activities are substituted. Supervision of children at school should be arranged, and schools may provide low-calorie lunches, if requested.

Growth should be closely monitored. Considering the dietary restrictions likely to be in place and the strong evidence of osteoporosis in these patients, supplemental vitamins and intake of the daily recommended allowance of calcium are important.

Growth hormone treatment has proven useful in the management of children with confirmed PWS and growth problems (see Figure 7–2). Benefits include improvement of height, increase in lean body mass, and improved mobility. Growth hormone therapy also helps with weight management. Treatment can be started in infancy or at the time of diagnosis (Höybye et al. 2005; Iughetti et al. 2008). Improvements in head circumference, height, and body composition and proportions, as well as in gross motor skills, language development, and cognition, have been documented in infants treated with growth hormone therapy (Cassidy et al. 2012). Adolescents treated with growth hormone therapy may also have improvements in behavior (Whitman et al. 2002). All individuals with a diagnosis of PWS should be referred to endocrinology for further discussion regarding the benefits and limitations of growth hormone therapy.

Cryptorchidism may resolve spontaneously or with the help of hormone and surgical treatments. Ophthalmological evaluation is very important for the treatment of strabismus, a common manifestation of PWS.

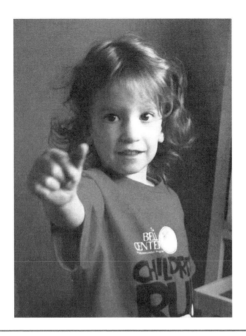

FIGURE 7–2. A young female with Prader-Willi syndrome who is treated with growth hormone therapy. Note the almond-shaped eyes, inner epicanthal folds, and thin upper lip.

Source. Image used with parental permission.

For baseline evaluation once the diagnosis of PWS is established, the following measures are recommended:

- Assess newborns and young infants for sucking problems and failure to thrive.
- Regardless of the child's age, measure and plot height and weight on either age-appropriate growth charts or charts developed specifically for PWS (Butler et al. 2006). Calculation of body mass index from weight and height (kg/m^2) may be helpful.
- Assess development in infants, and educational development as well as speech in children, to determine the need for appropriate intervention services.
- Refer for ophthalmological evaluation if strabismus is present and for assessment of visual acuity by age 1 year, or at diagnosis if later.
- Assess males for the presence of cryptorchidism regardless of age.
- Assess children with prolonged failure to thrive for hypothyroidism.
- Assess individuals, regardless of age, for the presence of scoliosis clini-

cally and, if indicated, radiographically. Very obese individuals cannot be adequately assessed clinically.

- Assess for the presence of behavior problems and obsessive-compulsive features after age 2 years, and for psychosis in adolescents and adults. Mental health professionals are a critical part of the treatment team.
- Evaluate respiratory status and perform a sleep study, regardless of age. These studies are specifically recommended prior to initiation of growth hormone therapy, along with assessment of the size of tonsils and adenoids, particularly in individuals who are obese.

Ongoing surveillance measures include careful monitoring of an exercise program and diet, evaluation for the presence of diabetes mellitus, monitoring for development of scoliosis, and dual-energy X-ray absorptiometry (DEXA) scans every 3–5 years to evaluate bone density. A sleep history should also be obtained during routine examinations to evaluate for sleep disturbances. Routine examinations should also assess for behavioral and psychiatric disturbances at least annually. Behavioral management programs may help with eating patterns as well as behavior problems. Family counseling and education of all individuals and educators in the patient's life are important for consistency. Behavioral interventions may be critical, and consistency in expectations at both school and home is key to successful behavioral modification.

Because individuals with PWS have developmental delays in motor, cognitive, and speech skills, early intervention services should be initiated as soon as possible. Educational intervention should include addressing individual strengths and weaknesses while taking into account the behavior difficulties. Most children require special education services. Speech, physical, and occupational therapies are often needed. Before individuals graduate from school, transition planning for vocational placement is essential. Involvement in PWS support groups helps many families cope with the challenges of a PWS diagnosis. Support and advocacy organizations include the Prader-Willi Syndrome Association (USA) (www.pwsausa.org), the International Prader-Willi Syndrome Organisation (www.ipwso.org), and the Foundation for Prader-Willi Research (http://fpwr.org).

Psychopharmacological Interventions

No medications are known to help with controlling hyperphagia. Elevated levels of ghrelin, a circulating orexigenic hormone produced mainly in the stomach, had been proposed as a potential hormonal abnormality to explain the hyperphagia that occurs in individuals with PWS; however, several studies investigating pharmacological reduction of ghrelin to normal levels found no effect on weight, height, or eating behavior (De Waele et al. 2008; Haqq et al. 2003; Tan et al. 2004).

The use of coenzyme Q10 (CoQ10) in individuals with PWS has also been studied, because decreased serum CoQ10 levels have been noted in obese individuals with and without PWS (Butler et al. 2003); however, two studies using CoQ10 supplementation in individuals with PWS for 1 year did not result in any improvement in body composition or growth (Eiholzer and Whitman 2004; Eiholzer et al. 2008). Individuals with PWS may need psychotherapy and pharmaceutical treatments for psychiatric problems; specific serotonin reuptake inhibitors have been used with relative success. In a study trial evaluating behavioral effects in individuals with PWS who received a single intranasal dose of oxytocin, Tauber et al. (2011) noted that oxytocin may increase trust in others and decease disruptive behaviors in individuals with PWS. Further studies looking at dose-related effects and long-term outcomes are needed.

New Research Directions

Although prior research focused on improving treatment of seizures in individuals with AS, as well as gaining a better understanding the behavioral phenotype and developing appropriate interventions, current attention has focused on better understanding *UBE*3A* function. Preferential expression of the maternal *UBE*3A* allele in the human fetal brain and adult frontal cortex has been well documented, leading to a research focus on the identification of *UBE*3A* protein targets, with the expectation that this will lead to therapies for AS.

Identifying the substrates that *UBE*3A* targets for degradation, as well as other *UBE*3A*-interacting proteins, and understanding the effect of *UBE*3A* loss on synaptic plasticity, neuron functions, and cell survival will add to our knowledge of the biological mechanisms of AS. Future research will rely heavily on the development of new mouse models of Angelman syndrome and the development of artificial transcription factors, drugs, and other agents that may improve *UBE*3A* expression (Philpot et al. 2011).

Continued research is imperative for determination of the causative molecular mechanism for the PWS phenotype, although research is complicated by the fact that PWS is thought to be a contiguous gene disorder, with the complete phenotype being due to the loss of expression of multiple genes. Genotype-phenotype correlations may provide additional clues into the underlying genetic mechanism. An imprinting center deletion mouse model for PWS has been developed, allowing further insight into the molecular and behavioral phenotype of PWS due to imprinting center defects (Relkovic et al. 2010). Additional animal models need to be developed for each underlying genetic mechanism (maternal UPD, paternal deletion) so that molecular and behavioral data can be compared.

PWS is a model disease in efforts to understand the mechanism of satiety and morbid obesity; however, no consistently identified hormonal abnormalities have been found that can account for the hyperphagia. Further research is needed to understand the metabolic correlates of hyperphagia.

Key Points

- Angelman syndrome (AS) is characterized by severe developmental delay, ataxic gait, seizures, and a distinct behavioral phenotype associated with happy demeanor coupled with bursts of laughter and excitability.

- Prader-Willi syndrome (PWS) is characterized by severe infantile hypotonia and feeding difficulties, followed by excessive eating behaviors in childhood, and a distinct behavioral phenotype that includes intellectual disability, obsessive-compulsive characteristics, and attention-deficit and hyperactivity disorders.

- AS is caused by loss of function of the maternally contributed AS/PWS region located at 15q11.2-q13. PWS is caused by loss of the paternally derived AS/PWS region located at 15q11.2-q13.

- Genetic counseling is recommended for families because the recurrence risk for siblings of an individual with AS or PWS typically varies between <1% and 50%, depending on the underlying genetic mechanism.

- All individuals with a diagnosis of PWS should be referred to endocrinology for discussion regarding growth hormone therapy; benefits have included improvements in weight management, increase of height, and improvements of gross motor skills, language development, cognition, and behavior.

- Management of individuals with AS is largely symptomatic, although current research focusing on the biological actions of UBE*3A is promising and has created speculation surrounding future therapeutic targets.

Recommended Readings

Buiting K: Prader-Willi syndrome and Angelman syndrome. Am J Med Genet Part C Semin Med Genet 154C:365-376, 2010

Cassidy SB, Schwartz S, Driscoll DJ: Prader-Willi syndrome. Genet Med 14:10–26, 2012

Dagli A, Williams CA: Angelman Syndrome. GeneReviews at GeneTests: Medical Genetics Information Resource (database online). Seattle, University of Washington, 1998–2011 (updated Jun 16, 2011). Available at: http://www.genetests .org. Accessed January 31, 2011.

References

Akefeldt A, Tornhage CJ, Gillberg C: A woman with Prader-Willi syndrome gives birth to a healthy baby girl. Dev Med Child Neurol 41:789–790, 1999

Angelman H: "Puppet children": a report of three cases. Dev Med Child Neurol 7:681–688, 1965

Butler JV, Whittington JE, Holland AJ, et al: Prevalence of, and risk factors for, physical ill-health in people with Prader-Willi syndrome: a population-based study. Dev Med Child Neurol 44:248–255, 2002

Butler MG, Bittel DC: Plasma obestatin and ghrelin levels in subjects with Prader-Willi syndrome. Am J Med Genet A 143:415–421, 2007

Butler MG, Dasouki M, Bittel D, et al: Coenzyme Q10 levels in Prader-Willi syndrome: comparison with obese and non-obese subjects. Am J Med Genet A 119A:168–171, 2003

Cassidy SB, Schwartz S: Prader-Willi syndrome. September 2009. Available at: http://www.ncbi.nlm.nih.gov/books/NBK1330/. Accessed March 26, 2012

Cassidy SB, Schwartz S, Miller JL, et al: Prader-Willi syndrome. Genet Med 14:10–26, 2012

Dagli A, Williams CA: Angelman Syndrome. GeneReviews at GeneTests: Medical Genetics Information Resource (database online). Seattle, University of Washington, 1998–2011 (updated Jun 16, 2011). Available at: http://www.genetests .org. Accessed January 31, 2011.

Descheemaeker MJ, Govers V, Vermeulen P, et al: Pervasive developmental disorders in Prader-Willi syndrome: the Leuven experience in 59 subjects and controls. Am J Med Genet A 140:1136–1142, 2006

de Smith AJ, Purmann C, Walters RG, et al: A deletion of the HBII-85 class of small nucleolar RNAs (snoRNAs) is associated with hyperphagia, obesity and hypogonadism. Hum Mol Genet 18:3257–3265, 2009

De Waele K, Ishkanian SL, Bogarin R, et al: Long-acting octreotide treatment causes a sustained decrease in ghrelin concentrations but does not affect weight, behaviour and appetite in subjects with Prader-Willi syndrome. Eur J Endocrinol 159:381–388, 2008

Duker AL, Ballif BC, Bawle EV, et al: Paternally inherited microdeletion at 15q11.2 confirms a significant role for the SNORD116 C/D box snoRNA cluster in Prader-Willi syndrome. Eur J Hum Genet 18:1196–1201, 2010

Dykens EM: Are jigsaw puzzle skills "spared" in persons with Prader-Willi syndrome? J Child Psychol Psychiatry 43:343–352, 2002

Dykens EM, Cassidy SB, King BH: Maladaptive behavior differences in Prader-Willi syndrome due to paternal deletion versus maternal uniparental disomy. Am J Ment Retard 104:67–77, 1999

Dykens EM, Lee E, Roof E: Prader-Willi syndrome and autism spectrum disorders: an evolving story. J Neurodev Disord 3:225–237, 2011

Eiholzer U, Whitman BY: A comprehensive team approach to the management of patients with Prader-Willi syndrome. J Pediatr Endocrinol Metab 17:1153–1175, 2004

Eiholzer U, Meinhardt U, Rousson V, et al: Developmental profiles in young children with Prader-Labhart-Willi syndrome: effects of weight and therapy with growth hormone or coenzyme Q10. Am J Med Genet A 146:873–880, 2008

Festen DA, de Weerd AW, van den Bossche RA, et al: Sleep-related breathing disorders in prepubertal children with Prader-Willi syndrome and effects of growth hormone treatment. J Clin Endocrinol Metab 91:4911–4915, 2006

Fiumara A, Pittalà A, Cocuzza M, et al: Epilepsy in patients with Angelman syndrome. Ital J Pediatr 36:31, 2010

Fridman C, Varela MC, Kok F, et al: Paternal UPD15: further genetic and clinical studies in four Angelman syndrome patients. Am J Med Genet 92:322–327, 2000

Gilmour J, Skuse D, Pembrey M: Hyperphagic short stature and Prader-Willi syndrome: a comparison of behavioural phenotypes, genotypes and indices of stress. Br J Psychiatry 179:129–137, 2001

Gunay-Aygun M, Heeger S, Schwartz S, et al: The changing purpose of Prader-Willi syndrome clinical diagnostic criteria and proposed revised criteria. Pediatrics 108:E92, 2001

Haqq AM, Stadler DD, Rosenfeld RG, et al: Circulating ghrelin levels are suppressed by meals and octreotide therapy in children with Prader-Willi syndrome. J Clin Endocrinol Metab 88:3573–3576, 2003

Hartley SL, Maclean WE Jr, Butler MG, et al: Maladaptive behaviors and risk factors among the genetic subtypes of Prader-Willi syndrome. Am J Med Genet A 136:140–145, 2005

Holm VA, Cassidy SB, Butler MG, et al: Prader-Willi syndrome: consensus diagnostic criteria. Pediatrics 91:398–402, 1993

Horsthemke B, Wagstaff J: Mechanisms of imprinting of the Prader-Willi/Angelman region. Am J Med Genet A 146A:2041–2052, 2008

Höybye C, Thorén M, Böhm B: Cognitive, emotional, physical and social effects of growth hormone treatment in adults with Prader-Willi syndrome. J Intellect Disabil Res 49:245–252, 2005

Iughetti L, Bosio L, Corrias A, et al: Pituitary height and neuroradiological alterations in patients with Prader-Labhart-Willi syndrome. Eur J Pediatr 167:701–702, 2008

Jin DK: Systematic review of the clinical and genetic aspects of Prader-Willi syndrome. Korean J Pediatr 54(2):55–63, 2011

Joshi G, Petty C, Wozniak J, et al: The heavy burden of psychiatric comorbidity in youth with autism spectrum disorders: a large comparative study of a psychiatrically referred population. J Autism Dev Disord 40:1361–1370, 2010

Ledbetter DH, Riccardi VM, Airhart SD, et al: Deletions of chromosome 15 as a cause of the Prader-Willi syndrome. N Engl J Med 304:325–329, 1981

Lossie AC, Driscoll DJ: Transmission of Angelman syndrome by an affected mother. Genet Med 1:262–266, 1999

Lossie AC, Whitney MM, Amidon D, et al: Distinct phenotypes distinguish the molecular classes of Angelman syndrome. J Med Genet 38:834–845, 2001

Lugtenberg D, Kleefstra T, Oudakker AR, et al: Structural variation in Xq28: MECP2 duplications in 1% of patients with unexplained XLMR and in 2% of male patients with severe encephalopathy. Eur J Hum Genet 17:444–453, 2009

Nicholls RD, Knoll JH, Butler MG, et al: Genetic imprinting suggested by maternal heterodisomy in nondeletion Prader-Willi syndrome. Nature 342:281–285, 1989

Nixon GM, Brouillette RT: Sleep and breathing in Prader-Willi syndrome. Pediatr Pulmonol 34:209–217, 2002

Nowicki ST, Tassone F, Ono MY, et al: The Prader-Willi phenotype of fragile X syndrome. J Dev Behav Pediatr 28:133–138, 2007

Ohta T, Gray TA, Rogan PK, et al: Imprinting-mutation mechanisms in Prader-Willi syndrome. Am J Hum Genet 64:397–413, 1999

Pagon RA, Bird TD, Dolan CR, et al (eds): GeneReviews (Internet). Seattle, University of Washington, 1993–. Available at: http://www.ncbi.nlm.nih.gov/books/NBK5191/. Accessed April 30, 2012.

Philpot BD, Thompson CE, Franco L, et al: Angelman syndrome: advancing the research frontier of neurodevelopmental disorders. J Neurodev Disord 3:50–56, 2011

Priano L, Grugni G, Miscio G, et al: Sleep cycling alternating pattern (CAP) expression is associated with hypersomnia and GH secretory pattern in Prader-Willi syndrome. Sleep Med 7:627–633, 2006

Relkovic D, Doe CM, Humby T, et al: Behavioral and cognitive abnormalities in an imprinting centre deletion mouse model for Prader-Willi syndrome. Eur J Neurosci 31:156–164, 2010

Sahoo T, del Gaudio D, German JR, et al: Prader-Willi phenotype caused by paternal deficiency for the HBII-85 C/D box small nucleolar RNA cluster. Nat Genet 40:719–721, 2008

Smith A, Marks R, Haan E, et al: Clinical features in four patients with Angelman syndrome resulting from paternal uniparental disomy. J Med Genet 34:426–429, 1997

Tan TM, Vanderpump M, Khoo B, et al: Somatostatin infusion lowers plasma ghrelin without reducing appetite in adults with Prader-Willi syndrome. J Clin Endocrinol Metab 89:4162–4165, 2004

Tauber M, Mantoulan C, Copet P, et al: Oxytocin may be useful to increase trust in others and decrease disruptive behaviours in patients with Prader-Willi syndrome: a randomised placebo-controlled trial in 24 patients. Orphanet J Rare Dis 6:47, 2011

Thibert RL, Conant KD, Braun EK: Epilepsy in Angelman syndrome: a questionnaire-based assessment of the natural history and current treatment options. Epilepsia 50:2369–2376, 2009

Varela MC, Kok F, Otto PA, et al: Phenotypic variability in Angelman syndrome: comparison among different deletion classes and between deletion and UPD subjects. Eur J Hum Genet 12:987–992, 2004

Veltman MW, Craig EE, Bolton PF: Autism spectrum disorders in Prader-Willi and Angelman syndromes: a systematic review. Psychiatr Genet 15:243–254, 2005

Whitman BY, Myers S, Carrel A, et al: The behavioral impact of growth hormone treatment for children and adolescents with Prader-Willi syndrome: a 2-year, controlled study. Pediatrics 109:E35, 2002

Whittington J, Holland A, Webb T, et al: Academic underachievement by people with Prader-Willi syndrome. J Intellect Disabil Res 48:188–200, 2004a

Whittington J, Holland A, Webb T, et al: Cognitive abilities and genotype in a population-based sample of people with Prader-Willi syndrome. J Intellect Disabil Res 48:172–187, 2004b

Wigren M, Hansen S: ADHD symptoms and insistence on sameness in Prader-Willi syndrome. J Intellect Disabil Res 49(pt 6):449-456, 2005

Williams CA: Neurological aspects of the Angelman syndrome. Brain Dev 27:88–94, 2005

Williams CA, Beaudet AL, Clayton-Smith J, et al: Angelman syndrome 2005: updated consensus for diagnostic criteria. Am J Med Genet A 140:413–418, 2006

C H A P T E R   8

WILLIAMS SYNDROME

Mary Beth Steinfeld, M.D.
Robin L. Hansen, M.D.

The unique contrasts found in individuals with Williams syndrome (WS), between their charming, even enviable sociability in the face of their significant difficulties succeeding socially, limited cognitive skills, and extremely compromised understanding of spatial concepts, have fascinated clinicians and neuroscientists since WS was clinically described in the 1950s. How is it possible that such delightful people struggle to really understand others? What does this dichotomy mean about being genuinely interested in and caring about others? Can we find answers regarding charm and personality and empathy in the genes or on functional magnetic resonance imaging? Intensive research by cognitive neuroscientists has resulted in an increasingly detailed delineation of the characteristic neuropsychological profile, as well as efforts to link underlying genetic and brain structure–function relationships to the cognitive and behavioral phenotype in WS.

WS is the result of a contiguous gene microdeletion at chromosome 7q11.23, affecting multiple organ systems. In 1964, Garcia et al. published a case report on a child with severe hypercalcemia, mental subnormality, unusual facial features, and supravalvular aortic stenosis (SVAS), thereby combining two previously described groups of associations (Beuren et al. 1962; Bongiovanni et al. 1957; Schlesinger et al. 1956; Williams et al. 1961) into a newly identified syndrome that has come to be known as Williams syndrome or Williams-Beuren syndrome. The microdeletion associated with WS was reported in 1993 (Ewart et al. 1993). The 1.5- to 1.8-megabase (Mb) deletion results in hemizygosity of 23–26 genes, all of which have been identified, although the function of only one deleted gene, *ELN*, is well understood. *ELN* codes for elastin, a protein responsible for the elastic properties of different tissues, such as lung, skin, ligaments, cartilage, and blood vessels. The *ELN* haploinsufficiency accounts for many but not all of the clinically relevant features in WS. In addition to their neurocognitive difficulties, both children and adults with WS are at risk for serious lifelong medical and psychiatric complications that need to be recognized and treated to maximize healthy and productive outcomes.

Epidemiology

WS has an estimated prevalence of 1 in 7,500 individuals (Stromme et al. 2002). The condition is almost always sporadic and occurs equally in males and females (Pober 2010). The microdeletion is due to a misalignment error during meiosis resulting in nonhomologous recombination, which can occur on either the maternal or paternal chromosome (Pober 2010). Some findings about WS suggest that the cardiac lesions are more prevalent and severe in males than in females (Sadler et al. 2001), that males are more severely affected intellectually (Fisch et al. 2010), and that females show greater degrees of externalizing behavior (Porter et al. 2009). The increasing availability of genomewide testing can be expected to lead to earlier diagnoses and more accurate estimates of incidence and prevalence.

Signs and Symptoms

Although WS is etiologically a relatively homogeneous disorder, the extent of medical and neurodevelopmental problems can be quite variable. Early detection of WS is most likely when SVAS or another clinically significant congenital heart defect leads to genetic testing, at an average age of 12–16 months (Carrasco et al. 2005; Ferrero et al. 2007). Intrauterine growth retardation, early feeding problems, colic, vomiting, gastroesophageal reflux, constipation, and failure to thrive may be present in infancy, with motor and language delays evident in the toddler years. As children develop language skills, their friendly, talkative personalities emerge, often resulting in an underestimate of the degree of intellectual impairment. In the absence of heart disease or other significant medical problems, WS may go undetected until the early grade school years when cognitive and behavioral deficits become apparent, delaying the average age at diagnosis to 5–10 years (Carrasco et al. 2005; Ferrero et al. 2007).

Dysmorphology

The characteristic dysmorphic facial features of WS include broad forehead, periorbital fullness of subcutaneous tissue, epicanthal folds, flat nasal bridge, short upturned nose with long and smooth philtrum, wide mouth, full lips and cheeks, and a small jaw. A stellate iris pattern may be seen in children with light irises. The cardiologists who first noted the association described an "elfin" or "pixielike" face (see Figure 8–1). The facial features are not present at birth but become more apparent in the second year of life. As the children age, their facial features coarsen, and older individuals commonly have prominent lips with an open mouth, a wide smile, and full nasal tip (Pober 2010). Adults with WS tend to have long faces and necks. Dental abnormalities are common, including increased frequency of dental caries, hypoplastic enamel, malocclusion, and unusual tooth shapes (Axelsson 2005). Hypoplastic nails, hallux valgus, and premature graying of the hair and wrinkling of the skin are also common (Jones 2006). Most individuals with WS have hoarse voices throughout their lives (Morris et al. 1988).

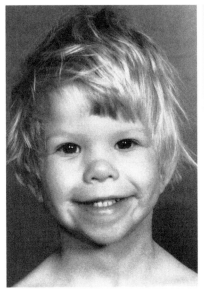 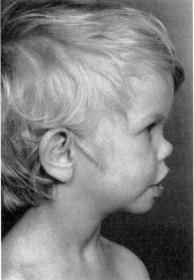

FIGURE 8–1.   Infant with Williams syndrome.

Left: Epicanthic fold and other typical features. *Right:* Periorbital fullness, bulbous nose, small chin, and long neck.

Source.   Reprinted from Kaplan P, Wang PP, Francke U: "Williams (Williams Beuren) Syndrome: A Distinct Neurobehavioral Disorder." *Journal of Child Neurology* 16:177–190, 2001, Figure 4, p. 179. Used with permission of Sage Publications and Paige Kaplan, M.B.B.Ch.

Growth Deficiency

Most children with WS are born at term, often with intrauterine growth restriction and relative sparing of head growth (Ferrero et al. 2007; Morris et al. 1988). The majority of infants have early-onset feeding problems associated with poorly coordinated suck and swallow skills and hypotonia. Prolonged irritability, sometimes attributed to hypercalcemia, gastroesophageal reflux, and delayed feeding skill progression, can contribute to the development of oral aversions and failure to thrive. Vomiting and constipation may also interfere with feeding and growth (Morris et al. 1988).

Children with WS tend to remain below the 5th percentile for the first 4 years of life, despite normal bone age, and then experience an average growth rate of about 75% of normal (Jones 2006). Head growth is proportional to height in childhood. Early puberty contributes to the short adult stature of most individuals with WS (Pober 2010). People with WS develop musculoskeletal problems with age, including progressive joint contractures as well as shoulder sloping, lordosis, thoracic kyphosis, and scoliosis, all of which also compromise adult height (Pober 2010). WS-specific growth charts are available (Committee on Genetics 2001; Martin et al. 2007). Truncal obesity is common in adulthood (Cherniske et al. 2004), and more than 50% of adults with WS are overweight or obese (Pober 2010).

Cardiovascular Disease

People with WS are missing one allele of the *ELN* gene, which codes for elastin, a protein that regulates the production of smooth muscle cells in the tunica media of medium- and large-sized arteries. The resulting lack of sufficient elastin leads to arterial smooth muscle cell proliferation and ultimately thickening and narrowing of the arteries. This is a diffuse process present in all systemic and pulmonary muscular arteries (Lacro and Smoot 2006); clinical symptoms depend on the severity of the arteriopathy. As noted in "Epidemiology" above, cardiovascular disease tends to be more severe in males than females (Sadler et al. 2001).

SVAS, the most common clinically relevant congenital heart disease occurring in WS, is otherwise a rare disorder. It occurs in approximately 70% of individuals with WS and ranges in degree from mild to severe (Eronen et al. 2002; Pober 2010). SVAS is caused by narrowing of the ascending aorta just distal to the origin of the coronary arteries, which may also be narrowed. An asymptomatic murmur may lead to an echocardiographic diagnosis of SVAS, and echocardiography may show either discrete narrowing of the aorta (~77% of the time) or involvement of the entire ascending aorta (~23% of the time) (Stamm et al. 1997). The stenosis can progress over time, especially in the first 5 years of life (Pober 2010), and requires ongoing cardiac monitoring.

Pulmonary artery stenosis (PAS) and peripheral pulmonary artery stenosis (PPAS) are also relatively common and often asymptomatic. Unlike SVAS, PAS and PPAS generally diminish in severity during childhood (Lacro and Smoot 2006; Pober 2010).

Early-onset, asymptomatic hypertension is also associated with WS, with a mean age at onset of 10 years (range 1–15 years) (Ferrero et al. 2007). Up to 55% of adults with WS are reported to have hypertension (Broder et al. 1999; Eronen et al. 2002; Pober 2010). Other potential cardiovascular complications include biventricular outflow tract obstruction, abdominal coarctation, renal artery obstruction, cerebrovascular accidents, myocardial infarction, dysrhythmias, and (very rarely) sudden death (Burch et al. 2008).

Cardiovascular-related mortality is increased 25–100 times, and cardiovascular complications are the major cause of death in patients with WS (Pober 2010; Wessel et al. 2004). Ferrero et al. (2007) found that 90% of individuals with confirmed WS who were identified based on neurocognitive profile had unrecognized cardiovascular pathology, supporting the recommendation that all individuals with WS be followed cardiologically on a regular basis across the life span (Cherniske et al. 2004; Committee on Genetics 2001; Pober 2010).

Idiopathic Hypercalcemia

The incidence of the idiopathic hypercalcemia of infancy associated with WS has been estimated at approximately 15% (Committee on Genetics 2001), but reports vary from 5% to 50% (Pober 2010). The hypercalcemia is generally mild (≤11.5 mg/dL), transient, and asymptomatic, or results in nonspecific symptoms such as infantile colic, irritability, feeding problems, vomiting, hypotonia, or constipation (Pober 2010). It usually resolves by age 4 years (Committee on Genetics 2001) and is rarely detected in children who are otherwise not considered to be in need of a calcium level check. However, the hypercalcemia can be severe and recurrent, requiring acute treatment (Cagle et al. 2004). WS should be considered in any infant with clinically significant hypercalcemia. The American Academy of Pediatrics recommends hypercalcemia monitoring throughout childhood for individuals with documented WS (Committee on Genetics 2001), and Cherniske et al. (2004) and Pober (2010) recommend ongoing monitoring every 1–2 years throughout adulthood.

Endocrine Issues

Adults with WS have high rates of impaired glucose tolerance, up to 90% in one series (Cherniske et al. 2004), as well as increased incidence of excessive weight gain and diabetes. Workup including fasting blood glucose

and hemoglobin A_{1c} levels in overweight teens and adults with WS is recommended, as is regular monitoring of glucose tolerance beginning at age
30 (Cherniske et al. 2004; Pober 2010). Thyroid hypoplasia on ultrasound
in infancy has been described in 60% of 45 patients in one series (Bedeschi
et al. 2011). Subclinical hypothyroidism has been found in 2%–40% of individuals with WS (Bedeschi et al. 2011; Cambiaso et al. 2007; Committee
on Genetics 2001; Ferrero et al. 2007; Stagi et al. 2005), although the clinical course is unknown. Regular thyroid function testing is currently recommended across the life span in individuals with WS (Pober 2010).
Decreased bone mineral density has been found in a substantial proportion
of adults with WS (Cherniske et al. 2004); therefore, assessment with dual-
energy X-ray absorptiometry (DEXA) should start at age 30 years and
should continue as clinically indicated thereafter (Cherniske et al. 2004;
Pober 2010).

Musculoskeletal Disorders

Approximately 80%–90% of infants and children with WS have central hypotonia and joint hypermobility (Committee on Genetics 2001). Progressive contractures in upper-extremity joints occur with age in approximately
50% of cases (Committee on Genetics 2001), and radioulnar synostosis developed in over 50% of cases in one series (Cherniske et al. 2004). Kyphosis, lordosis, and scoliosis develop with age, contributing to shortened adult
height and stiff walking gait (Cherniske et al. 2004; Committee on Genetics 2001). Up to 80% of young adults with WS had orthopedic abnormalities in one series (Bedeschi et al. 2011). Early and ongoing physical therapy
to maintain strength and joint mobility is recommended (Pober 2010).

Gastrointestinal Disorders

Early feeding problems, including oral motor delays, gastroesophageal reflux, vomiting, and constipation, occur in about 70% of infants (Committee on Genetics 2001). Chronic constipation beginning in infancy may be
present in up to 25% of adults with WS (Bedeschi et al. 2011), and difficulties with gastroesophageal reflux, chronic abdominal pain, and diarrhea are
reported in adults as well (Cherniske et al. 2004). Intestinal diverticular disease and rectal prolapse, both associated with constipation, are not uncommon and may be the result of the elastin haploinsufficiency (Bedeschi et al.
2011; Cherniske et al. 2004; Committee on Genetics 2001). Inguinal hernias are another common occurrence (Carrasco et al. 2005).

Elevated rates of celiac disease have been found in individuals with WS
(Pober 2010). Approximately 10% of individuals with WS were found to

be serum antibody and biopsy positive for celiac disease in one study (Giannotti et al. 2001).

Integument Differences

Between 50% and 90% of individuals with WS were reported to have soft skin with premature wrinkling (Cherniske et al. 2004; Committee on Genetics 2001; Pober 2010), and about 90% were reported to have premature graying of the hair (Cherniske et al. 2004; Committee on Genetics 2001).

Renal Disorders

Individuals with WS have delayed toilet training, as well as increased incidence of urinary urgency, enuresis, renal structural defects, and urinary tract infections (Committee on Genetics 2001). Nephrocalcinosis due to hypercalcemia may be a presenting sign of WS in rare individuals (Cagle et al. 2004; Ferrero et al. 2007). Urinary frequency is common at all ages (Cherniske et al. 2004). Bladder diverticula have been described as well (Bedeschi et al. 2011; Committee on Genetics 2001; Pober 2010). Regular monitoring of renal function across the life span is recommended (Pober 2010).

Auditory Problems

Audiological problems are common in individuals with WS (Bedeschi et al. 2011). Recurrent otitis media has been reported in approximately 50% of children with WS (Committee on Genetics 2001). Presbycusis, a type of sensorineural hearing loss, has been described in up to 75% of individuals with WS and begins in early adulthood (Pober 2010). Audiological testing of individuals with WS is recommended at age 1 year and every 2 years thereafter in childhood, with more frequent testing recommended if clinically indicated (e.g., in individuals with recurrent otitis media). At least one objective hearing test is recommended during adolescence, another at about 30 years of age, and later tests as clinically indicated (Pober 2010).

Patients with WS have characteristic and unusual sound sensitivities and preferences. Although previously described as experiencing hyperacusis, meaning abnormal sensitivity to sound, people with WS in fact do not generally have a lowered hearing threshold. Rather, they often have odynacusis, which means that compared with control subjects, they experience loud sounds as unusually uncomfortable (Levitin et al. 2005). Additionally, they may exhibit auditory allodynia, the aversion to or fear of specific sounds not normally considered aversive (Levitin et al. 2005). Finally, they may be fascinated with certain sounds (Levitin et al. 2005). Levitin et al. (2003) reported diffuse and variable activations on functional magnetic resonance imaging (fMRI) throughout the brain in response to auditory stimuli of various types in individuals with WS compared to control subjects.

Children and adults with WS are often attracted to and soothed by music. They have a relative strength in the area of rhythmic ability (Levitin and Bellugi 2006). Music may be successfully combined with other interventions to facilitate learning in individuals with WS (Levitin and Bellugi 2006).

Ophthalmological Impairments

Visual impairments are common in WS. Half of infants with WS have esotropia (Committee on Genetics 2001), and up to 100% of adults have some visual impairment, including esotropia, hyperopia, myopia, cataracts, and presbyopia. Ongoing vision screening is recommended, with formal ophthalmological evaluations recommended periodically and as clinically indicated (Pober 2010).

Central Nervous System Problems

Although infants with WS present with hypotonia and delayed motor skills, distal tone increases with age, resulting in brisk deep tendon reflexes in up to 50% of children who are of preschool to early school age (Committee on Genetics 2001; Gagliardi et al. 2007; Morris 2010a; Pober 2010). Tightening of the heel cords and hamstrings begins in childhood (Morris 1988). Poor balance and coordination and abnormal gaits were found in 60%–100% of patients (Cherniske et al. 2004; Committee on Genetics 2001). Mild cerebellar signs (intention and resting tremors) have also been described (Cherniske et al. 2004; Gagliardi et al. 2007). Soft extrapyramidal signs, specifically dystonia and rigidity, increase with age, contributing to clumsiness; poor balance; awkward, slow gaits; and difficulty with complex gross and fine motor tasks (Gagliardi et al. 2007).

Infantile spasms have been rarely reported and are associated with larger deletions (Rothlisberger et al. 2010; Wu et al. 1999). Asymptomatic Chiari type I malformations have been found during neuroimaging research studies in about 10% of children with WS (Cherniske et al. 2004; Committee on Genetics 2001; Pober and Filiano 1995).

Sleep problems were identified in 57% of 28 children with WS, and subsequently 7 of those children (ages 1.8–7 years) underwent polysomnography and were found to have more wake time, less efficient sleep, and more frequent periodic limb movements compared with a group of control children (Mason and Arens 2006). A study of sleep patterns in 23 older individuals (ages 17–35 years) with WS has documented, using actigraphy, ongoing sleep disruptions including sleep onset delays, more wake time, and increased restlessness, as well as subjective complaints of excessive daytime sleepiness (Goldman et al. 2009). Screening for sleep disturbances throughout the life span is a recommended addition to the medical monitoring schedule for WS.

Development

Gross Motor Development

Global developmental delay in early childhood is a universal feature of WS. Early hypotonia leads to delayed gross motor skills, with the mean age of rolling over at 11 months, sitting at about 12 months, and walking at 21–28 months of age (Morris et al. 1988; Plissart and Fryns 1999).

Fine Motor Development

Fine motor skills are more significantly delayed. Transferring objects from one hand to the next emerges on average at 18 months, a neat pincer grasp by 25 months, and building a tower of two cubes by 36 months (Plissart and Fryns 1999).

Nonverbal Cognitive Development

Delays of up to 16–20 months became apparent in the second and third years of life in one series of children tested with the Bayley Scales of Infant Development. Object permanence emerged at 28 months, shape recognition at 36 months, and color sorting at 45 months (Plissart and Fryns 1999).

Language Development

Early language delays are very common in WS, with early language comprehension more significantly impaired than expressive language. For example, children with WS were able to give an object on purely verbal request on average at 36 months, compared to 10–11 months in typical control subjects (Plissart and Fryns 1999), with first words emerging between 21 and 28 months. Once their language skills emerge, children with WS develop strong concrete vocabularies with fluent language production that is comparable to their overall nonverbal reasoning skills (Morris 2010a). While their receptive and expressive concrete vocabularies are areas of relative strength, their vocabularies for spatial, temporal, and quantitative relationships are very weak and are commensurate with their limited spatial conceptual skills, suggesting a single processing center for such spatially related constructs (Mervis and John 2010). Grammatical complexity matures in the typical order but is delayed, with scores falling in the borderline range for most children with WS (Mervis and John 2010). Interestingly, compared to typically developing children, children with WS rely more heavily on their verbal working memory on tests of receptive grammatical skill (Robinson et al. 2003). Although children with WS generally have delayed reading skills, with one study finding an average 2nd grade reading level in individuals 10–20 years old (Pagon et al. 1987), some individuals with WS can read and comprehend at grade level. Notably, children with WS benefit from being taught to read using phonics rather than whole-word or sight-word approaches (Levy et al. 2003).

Despite their extreme sociability and relative strengths in rich, descriptive, expressive language, vocabulary, fluency, verbal short-term memory, and pronunciation, individuals with WS have significant ongoing pragmatic language deficits that affect their social success. Pragmatic deficits include conversational difficulties, such as poor topic maintenance (Mervis and John 2010), stereotyped phrases, perseverative responses, and poor perspective taking (Järvinen-Pasley et al. 2008; Laws and Bishop 2004; Morris 2010a). Due to their frequent use of "audience hookers" and use of words that build attention and interest in their listeners, such as "lo and behold" (Losh et al. 2004), individuals with WS often give the impression that they are more verbally adept than they actually are (Järvinen-Pasley et al. 2008).

Cognitive Function

Most individuals with WS have full scale IQ scores in the range of mild to moderate intellectual disability, although IQ scores from 40 to 100 have been reported (Martens et al. 2008). Bennett et al. (1978) first confirmed and quantified the unique psychological profile of children with WS by showing that relative to their verbal performance, they struggled with gross motor and performance items, such as drawing, puzzle completion, and cube-building skills, on the McCarthy Scales of Children's Abilities. The relatively consistent and unique pattern of strengths and weaknesses in the neuropsychological profile of individuals with WS has been described as the Williams syndrome cognitive profile (Mervis et al. 2000). This profile is characterized by relative strengths in auditory short-term memory (digit recall), uneven verbal skills as outlined in "Language Development" above, and extreme difficulties in visuospatial and visuomotor construction skills (e.g., the ability to visualize the relationship of parts to whole and/or to construct a whole from parts, such as required by pattern construction and drawing tasks) (Mervis et al. 2000). Mervis and John (2010) point out that IQ tests vary in the way various skills are clustered into verbal and performance scores, and that an uneven cognitive profile may not be apparent when spatial abilities are not parsed from other performance or nonverbal reasoning skills.

Study results regarding long-term cognitive trajectories are inconsistent, with one study showing improvements in IQ scores from teenage years to young adulthood (Udwin et al. 1996), another showing no change (Cherniske et al. 2004), and two others showing a decrease (Fisch et al. 2010; Gosch and Pankau 1996). Although Udwin et al. (1996) found an increase in IQ scores, they did not find improvements in reading, spelling, or math achievement scores, suggesting little educational progress after the early teenage years.

Social-Emotional Development

Individuals with WS are known for their overly friendly and social personalities, which are apparent very early on. Although typically developing infants attend preferentially to faces, by age 6 months they are also fascinated by objects. Infants and toddlers with WS attend preferentially and intensely to social versus nonsocial stimuli (Mervis et al. 2003) well beyond age 6 months. They look at people's faces (particularly the eyes), including strangers' faces, more intently and for much longer periods of time than do typically developing children. This was true up to age 31 months in a group of infants and toddlers with WS whose social attention was compared with that of typically developing control subjects (Mervis et al. 2003). WS toddlers were found to engage with an unfamiliar examiner rather than with a familiar adult or experimental objects (Järvinen-Pasley et al. 2008). Additionally, triadic interactions became dyadic with a novel experimenter, resulting in less joint attention behavior (Järvinen-Pasley et al. 2008; Mervis et al. 2003). The decreased joint attention may contribute to the early language delays and later pragmatic language and learning deficits in children with WS (Järvinen-Pasley et al. 2008; Mervis et al. 2003). In addition to their continuing intense, indiscriminate social interest in strangers, toddlers and preschoolers with WS initiate frequent social interaction and are more empathetic than typically developing children (Mervis et al. 2003). Despite their extreme sociability and strong interest in others, individuals with WS, by middle childhood, have difficulties making and keeping friends and exhibit poor social judgment. Difficulties in accurately perceiving social cues (Gosch and Pankau 1997; Meyer-Lindenberg et al. 2005; Santos et al. 2010), pragmatic language deficits, and poor theory of mind underlie their social difficulties (Järvinen-Pasley et al. 2008; Plesa-Skwerer and Tager-Flusberg 2006).

The social disinhibition seen in WS has also been argued to reflect a frontal lobe–associated executive function deficit. In a study using standardized executive function measures, Rhodes et al. (2010) compared adolescents and young adults with WS to an age-matched control group and a verbal-age-matched control group. The authors reported frontal lobe–related executive function impairments in subjects with WS, including poor attentional set-shifting, working memory, and planning skills. In addition, delayed short-term memory was impaired.

Adaptive Skills

Mervis et al. (2001) found that children ages 4–8 years with WS demonstrated delays in adaptive skills on the Vineland Adaptive Behavior Scales (VABS) commensurate with their cognitive scores on the Differential Abilities Scales. Not surprisingly, the VABS subscale scores showed an uneven profile, with greater delays on subscales involving independent daily living and motor skills than socialization and communication skills. A study of adults with WS (Cherniske et al. 2004) found continuing delays in adaptive skills. Compared to an average full scale IQ of 68, the VABS composite score was 55, and the mean scores for communication, daily living skills, and socialization were 46, 61, and 66, respectively. Most of the adults were living at their parents' homes or in group homes or supervised apartments. Only one of the 20 adults studied had competitive employment.

Behavior and Psychiatric Disturbances

In addition to being described as overly friendly, talkative, sensitive, and empathetic, individuals with WS are also described by parents and caregivers as excessively worried and anxious. Based on parent questionnaire data, Klein-Tasman and Mervis (2003) documented a WS personality profile met by 96% of their sample of 23 children ages 8–10 years with WS. Compared to an age-matched group of children with mixed etiologies for intellectual disability, the children with WS showed a pattern of high sociability, empathy, gregariousness, people orientation, and sensitivity, and were more visible in a crowd (Klein-Tasman and Mervis 2003). This pattern has been described by other groups studying WS as well (Gosch and Pankau 1997; Sarimski 1997; Tomc et al. 1990). High intensity and negative mood, described by others as characteristic of WS, were not confirmed as unique to that disorder by Klein-Tasman and Mervis (2003). Similarly, Sarimski (1997) found that attention problems were not unique to WS but were common in children with developmental disabilities in general.

Leyfer et al. (2006) interviewed the parents of 119 children (ages 4–16 years) with WS using the Anxiety Disorders Interview Schedule for DSM-IV: Parent Interview Schedule (ADIS-P) by Silverman and Albano (1996).

In addition to assessing anxiety disorders, the ADIS-P also assesses attention-deficit/hyperactivity disorder (ADHD), oppositional defiant disorder, conduct disorder, major depressive disorder, and dysthymia. ADHD was the most common psychiatric condition, occurring in about 65% of the children, with the inattentive subtype being the most common (69%), followed by the combined subtype (27%). Specific phobia was the next most common disorder, reported in 54% of the children; loud noises were the most common specific phobia, occurring in 28% of the group. Generalized anxiety disorder was reported in 12% of the children. Only 22% of the subjects did not have a psychiatric disorder. Although there was no significant gender difference in the occurrence of the disorders, there were differences by age. ADHD was most common in children ages 7–10 years, and generalized anxiety disorder was most common in children ages 11–16 years. No significant age difference was found for the rate of specific phobia. These behavioral findings are consistent with previous reports of inattention, for which stimulants are likely effective (Carrasco et al. 2005; Green et al. 2011; Greer et al. 1997), as well as hyperactivity with oppositional behaviors, anxiety, and phobias (Carrasco et al. 2005).

Behavioral descriptions of adults with WS are consistent with Leyfer et al.'s (2006) findings in children. Cherniske et al. (2004) interviewed caregivers of 20 adults with WS and found that 13 had significant levels of anxiety, most commonly specific phobia, followed by generalized anxiety. Several other psychiatric disorders were found in much smaller numbers, and four individuals had required psychiatric hospitalizations. Selective serotonin reuptake inhibitors (SSRIs) were the most commonly used medications reported by this group; however, symptoms of disinhibition related to SSRI use should be monitored (Pober 2010). Pober (2010) describes increasing levels of anxiety and social isolation in adolescents and adults with WS.

Davies et al. (1998) used the Social and Emotional Functioning Interview with parents and other caregivers of 70 adults with WS. Fifty percent of the individuals were reported to have disruptive preoccupations/obsessions (commonly related to cars, electrical appliances, tools, and machinery), and 69% had disruptive levels of distractibility. Sixteen percent had disruptive levels of anxiety, whereas 73% exhibited anxiety at a lower level. The excessive anxiety was described as anticipatory and related to perceived threats, inappropriate demands, uncertainty, or changes in routine, rather than being related to social anxiety. Significant life changes were risk factors for prolonged anxiety or depression, reported in 10%. Nearly half had disruptive stereotyped/repetitive movements, and 41% had frequent anger outbursts. Psychological counseling, support, and preparation for anticipated and even unanticipated change were recommended.

Although individuals with WS are known for their extreme social interest, and individuals with autism for their social avoidance, there are overlapping features of the two disorders. Lincoln et al. (2007) found that young children with autism spectrum disorder (ASD) and young children with WS share impairments in joint attention and attention shifting, delays in language development, decreased use of communicative gestures, sensitivity to sounds, and other sensory processing difficulties. Ten percent of their study sample of subjects with WS met Autism Diagnostic Observation Schedule or DSM-IV-TR criteria for autistic disorder. However, on formal autism testing between age- and IQ-matched children with ASD and children with WS, the differing social orientations between the subject groups were evident, in that children with WS made social overtures, shared enjoyment, directed facial expressions and vocalizations, and had normal eye contact. Another study (Klein-Tasman et al. 2009) documented that many young children with WS have social communication deficits consistent with a diagnosis of pervasive developmental disorder not otherwise specified. Diagnosis of an ASD when clinically appropriate, followed by appropriate intensive intervention, is strongly recommended (Klein-Tasman et al. 2009). In older individuals with WS, ongoing difficulties with pragmatic language and peer interactions are common and consistent with difficulties along the autism spectrum. Individuals with WS who have behavioral concerns suggestive of an ASD should be comprehensively evaluated to determine the possibility of both diagnoses, and when both are present, ongoing intensive intervention services should be provided.

Definite difficulties with sensory modulation were found on the Short Sensory Profile (McIntosh et al. 1999) in over half of a group of 78 children with WS, and probable sensory differences were found in an additional 34% of this group (John and Mervis 2010). Poor muscle tone and postural awareness, over- or underresponsiveness to sensory events, and hypo- or hyperresponsiveness to sound were the most common sensory differences found. The children in this sample who were reported to have severe impairment in sensory modulation also had poorer executive functioning, more negativity, more attention problems, and more anxiety than children with milder impairments (John and Mervis 2010).

Etiologies

WS is the result of a 1.5- to 1.8-Mb deletion at chromosome 7q11.23 (Williams-Beuren syndrome critical region, or WBSCR), resulting in hemizygosity of 23–26 genes in that region. Although WS was initially hypothesized to be related to vitamin D toxicity due to the common association with hypercalcemia (Friedman and Mills 1969; Garcia et al. 1964), the genetic etiology was discovered in 1993 by Ewart et al., who studied SVAS families by echocardiography and recombinant DNA technology, establishing the *ELN* deletion as causative of SVAS. Although all the missing genes have been identified, only the function of the *ELN* gene deletion is well understood. Other genotype-phenotype correlations, particularly related to the neurocognitive profile, are actively being researched, with single genes *LIMK1*, *GTF21*, *GTF21RD1*, and *CYLN2* linked to cognitive as well as to craniofacial features of WS (Järvinen-Pasley et al. 2008). The variability in characteristics seen in individuals with WS is not completely explained by variations in size of the deletion, and it is probable that polymorphisms in nondeleted copies of the genes, effects of neighboring or modifier genes in other regions of the genome, including epigenetic alterations, account for much of the variation (Pober 2010).

The deletion is usually the result of a de novo nonallelic homologous recombination (NAHR) in meiosis, resulting in a 23- to 26-gene deletion in 98% of individuals clinically diagnosed with WBS (Pober 2010). The deleted genes are flanked by low copy repeats, implicated as the basis for NAHR, which can result in deletion, duplication, or inversion of the WBSCR segment. The deletion can occur on either the maternally or paternally inherited chromosome. There is some evidence of symptomatic differences related to parent of origin (Collette et al. 2009). The deletion is sporadic in almost all cases, so that the risk to parents of having another child with WS is <1%. Genetic testing of parents may be indicated, and genetic counseling is advised (Cusco 2008). Adults with WS have a 50:50 risk of having a child who inherits the deletion (Pober 2010). The deletion can be detected by fluorescent in situ hybridization (FISH), targeted mutation analysis, or chromosomal microarray (CMA).

Duplication at the WBSCR results in a milder phenotype (Merla et al. 2010), which includes congenital heart defects, hypotonia, speech and language delay, intellectual impairment (with sparing of visuospatial skills), ADHD, and ASDs. Because the facial features are less distinctive than those of WS, this duplication syndrome is likely underdiagnosed (Merla et al. 2010). Inversion of the segment results in asymptomatic individuals, who have an increased risk of transmitting WS to their offspring (1 in 2,000 vs. 1 in 9,500 in the noninversion general population) (Pober 2010).

Environmental Impacts

Few studies have looked systematically at environmental impacts on the phenotypic presentation or variability in WS. Zitzer-Comfort et al. (2007)

studied parent reports of sociability in children with WS from the United States and Japan, matched in each group with typically developing control subjects. Compared with their typically developing cultural control groups, both Japanese and American children with WS were rated significantly higher on the Approach Strangers subscale of the Salk Institute Sociability Questionnaire (Jones et al. 2000). However, both American children with WS and controls were rated as more sociable than the Japanese children, highlighting the mediating influence that culture has on the expression of social behavior. In a study of social evaluative language (narrative) and morphology-syntax across French, Italian, and U.S. children and adolescents with WS, compared with typically developing controls from each country, individuals with WS across all three cultures used significantly more social evaluative language (Reilly et al. 2003), with Italians exceeding Americans, who exceeded French subjects, again demonstrating the moderating effect of culture.

Diagnostic Evaluation and Differential Diagnosis

A high index of suspicion is important when any of the physical, developmental, or behavioral manifestations of WS are present, and genetic testing therefore should be completed. For example, children with symptomatic SVAS should all be tested for WS. In infancy, early feeding problems, slow growth with failure to thrive, extreme fussiness, and hypotonia should prompt an etiological workup, including metabolic panel with calcium level, which may lead to a diagnosis of hypercalcemia and further evaluation for possible WS. Extreme social interest at a very young age in a child with other delays, hypotonia, or both may trigger the pediatric clinician to think further about the possibility of WS, as should learning problems in school associated with an overly friendly, loquacious personality and characteristic facial features.

Genetic testing for confirmation of WS can be done using either FISH or CMA testing to identify the deleted segment. FISH testing can identify the deletion of the *ELN* gene or the WS chromosomal region, which includes *ELN*, *LIMK1*, and the D7S613 locus in 98%–99% of individuals with WS (Morris 2006). The growing availability of CMA is likely to increase detection of WS, and CMA may be the test of choice if an individual's features are not classic. CMA testing will detect DNA copy number changes in the deleted genes. When the diagnosis is made, a clinician should comprehensively assess for the other associated medical, cognitive, and behavioral characteristics for which individuals with WS are at risk.

Management and Interventions

Over their lifetime, individuals with WS generally have multiple specialists involved in their care to provide medical assessment and management, anticipatory guidance and monitoring, psychoeducational assessment and intervention, and ongoing behavioral and mental health assessment and treatment. The American Academy of Pediatrics Committee on Genetics prepared a comprehensive guideline for both the initial evaluation and ongoing monitoring of children with WS (Committee on Genetics 2001). Other resources for the initial evaluation and the ongoing monitoring of individuals with WS can be found on the GeneReviews Web site (www.ncbi.nlm.nih.gov/books/NBK1249) and in the supplemental appendix to Pober's (2010) Williams-Beuren syndrome review article.

Medical Management

Close cardiovascular assessment and monitoring is required even if an individual with WS has no cardiac symptomatology at the time of diagnosis. Surgery or angioplasty may be required at any point during a person's life, not only related to the severity of the arteriopathy but also for strabismus, P-E tubes, hernia repair, or other reasons. Individuals with WS are at increased risk from anesthesia, though problems are uncommon. Preoperative assessment with an anesthesiologist prior to surgery to review physiological implications of the patient's cardiac status, arteriopathy, mandibular and dental variables, calcium levels, possible joint contractures, and neurodevelopmental and emotional well-being is very important. Regular blood pressure monitoring is also required to detect and treat hypertension.

Gastroenterologists, speech and occupational therapists, dietitians, and other feeding specialists may need to be involved in managing feeding difficulties related to weak suck due to hypotonia; poorly coordinated suck and swallow; gastroesophageal reflux with vomiting and irritability; irritability and feeding refusal due to esophagitis; constipation; irritability due to hypercalcemia; and tactile defensiveness. Bowel hypotonia may contribute to constipation, and patients with WS have increased risk for diverticula and rectal prolapse. Inguinal and umbilical hernias can develop in children as well as adults. Individuals with WS should routinely be screened for celiac disease and hypothyroidism, particularly when growth failure is present (Committee on Genetics 2001; Pober 2010). The American Academy of Pediatrics has developed WS-specific growth charts (Committee on Genetics 2001).

Physical and occupational therapy are important to initiate as soon after diagnosis as possible. Physical therapy should address early hypotonia and emerging difficulties with gait and balance that may be associated with evolving hypertonia and developing joint contractures. Heel cord release surgery should only be considered after brain imaging has been performed to assess for Chiari malformation. Occupational therapy is needed to address a range of difficulties, including fine motor coordination difficulties, visuospatial deficits, tone abnormalities, and contractures of small joints that affect daily living skills. For individuals with handwriting difficulties, accommodations such as keyboard skill training and access to computers are beneficial. Interventions to support sensory processing and integration may also be helpful for overall functioning both in the classroom and at home.

Endocrine function also needs to be followed, especially thyroid and glucose homeostasis, given the high prevalence of glucose intolerance in adults with WS. Healthy eating habits and regular physical exercise need to be supported and monitored, particularly given the difficulties with gait that develop and increase the risk for obesity.

Children with WS should not be given multivitamins because all contain vitamin D and many contain calcium. Liberal and consistent use of sunscreen is also important to reduce vitamin D exposure. Calcium levels need to be followed throughout life; treatment of hypercalcemia through dietary restriction or bisphosphonate therapy may be necessary. Monitoring for osteopenia is also important beginning in early adulthood, with DEXA scans recommended starting at age 30. Early pubertal development needs to be anticipated and management strategies discussed with families and children prior to onset of menses in females.

Parents of children with WS experience a level of stress similar to that of parents of children with other intellectual disability syndromes (Sarimski 1997). Perceived social support and individual coping skills are important to cultivate. The Williams Syndrome Association (www.williams-syndrome.org) is a parent support group that provides detailed online information for families, as well as links to other helpful resources.

Transition from pediatric to adult health care providers is often problematic for families and individuals with WS; helping families with this transition is an important role for both primary care and pediatric subspecialists. Pober's (2010) appendix to her review of Williams-Beuren syndrome lists several helpful Web sites for young adults with WS transitioning into adulthood, their parents, and medical and other support professionals.

Behavioral and Educational Interventions

Educational interventions should be based on a comprehensive psychological assessment that identifies areas of both strength and weakness for intervention, rather than summary full scale IQ or achievement scores. For example, although individuals with WS typically have full scale IQ scores in the borderline to moderate range of intellectual disability; their cognitive profile is uneven, with relative strengths in concrete language and concrete nonverbal and short-term memory skills and weaknesses in visual-spatial construction, pragmatic language, and relational language (Morris et al. 2010). Guidance from a professional with expertise in the behavioral and educational needs of children with WS, when available, can be very helpful in determining special education needs. Visuospatial and visuomotor skill deficits will need intervention and accommodations in the classroom. Preferential seating for individuals with hearing deficits is recommended. Monitoring for anticipatory anxiety, phobias, and social difficulties with peers is important. Some individuals with WS who have relatively strong concrete verbal skills may benefit from cognitive-behavioral strategies to reduce anxiety. Applied behavior analysis for adaptive skills development and social skills training can be helpful as well. Semel and Rosner (2003) provide a wealth of specific and problem-focused educational and behavioral guidance related to the various challenges facing students with WS.

Psychopharmacological Interventions

Stimulants were reported to be effective for the symptoms of ADHD in approximately 70% of the children with WS who also had ADHD (Green et al. 2011). Approximately half of adolescents and adults with WS are treated at some point with an anxiolytic agent (Pober 2010), typically an SSRI. Because patients with WS are reported to be particularly sensitive to the disinhibiting effects of SSRIs, careful monitoring is important (Pober 2010). Antipsychotic medications are also used, but no systematic data are available on their use in individuals with WS.

Outcomes

The quality of life for individuals with WS is primarily determined by cognitive and adaptive skills limitations, emotional and behavioral difficulties, and family and community supports. Health problems due to various organ system involvements are common; individuals may have needs related to cardiac, renal, orthopedic, gastrointestinal, endocrine, vision, and hearing systems. Although statistics on the average life expectancy are not available, the increasing availability of genome-wide testing can be expected to lead to earlier diagnosis and receipt of early and ongoing medical and mental health monitoring and treatment.

In one outcome study performed by parent survey, most individuals with WS (62%) were living with their parents into adulthood, and only 16% were living semi-independently or independently (Howlin and Udwin 2006). Access to professional medical services for the recommended ongoing medical monitoring and management was inadequate. Although 71% had attended some form of college, only 33% had achieved an academic or vocational certificate or qualification. Just over one-third were employed, mostly either part time or in a sheltered work setting, with only 4 of the 239 individuals in full-time independent employment. Difficulties with functional literacy and money concepts persisted. Most managed simple hygiene needs but required assistance with more complicated tasks. Mental health treatment for anxiety and depression was required for approximately one-third of the sample. Parent support resources are an important ongoing need for families of individuals with intellectual disability, including those with WS.

New Research Directions

The identification of the genetic etiology of WS and the specific genes in the deleted segment, along with advances in neuroimaging technology, has focused research in the field on better understanding of the gene-brain-behavior links underlying the unique cognitive-behavioral phenotype in WS, as well as the variability within the phenotype.

Animal Models

Similarities in the WS chromosome region in humans and its corresponding region in mice have helped to identify specific gene functions and contributions to the WS phenotype. Both single-gene and multigene knockout mice strains have been developed (Li et al. 2009; Schubert 2009). Mouse models have suggested a putative effect of the gene *FXC9* on osteopenia; *BAZ1B* on hypercalcemia and cardiac malformations; *STX1A* on glucose tolerance; *LIMK1* on impairments in visuospatial abilities; *CLIP2* on visuospatial and motor deficits; and the *GTF21* family of genes on craniofacial, dental, and growth abnormalities and on intellectual disability, WS cognitive profile, and impaired visual responses (Pober 2010).

Neuroimaging

Structural imaging (MRI) shows that individuals with WS have a reduction in cerebral volume that includes both white and gray matter, with preserved cerebellar volume (Cherniske et al. 2004; Reiss et al. 2000). Functional imaging studies have begun to provide better understanding of links between brain and behavior in WS. For example, fMRI studies have shown that subjects with WS have normal activation compared to controls in the visual pathway's ventral stream circuit during matching tasks; however, the same patients showed significantly reduced cortical activation in the dorsal visual stream during visuospatial constructive and attention to location tasks, along with adjacent gray matter reductions in the parieto-occipital/intraparietal sulcus. These findings help to explain the deficits in visuospatial skills characteristic in WS (Boddaert et al. 2006; Meyer-Lindenberg et al. 2004). fMRI studies have also shown that compared to controls, individuals with WS have decreased reactivity in the amygdala to angry or fearful faces but show exaggerated amygdala activation in response to threatening nonsocial scenes (Meyer-Lindenberg et al. 2005; Santos et al. 2010). Meyer-Lindenberg et al. (2006) also showed impaired regulation of the amygdala by the orbitofrontal cortex, suggesting that impaired function of the orbitofrontal cortex and limbic circuitry contributes to the social disinhibition and impaired social judgment in WS, as well as to the characteristic anxiety profile.

Future Directions

Significant progress has been made in elucidating both structural and functional differences in neural systems underlying social-affective processing in WS. However, longitudinal studies of individuals with WS identified in infancy will be important to understand the early origins of the cognitive-behavioral phenotype in terms of biological and environmental factors that affect further development, which in turn will help in identifying areas of function sensitive to early intervention (Järvinen-Pasley et al. 2008). Further identification of the contribution of specific genes deleted in the WS segment to the many varied aspects of the syndrome, both physical and neurodevelopmental, will require comprehensive comparisons of individuals with differing gene segment deletions across developmental time and domains, as well as comparisons of animal models with specific gene deletions.

Summary

WS is a relatively rare but clinically well-characterized contiguous gene microdeletion syndrome with a wide range of neurodevelopmental, behavioral, and medical features. Early recognition of the characteristic, although sometimes nonspecific, medical symptoms in infancy, related to cardiac findings and feeding and growth difficulties, and of the unique developmental-behavioral constellation of intense, prolonged eye contact and sociability in the presence of language and motor delay is important to early diagnosis and intervention. Advances in the understanding of specific gene functions relative to the neurodevelopmental and medical aspects of WS, along with the increasing availability of confirmatory genetic testing, are likely to contribute to better outcomes for individuals with WS as a result of earlier, specific treatments and available published guidelines for comprehensive, focused monitoring. Although many of the medical and psychiatric complications are familiar to most health care professionals, providing care to individuals with WS requires an appreciation of the unique challenges facing them, as well as collaboration across many disciplines and with care providers to ensure that individuals with WS are provided the support and opportunities they need to achieve healthy, productive lives in the community.

Key Points

- Williams syndrome is a multisystem disorder requiring a medical home and a life span approach to treatment.

- Individuals with Williams syndrome experience a high rate of social difficulties and psychopathology, despite their sociability.

- Significant cognitive deficits may be masked by these individuals' approaching and pleasing personalities.

Recommended Readings

Committee on Genetics: American Academy of Pediatrics: health care supervision for children with Williams syndrome. Pediatrics 107:1192–1204, 2001

Morris CA: Williams Syndrome (Williams-Beuren Syndrome). GeneReviews-NCBI Bookshelf, 2006. Available at: http://www.ncbi.nlm.nih.gov/books/NBK1249. Accessed August 24, 2012.

Pober BR: Williams-Beuren syndrome. N Engl J Med 362:239–252, 2010 [see Appendix]

References

Axelsson S: Variability of the cranial and dental phenotype in Williams syndrome. Swed Dent J Suppl (170):3–67, 2005

Bedeschi MF, Bianchi V, Colli AM, et al: Clinical follow-up of young adults affected by Williams syndrome: experience of 45 Italian patients. Am J Med Genet A 155A:353–359, 2011

Bennett FC, LaVeck B, Sells CJ: The Williams elfin facies syndrome: the psychological profile as an aid in syndrome identification. Pediatrics 61:303–306, 1978

Beuren AJ, Apitz J, Harmjanz D: Supravalvular aortic stenosis in association with mental retardation and a certain facial appearance. Circulation 26:1235–1240, 1962

Boddaert N, Mochel F, Meresse I, et al: Parieto-occipital grey matter abnormalities in children with Williams syndrome. Neuroimage 30:721–725, 2006

Bongiovanni AM, Eberlein WR, Jones IT: Idiopathic hypercalcemia of infancy, with failure to thrive; report of three cases, with a consideration of the possible etiology. N Engl J Med 257:951–958, 1957

Broder K, Reinhardt E, Pober B: Elevated ambulatory blood pressure in 20 subjects with Williams syndrome. Am J Med Genet 83:356–360, 1999

Burch TM, McGowan FX Jr, Kussman BD, et al: Congenital supravalvular aortic stenosis and sudden death associated with anesthesia: what's the mystery? Anesth Analg 107:1848–1854, 2008

Cagle AP, Waguespack SG, Buckingham BA, et al: Severe infantile hypercalcemia associated with Williams syndrome successfully treated with intravenously administered pamidronate. Pediatrics 114:1091–1095, 2004

Cambiaso P, Orazi C, Digilio MC, et al: Thyroid morphology and subclinical hypothyroidism in children and adolescents with Williams syndrome. J Pediatr 150:62–65, 2007

Carrasco X, Castillo S, Aravena T, et al: Williams syndrome: pediatric, neurologic, and cognitive development. Pediatr Neurol 32:166–172, 2005

Cherniske EM, Carpenter TO, Klaiman C, et al: Multisystem study of 20 older adults with Williams syndrome. Am J Med Genet A 131:255–264, 2004

Collette JC, Chen XN, Mills DL, et al: William's syndrome: gene expression is related to parental origin and regional coordinate control. J Hum Genet 54:193–198, 2009

Committee on Genetics: American Academy of Pediatrics: health care supervision for children with Williams syndrome. Pediatrics 107:1192–1204, 2001

Cuscó I, Corominas R, Bayés M, et al: Copy number variation at the 7q11.23 segmental duplications is a susceptibility factor for the Williams-Beuren syndrome deletion. Genome Res 18:683–694, 2008

Davies M, Udwin O, Howlin P: Adults with Williams syndrome: preliminary study of social, emotional and behavioural difficulties. Br J Psychiatry 172:273–276, 1998

Eronen M, Peippo M, Hiippala A, et al: Cardiovascular manifestations in 75 patients with Williams syndrome. J Med Genet 39:554–558, 2002

Ewart AK, Morris CA, Atkinson D, et al: Hemizygosity at the elastin locus in a developmental disorder, Williams syndrome. Nat Genet 5:11–16, 1993

Ferrero GB, Biamino E, Sorasio L, et al: Presenting phenotype and clinical evaluation in a cohort of 22 Williams-Beuren syndrome patients. Eur J Med Genet 50:327–337, 2007

Fisch GS, Carpenter N, Howard-Peebles PN, et al: The course of cognitive-behavioral development in children with the FMR1 mutation, Williams-Beuren syndrome, and neurofibromatosis type 1: the effect of gender. Am J Med Genet A 152A:1498–1509, 2010

Friedman WF, Mills LF: The relationship between vitamin D and the craniofacial and dental anomalies of the supravalvular aortic stenosis syndrome. Pediatrics 43:12–18, 1969

Gagliardi C, Martelli S, Burt MD, et al: Evolution of neurologic features in Williams syndrome. Pediatr Neurol 36:301–336, 2007

Garcia RE, Friedman WF, Kaback MM, et al: Idiopathic hypercalcemia and supravalvular aortic stenosis: documentation of a new syndrome. N Engl J Med 271:117–120, 1964

Giannotti A, Tiberio G, Castro M, et al: Coeliac disease in Williams syndrome. J Med Genet 38:767–768, 2001

Goldman SE, Malow BA, Newman KD, et al: Sleep patterns and daytime sleepiness in adolescents and young adults with Williams syndrome. J Intellect Disabil Res 53:182–188, 2009

Gosch A, Pankau R: Longitudinal study of the cognitive development in children with Williams-Beuren syndrome. Am J Med Genet 61:26–29, 1996

Gosch A, Pankau R: Personality characteristics and behaviour problems in individuals of different ages with Williams syndrome. Dev Med Child Neurol 39:527–533, 1997

Green T, Avda S, Dotan I, et al: Phenotypic psychiatric characterization of children with Williams syndrome and response of those with ADHD to methylphenidate treatment. Am J Med Genet B Neuropsychiatr Genet 159B:13–20, 2011

Greer MK, Brown FR 3rd, Pai GS, et al: Cognitive, adaptive, and behavioral characteristics of Williams syndrome. Am J Med Genet 74:521–525, 1997

Howlin P, Udwin O: Outcome in adult life for people with Williams syndrome: results from a survey of 239 families. J Intellect Disabil Res 50:151–160, 2006

Järvinen-Pasley A, Bellugi U, Reilly J, et al: Defining the social phenotype in Williams syndrome: a model for linking gene, the brain, and behavior. Dev Psychopathol 20:1–35, 2008

John AE, Mervis CB: Sensory modulation impairments in children with Williams syndrome. Am J Med Genet C Semin Med Genet 154C:266–276, 2010

Jones KL: Smith's Recognizable Patterns of Human Malformation. Philadelphia, PA, Elsevier Saunders, 2006, pp 120–123

Jones W, Bellugi U, Lai Z, et al: Hypersociability in Williams syndrome. J Cogn Neurosci 12:30–46, 2000

Klein-Tasman BP, Mervis CB: Distinctive personality characteristics of 8-, 9-, and 10-year-olds with Williams syndrome. Dev Neuropsychol 23:269–290, 2003

Klein-Tasman BP, Phillips KD, Lord C, et al: Overlap with the autism spectrum in young children with Williams syndrome. J Dev Behav Pediatr 30:289–299, 2009

Lacro RV, Smoot LB: Cardiovascular disease in Williams-Beuren syndrome, in Williams-Beuren Syndrome: Research, Evaluation, and Treatment. Edited by Morris CA, Lenhoff HM, Wang PP. Baltimore, MD, Johns Hopkins University Press, 2006, pp 107–124

Laws G, Bishop D: Pragmatic language impairment and social deficits in Williams syndrome: a comparison with Down's syndrome and specific language impairment. Int J Lang Commun Disord 39:45–64, 2004

Levitin DJ, Bellugi U: Rhythm timbre and hyperacusis in Williams-Beuren syndrome, in Williams-Beuren Syndrome: Research, Evaluation, and Treatment. Edited by Morris CA, Lenhoff HM, Wang PP. Baltimore, MD, Johns Hopkins University Press, 2006, pp 343–358

Levitin DJ, Menon V, Schmitt JE, et al: Neural correlates of auditory perception in Williams syndrome: an fMRI study. Neuroimage 18:74–82, 2003

Levitin DJ, Cole K, Lincoln A, et al: Aversion, awareness, and attraction: investigating claims of hyperacusis in the Williams syndrome phenotype. J Child Psychol Psychiatry 46:514–523, 2005

Levy Y, Smith J, Tager-Flusberg H: Word reading and reading-related skills in adolescents with Williams syndrome. J Child Psychol Psychiatry 44:576–587, 2003

Leyfer OT, Woodruff-Borden J, Klein-Tasman BP, et al: Prevalence of psychiatric disorders in 4 to 16-year-olds with Williams syndrome. Am J Med Genet B Neuropsychiatr Genet 141B:615–622, 2006

Li HH, Roy M, Kuscuoglu U, et al: Induced chromosome deletions cause hypersociability and other features of Williams-Beuren syndrome in mice. EMBO Mol Med 1:50–65, 2009

Lincoln AJ, Searcy YM, Jones W, et al: Social interaction behaviors discriminate young children with autism and Williams syndrome. J Am Acad Child Adolesc Psychiatry 46:323–331, 2007

Losh M, Bellugi U, Anderson JD: Narrative as a social engagement tool: the excessive use of evaluative narratives from children with Williams syndrome. Narrative Inquiry 10:265–290, 2000

Martens MA, Wilson SJ, Reutens DC, et al: Research review: Williams syndrome: a critical review of the cognitive, behavioral, and neuroanatomical phenotype. J Child Psychol Psychiatry 49:576–608, 2008

Martin ND, Smith WR, Cole TJ, et al: New height, weight and head circumference charts for British children with Williams syndrome. Arch Dis Child 92:598–601, 2007

Mason TBA, Arens R: Sleep patterns in Williams Beuren syndrome, in Williams-Beuren Syndrome: Research, Evaluation, and Treatment. Edited by Morris CA, Lenhoff HM, Wang PP. Baltimore, MD, Johns Hopkins University Press, 2006, pp 294–308

McIntosh DN, Miller LJ, Shyu V, et al: Short Sensory Profile. New York, The Psychological Corporation, 1999

Merla G, Brunetti-Pierri N, Micale L, et al: Copy number variants at Williams-Beuren syndrome 7q11.23 region. Hum Genet 128:3–26, 2010

Mervis CB, John AE: Cognitive and behavioral characteristics of children with Williams syndrome: implications for intervention approaches. Am J Med Genet C Semin Med Genet 154C:229–248, 2010

Mervis CB, Robinson BF, Bertrand J, et al: The Williams syndrome cognitive profile. Brain Cogn 44:604–628, 2000

Mervis CB, Klein-Tasman BP, Mastin ME: Adaptive behavior of 4- through 8-year-old children with Williams syndrome. Am J Ment Retard 106:82–93, 2001

Mervis CB, Morris CA, Klein-Tasman BP, et al: Attentional characteristics of infants and toddlers with Williams syndrome during triadic interactions. Dev Neuropsychol 23:243–268, 2003

Meyer-Lindenberg A, Kohn P, Mervis CB, et al: Neural basis of genetically determined visuospatial construction deficit in Williams syndrome. Neuron 43:623–631, 2004

Meyer-Lindenberg A, Hariri AR, Munoz KE, et al: Neural correlates of genetically abnormal social cognition in Williams syndrome. Nat Neurosci 8:991–993, 2005

Meyer-Lindenberg A, Mervis CB, Berman KF: Neural mechanisms in Williams syndrome: a unique window to genetic influences on cognition and behaviour. Nat Rev Neurosci 7:380–393, 2006

Morris CA: Williams Syndrome (Williams-Beuren Syndrome). 2006. Available at: http://www.ncbi.nlm.nih.gov/books/NBK1249. Accessed August 24, 2012.

Morris CA: The behavioral phenotype of Williams syndrome: a recognizable pattern of neurodevelopment. Am J Med Genet C Semin Med Genet 154C:427–431, 2010a

Morris CA: Introduction: Williams syndrome. Am J Med Genet C Semin Med Genet 154C:203–208, 2010b

Morris CA, Demsey SA, Leonard CO, et al: Natural history of Williams syndrome: physical characteristics. J Pediatr 113:318–326, 1988

Pagon RA, Bennett FC, LaVeck B, et al: Williams syndrome: features in late childhood and adolescence. Pediatrics 80:85–91, 1987

Plesa-Skwerer D, Tager-Flusberg H: Social cognition in Williams-Beuren syndrome, in Williams-Beuren Syndrome: Research, Evaluation, and Treatment. Edited by Morris CA, Lenhoff HM, Wang PP. Baltimore, MD, Johns Hopkins University Press, 2006, pp 237–253

Plissart L, Fryns JP: Early development (5 to 48 months) in Williams syndrome: a study of 14 children. Genet Couns 10:151–156, 1999

Pober BR: Williams-Beuren syndrome. N Engl J Med 362:239–252, 2010 [see Appendix]

Pober BR, Filiano JJ: Association of Chiari I malformation and Williams syndrome. Pediatr Neurol 12:84–88, 1995

Porter MA, Dodd H, Cairns D: Psychopathological and behavior impairments in Williams-Beuren syndrome: the influence of gender, chronological age, and cognition. Child Neuropsychol 15:359–374, 2009

Reiss AL, Eliez S, Schmitt JE, et al: IV: Neuroanatomy of Williams syndrome: a high-resolution MRI study. J Cogn Neurosci 12 (suppl 1):65–73, 2000

Rhodes SM, Riby DM, Park J, et al: Executive neuropsychological functioning in individuals with Williams syndrome. Neuropsychologia 48:1216–1226, 2010

Robinson BF, Mervis CB, Robinson BW: The roles of verbal short-term memory and working memory in the acquisition of grammar by children with Williams syndrome. Dev Neuropsychol 23:13–31, 2003

Rothlisberger B, Hoigné I, Huber AR, et al: Deletion of 7q11.21-q11.23 and infantile spasms without deletion of MAGI2. Am J Med Genet A 152A:434–437, 2010

Sadler LS, Pober BR, Grandinetti A, et al: Differences by sex in cardiovascular disease in Williams syndrome. J Pediatr 139:849–853, 2001

Santos A, Silva C, Rosset D, et al: Just another face in the crowd: evidence for decreased detection of angry faces in children with Williams syndrome. Neuropsychologia 48:1071–1078, 2010

Sarimski K: Behavioural phenotypes and family stress in three mental retardation syndromes. Eur Child Adolesc Psychiatry 6:26–31, 1997

Schlesinger BE, Butler NR, Black JA: Severe type of infantile hypercalcaemia. Br Med J 1:127–134, 1956

Schubert C: The genomic basis of the Williams-Beuren syndrome. Cell Mol Life Sci 66:1178–1197, 2009

Semel EM, Rosner SR: Understanding Williams Syndrome: Behavioral Patterns and Interventions. Mahwah, NJ, Erlbaum, 2003

Silverman WK, Albano AM: Anxiety Disorders Interview Schedule for DSM-IV: Parent Interview Schedule. San Antonio, TX, Graywind Publications, 1996

Stagi S, Bindi G, Neri AS, et al: Thyroid function and morphology in patients affected by Williams syndrome. Clin Endocrinol (Oxf) 63:456–460, 2005

Stamm C, Li J, Ho SY, et al: The aortic root in supravalvular aortic stenosis: the potential surgical relevance of morphologic findings. J Thorac Cardiovasc Surg 114:16–24, 1997

Stromme P, Bjørnstad PG, Ramstad K: Prevalence estimation of Williams syndrome. J Child Neurol 17:269–271, 2002

Tomc SA, Williamson NK, Pauli RM: Temperament in Williams syndrome. Am J Med Genet 36:345–352, 1990

Udwin O, Davies M, Howlin P: A longitudinal study of cognitive abilities and educational attainment in Williams syndrome. Dev Med Child Neurol 38:1020–1029, 1996

Wessel A, Gravenhorst V, Buchhorn R, et al: Risk of sudden death in the Williams-Beuren syndrome. Am J Med Genet A 127A:234–237, 2004

Williams JC, Barratt-Boyes BG, Lowe JB: Supravalvular aortic stenosis. Circulation 24:1311–1318, 1961

Wu YQ, Nickerson E, Shaffer LG, et al: A case of Williams syndrome with a large, visible cytogenetic deletion. J Med Genet 36:928–932, 1999

Zitzer-Comfort C, Doyle T, Masataka N, et al: Nature and nurture: Williams syndrome across cultures. Dev Sci 10:755–762, 2007

CHAPTER 9

SEX CHROMOSOME ANEUPLOIDY

Jeannie Visootsak, M.D.
Nicole Tartaglia, M.D.

Sex chromosome aneuploidy (SCA) is the term used to describe a group of chromosomal disorders in which individuals are born with an atypical number of sex (X and Y) chromosomes. As a group, SCA conditions are also often known as sex chromosome abnormalities, sex chromosome variations, or sex chromosome anomalies. The missing or extra sex chromosomes lead to a variety of conditions, such as 47,XXY (Klinefelter syndrome) and 47,XYY in males, or 45,X (Turner syndrome [TS]) and 47,XXX (also called trisomy X, triple X, or triplo-X) in females. Less common conditions are tetrasomy (48,XXYY, 48,XXXY, 48,XYYY in males; 48,XXXX in females) and pentasomy (49,XXXXY in males; 49,XXXXX in females).

As a group, SCA conditions are estimated to occur in 1 in 400 births, making them the most common chromosomal abnormalities in humans. This prevalence rate has been established based on studies in which large cohorts of newborns were screened at birth, and the rate has been replicated in different studies across the United States, Europe, and Australia (Coffee et al. 2009; Nielsen and Wohlert 1990; Robinson et al. 1982). However, current newborn screening practices do not include screening for chromosomal abnormalities; therefore, cases of SCA are identified either through prenatal genetic testing or by genetic testing of individuals presenting with signs or symptoms of these conditions. Based on a comparison of the number of cases ascertained by clinical genetic testing to the estimated prevalence of 1 in 400, it is estimated that no more than 25% of individuals with SCA are diagnosed in their lifetime.

This low rate of ascertainment is due to a variety of factors. First, significant variability occurs in the clinical phenotype of the SCA conditions, and most cases of SCA are missing distinct dysmorphic features or congenital malformations that would trigger genetic testing. Girls with Turner syndrome have short stature and have increased risks for congenital heart defects or renal malformations, although this presentation is quite variable and many girls with Turner syndrome have very mild physical findings. In contrast, males and females with extra sex chromosomes tend to be tall with long limbs, and facial dysmorphic features are subtle, if present. The neurodevelopmental phenotypes are also quite variable. Individuals with SCA often present with mild developmental delays, low muscle tone, learning disabilities (rather than intellectual disability), or other difficulties such as anxiety or attention-deficit/hyperactivity disorder (ADHD) symptoms, but in many cases these milder presentations do not trigger genetic testing by physicians. Even though the presentation can be nonspecific in many cases, there continues to be little awareness of the features of SCA by most health care professionals, and, coupled with low public awareness, this leads to the low rates of suspicion and of genetic testing.

In this chapter, we review the most common SCA variations in males and females, providing information about epidemiology, physical and psychological features, recommendations for treatments, and areas of new research.

XXY/Klinefelter Syndrome

Epidemiology

XXY is the most common SCA, with a prevalence estimated between 1 in 581 and 1 in 917 male births based on newborn screening studies (Coffee et al. 2009; Morris et al. 2008). However, a much lower rate of diagnosis occurs in the general population, with up to 65% of males with XXY remaining undiagnosed throughout their lifetime.

Etiology

The extra X chromosome in XXY arises sporadically by nondisjunction either during meiotic divisions occurring in germ-cell development or in early embryonic mitotic cell divisions (Schwartz and Root 1991). XXY of paternal origin arises from formation of sperm with both X and Y chromosome material (24,XY), which joins with a normal 23,X ovum, resulting in 47,XXY. In maternally derived cases, a maternal 24,XX ovum may combine with a normal 23,Y sperm. Based on polymorphic DNA markers, the additional X chromosome has been shown to be of paternal origin in approximately half of all cases and maternal in origin in the other half (Lorda-Sanchez et al. 1992).

There appears to be an association with increasing maternal age; the estimated risk for a woman age 40 to have a child with XXY is two to three times that of a woman age 30 (Carothers and Filippi 1988). Some reports have revealed evidence of higher frequencies of sperm aneuploidy with advancing paternal age, although this research is not conclusive (Fonseka and Griffin 2011).

Researchers have proposed many genetic factors that may contribute to the phenotypic variation among individuals with XXY. One proposal is that the parent-of-origin of the extra X chromosome may account for some of the variability; however, studies have not conclusively demonstrated a consistent difference in phenotype between paternally and maternally derived cases of XXY (Harvey et al. 1990; Ross et al. 2008; Wikstrom et al. 2006). Another genetic mechanism involved in the phenotypic expression may be the pattern of X-inactivation of the extra X chromosome, and there may be a high frequency of skewed X-inactivation (>80%), which may be a factor in some males with XXY presenting with behavioral or learning problems (Iitsuka et al. 2001). Newer studies have identified a possible role for different polymorphisms (small variations of a gene) in the X-linked androgen receptor gene that carries a polymorphism in the number of CAG base repeats in the gene sequence. In some studies, the length of the CAG repeat has been found to be inversely associated with androgen action and associated with the phenotypic variation (Ross et al. 2005; Zinn et al. 2005).

Current research is seeking to identify the specific genes underlying the phenotypic features of XXY in humans; these genes remain largely unknown. One exception is the short stature homeobox-containing gene *SHOX*, which is located on the X and Y chromosomes; overexpression is related to the tall stature associated with XXY (Ottesen et al. 2010). Mouse models of XXY have been shown to share many features of the condition in humans, including testicular pathology, testosterone deficiency, impairment in spermatogenesis, osteopenia, and learning difficulties (Swerdloff et al. 2011). Further research on the animal models is important to inform further research in humans.

Signs and Symptoms

Growth Differences

Infants with XXY usually have normal weight and length, with head circumference typically between the 15th and 25th percentiles. Their average height increases from the 30th percentile before age 2 to the 60th percentile by age 8, reaching the 75th percentile by age 18. The mean final adult height is 179.2 ±6.2 cm, or approximately 8 cm greater than the mean midparental height (Stewart et al. 1991). In addition to being tall in stature, adult males with XXY often have relatively long legs, an increased arm span, narrowed shoulders, wider hips, and higher rates of scoliosis, kyphosis, and flat feet secondary to ligamentous laxity. They may also have features such as hypertelorism or clinodactyly (Figure 9–1A). The tall stature in XXY is likely related to the presence of three copies of the X and Y chromosome height-determining gene *SHOX* and to delayed epiphyseal fusion caused by decreased testosterone levels (Ottesen et al. 2010; Simpson et al. 2003).

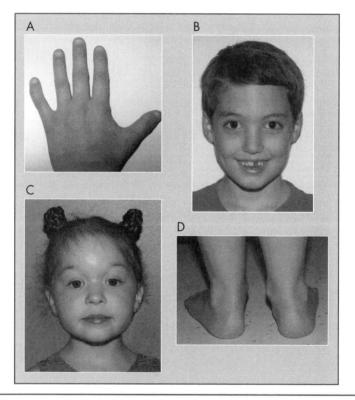

FIGURE 9–1.   Physical and facial features associated with XXY, XYY, and XXX syndromes are uncommon and often subtle.

An 8-year-old boy with XXY with fifth-digit clinodactyly (A), a 9-year-old boy with XYY syndrome with no dysmorphic features (B), and a 3½-year-old girl with XXX syndrome with small epicanthal folds (C) and flat feet with ankle pronation (D).

Source.   Images used with parental permission.

Endocrine and Fertility Complications

Males with XXY may have deficient testosterone synthesis in utero and may lack the normal infant male postnatal surge in testosterone that peaks at age 2–4 months, as is suggested by their increased rates of undescended testicles and somewhat shorter phallic lengths (Ross et al. 2005). Following infancy, testosterone levels remain at normal prepubertal levels until adolescence, when levels of the gonadotropins follicle-stimulating hormone and luteinizing hormone become elevated and serum testosterone levels decrease to the low-normal or below-normal range, resulting in hypergonadotropic hypogonadism (Ross et al. 2005). Elevated luteinizing hormone further stimulates testicular aromatization of testosterone to estradiol; therefore, the estradiol-to-testosterone ratio is further increased, and this may contribute to the gynecomastia found in approximately 20% of adolescent and adult males with XXY (Becker 1972). Delayed or incomplete progression through puberty, accompanied by decreased secondary sexual development (decreased body and facial hair, decreased male muscular development), is often observed in adolescent and adult males with XXY until testosterone replacement therapy is initiated.

The testes are initially normal in size but do not enlarge with increasing age or with testosterone replacement therapy. Adult testes of men with XXY are usually less than 2.5 cm in diameter, and testicular volume is less than 10 cc (Laron and Hochman 1971).

Infertility is almost universal in nonmosaic males with XXY, although there have been a few reported cases of unassisted pregnancy of partners. However, with advanced reproductive techniques utilizing microsurgical testicular sperm extraction followed by intracytoplasmic sperm injection (ICSI) and in vitro fertilization, the success rate for males with XXY in fathering a biological child is now approximately 50% at experienced centers. Other new studies show that the testes may produce some sperm at the beginning of puberty; the sperm may be able to be retrieved in some adolescents for cryopreservation for use in ICSI in adulthood.

Developmental, Cognitive, and Behavioral Issues

Males with XXY have wide variability of neurodevelopmental and psychological features. Hypotonia is often noted during infancy, and the boys may have delayed and/or uncoordinated motor development (Ross et al. 2008; Samango-Sprouse 2001). Longitudinal studies have consistently revealed speech delays, with delay of expressive language more significant than that of receptive language. By age 12 months, expressive language delay is apparent, with decreased vocalizations and deficits in phonemic development and motor imitation. In contrast, age-appropriate receptive language and cognitive skills are often present (Samango-Sprouse 2001). As the children grow older, deficits in oral language production become more evident (including deficits in morphology, word retrieval abilities, syntactic production, and oral narrative construction), as do deficits in written composition (Graham et al. 1988). As a consequence, language-based reading and learning disabilities often occur during school age, and approximately 70%–80% of males with XXY require special education supports of various intensities in the school setting. They may also have secondary problems involving attentional difficulties, executive function problems, anxiety and other socioemotional disorders, and some maladaptive behaviors (Tartaglia et al. 2010; Visootsak and Graham 2009).

According to a systematic review of neurocognitive outcomes in males with XXY ascertained at birth by newborn screening, the overall mean IQ is in the average range, with a profile typically showing verbal scores approximately 10 points lower than visuospatial scores (Leggett et al. 2010). Other studies of cohorts ascertained by clinical genetic testing (rather than newborn screening) have shown more variability in cognitive abilities and associated neurodevelopmental disorders. For example, a study of 51 males with XXY ages 5–19 (with an average overall IQ of 80) suggested an ADHD rate of 63% (with predominantly inattentive symptoms) and autism spectrum disorder rate of 27% (Bruining et al. 2009). By comparison, a study of 57 males with XXY ages 6–21 (with an average IQ of 95) revealed an ADHD rate of 36% and autism spectrum disorder rate of 5%. Thus, cognitive impairments are likely associated with more emotional and behavioral problems in XXY (Tartaglia et al. 2010).

The language difficulties of males with XXY may also be associated with emotional disorders and/or deficits in social interactions. In the study of 57 males with XXY ages 6–21 (mean age 12.26), 25% reported concerns of anxiety, depression, and somatic complaints, and more than 50% reported social withdrawal (Tartaglia et al. 2010). Hyperactivity and aggressive behaviors were not commonly reported. The anxiety and withdrawal that are more frequent in some males with XXY may also influence their self-esteem and social functioning.

Interestingly, an evaluation of strengths and weaknesses in different domains of social skills revealed that the majority of males with XXY showed strengths in the domains of social awareness and social motivation, including areas such as recognizing social differences from others and being motivated to engage in social interactions. However, weaknesses in the domains of social communication and social cognition were found in more than 40% of the group, suggesting that these areas may underlie the social difficulties seen in some males with XXY. Studies in adults with XXY have revealed an increased risk for deficits in social cognition, with decreased perception of socioemotional cues and increased autistic traits (van Rijn et al. 2006, 2008). Individuals with XXY may be prone to autistic traits because of their deficits in the perception of socioemotional cues and difficulty identifying and verbalizing their emotions in comparison to the general population (van Rijn et al. 2006). We again emphasize the importance of recognizing the wide variability across individuals with XXY, because many males with XXY do not have significant socioemotional difficulties.

Diagnostic Evaluation and Differential Diagnosis

XXY diagnosis is confirmed by a chromosome analysis or karyotype demonstrating at least one extra X chromosome. Testing may be carried out on peripheral blood lymphocytes, skin fibroblasts, amniocytes, or chorionic villi. Fluorescence in situ hybridization (FISH) studies with chromosome-specific probes and array comparative genomic hybridization can also be used to identify the sex chromosomal conditions.

Before puberty, the characteristics associated with XXY, such as speech delays and reading difficulties, may be variable and nonspecific, and most cases are not identified until adolescence or adulthood, when endocrine symptoms associated with testosterone deficiency become more apparent. For these reasons, a chromosome analysis should be considered for males who present with motor delays, speech and language deficits, and learning problems (including dyslexia), reading dysfunction, school failure, and behavioral or psychological issues (e.g., attention deficits and autism). In addition, males who present with endocrinological manifestations—small testes, hypergonadotropic hypogonadism (testosterone deficiency), lack of progression through puberty, infertility, gynecomastia—or osteoporosis also have genetic testing.

Conditions that should be considered as part of the differential diagnosis include disorders characterized by hypogonadotropic hypogonadism (e.g., Kallmann syndrome) or those associated with developmental delay (e.g., fragile X syndrome, other SCA variations such as XYY or XXYY). Kallmann syndrome includes features of hypogonadotropic hypogonadism with deficient olfaction. Other common disorders associated with hypogonadotropic hypogonadism include Prader-Willi syndrome and Bardet-Biedl syndrome, which are characterized by hypotonia, obesity, and cognitive disability that are typically more marked than in XXY. Fragile X syndrome is associated with a normal chromosome analysis, and molecular analysis of the fragile X gene is needed to make the diagnosis; however, cognitive abilities are usually more impaired, and postpubertal males with fragile X syndrome usually have large testicles instead of the small testicles seen in XXY. Other conditions associated with tall stature and joint hyperextensibility should also be considered, including Marfan syndrome and homocystinuria.

Evaluation and Treatment

Upon diagnosis, individuals with XXY should receive comprehensive assessments to evaluate for medical and neurodevelopmental features of these conditions. Physical and occupational therapists should assess the individual's gross and fine motor skills. Physical therapy is indicated if a child with XXY presents with hypotonia, gross motor delay, and/or poor coordination, and it may also be helpful in adolescents with decreased strength and coordination. Occupational therapy should be considered for individuals with fine motor deficits, delays in self-care skills, and sensory sensitivities. Other activities that may be helpful in developing strength, tone, and coordination include gymnastics, martial arts, and swimming. Sports activities are beneficial for muscle development, as well as for enhancement of social skills and self-esteem. Speech-language evaluation is important to evaluate for speech-language delays and features of apraxia of speech, and ongoing speech-language therapies should address language delays and intelligibility, with consideration that these issues may also influence social skills, self-esteem, and learning. Additional social skills therapy may help enhance abilities in pragmatic communication, conversation skills, and interpretation of social cues.

For school-age children and adolescents, a comprehensive psychoeducational evaluation should be considered to assess cognition, achievement, executive function, and adaptive functioning, with the goals of identifying learning disabilities and areas of strength and weakness and then planning appropriate educational strategies and resources to optimize the child's learning potential. Psychological and/or psychiatric evaluation may be needed in individuals with socioemotional problems, such as anxiety or depression, or other psychological issues. Because males with XXY are at a risk for autism spectrum disorder, parents and clinicians should be aware of signs of delayed and/or atypical social development. Appropriate referrals to developmental-behavioral specialists, neurologists, or child psychiatrists may be required. In some cases, psychopharmacological intervention should be combined with interventional strategies, including speech therapy, sensory integration therapy, behavioral therapy, and psychological counseling.

Medically, evaluation by an endocrinologist to assess the need for testosterone replacement therapy starting in early adolescence is essential, because testicular failure occurs in XXY and low levels of testosterone lead to lack of secondary sexual development and pubertal progression. Testosterone replacement therapy can improve bone density, increase muscle mass and strength, produce a more masculine body shape, and help produce adequate pubertal maturation with increased body hair, penile enlargement, and male distribution of facial and body hair. Furthermore, testosterone replacement therapy may improve some aspects of self-esteem, attention, endurance, mood, and motor skills. Several types of testosterone formulations are available, including testosterone injections, patches, and gels. Dosage and route of testosterone replacement depend on age and treatment goals, and should be discussed with an endocrinologist.

Testosterone replacement therapy does not lead to improvement of the infertility associated with XXY, and consultation with a reproductive endocrinologist or urologist is recommended to discuss options related to reproduction. In some cases, sperm may be found in the ejaculate of adolescents and frozen for future use. For adults who are ready to have children, it may be possible to extract chromosomally normal sperm cells from testicular tissue by surgical microdissection for use for ICSI. Because these advanced reproductive techniques are not successful for all individuals with XXY, the use of donor sperm and adoption are also options that should be emphasized. Prenatal genetic counseling is also recommended to discuss risk for possible recurrence of sex chromosome aneuploidies; the risk is low, but higher than in the general population.

Other medical evaluations that may be necessary include evaluations for scoliosis, flat feet, tremor, thyroid problems, type 2 diabetes, sleep apnea, and seizures, all of which occur slightly more often in individuals with XXY than in the general population and which can affect motor skills, overall well-being, endurance, and emotional functioning.

Resources for ongoing support and advocacy should be provided for families. Helpful Web sites include those of the following groups: in the United States, Knowledge, Support & Action (KS&A; www.genetic.org) and the American Association for Klinefelter Syndrome Information and Support (www.AAKSIS.org); and in the United Kingdom, Unique (www.rarechromo.org). Local support organizations serving individuals with general developmental disabilities, learning disabilities, or mental health problems can also assist by helping families identify local resources.

XYY Syndrome

Epidemiology

XYY syndrome occurs in approximately 1 in 1,000 male births, based on newborn screening studies. However, there is a much lower rate of diagnosis in the general population, with up to 90% of males with XYY remaining undiagnosed in their lifetime (Abramsky and Chapple 1997).

Etiology

XYY syndrome occurs due to a nondisjunction event in which a sperm with YY chromosomes fertilizes a typical X egg or, less often, due to postzygotic nondisjunction. Studies have not identified factors that increase the risk of XYY, such as paternal age or environmental exposures.

Signs and Symptoms

Few physical findings are associated with XYY syndrome. Tall stature is the most common physical feature, and individuals with XYY are typically taller than expected for their family history. Compared to individuals with XXY, those with XYY usually have normal pubertal development, testicular size, and testosterone levels. Fertility problems are slightly increased compared to the general population, although in most cases fertility is normal. Other dysmorphic features or congenital malformations are rare, although mild hyperextensibility, scoliosis, flat feet, clinodactyly, and radioulnar synostosis (fusion of the radius and ulna bones of the forearm) are more common than in the general population. See Figure 9–1 for photographs of common physical features in XYY other SCA conditions.

Neurological findings can include hypotonia, fine and gross motor delays, and motor coordination problems (Salbenblatt et al. 1987). Motor tics, intention tremor, and seizures are also present in some patients with XYY (Boisen and Rasmussen 1978; Geerts et al. 2003).

With XYY, as with the other SCA conditions, there is significant variability in the phenotype across males. Some males with XYY have minimal features, whereas others are more affected by the neurodevelopmental or psychological problems that can be associated with the genotype. Males with XYY may have early developmental delays in motor or speech and language skills. Learning disabilities can vary as well, with some individuals requiring minimal supports in the school setting and others requiring more intensive therapies. Prospective studies of males with XYY diagnosed by newborn screening showed that their mean cognitive abilities are within the average range (mean full scale IQs of 90–100); however, overall their cognitive skills are typically approximately 10 points lower than those of their siblings (Bender et al. 1986; Ratcliffe et al. 1990). A cognitive profile with weaknesses in verbal skills compared to nonverbal/visuospatial skills is shared with that of XXY, and rates of learning disabilities and the need for academic supports ranged from 40% to 55% in patients identified at birth (Leggett et al. 2010; Ratcliffe 1999).

Behaviorally, males with XYY may show ADHD symptoms, including difficulties with attention span, distractibility, and impulsivity (Hagerman 1999; Walzer et al. 1990). Some patients with XYY also show features of behavioral dysregulation or emotional difficulties, with susceptibility to depression and anxiety symptoms, especially when compounded by psychosocial stressors or family dysfunction (Ratcliffe et al. 1990). Increased rates of autism spectrum disorders have also been reported in individuals with XYY (Geerts et al. 2003). Early studies suggesting a link between XYY and antisocial or criminal behaviors have not been supported by population-based prospective studies, and this association is now considered to be inaccurate and stigmatizing.

Diagnostic Evaluation and Differential Diagnosis

XYY diagnosis is confirmed by a chromosome analysis or karyotype demonstrating an extra Y chromosome. As for XXY, XYY testing may be carried out on peripheral blood lymphocytes, skin fibroblasts, amniocytes, or chorionic villi. FISH studies with chromosome-specific probes and array comparative genomic hybridization can also be used to identify the sex chromosomal conditions.

Cases of XYY may be identified by prenatal genetic testing or by genetic testing in response to clinical features in the postnatal period. The features associated with XYY, such as speech or motor delays, learning disabilities, autism spectrum disorders, or behavioral disorders, may be variable and nonspecific, and most cases that are identified postnatally are ascertained when genetic testing is conducted in early childhood due to the presence of these early problems. After early childhood, although the learning or behavioral problems may be present, it is less likely for physicians to order the genetic testing unless they have suspicion of SCA or they are considering a different genetic disorder. We suggest that a chromosome analysis be considered for males who present with motor delays, speech and language deficits, learning problems, school failure, and behavioral or psychological issues (e.g., attention deficits and autism spectrum disorders).

Other conditions that should be considered as part of the differential diagnosis include disorders associated with developmental delay or autism spectrum disorders (e.g., fragile X syndrome, other SCA variations such as XXY or XXYY). As with XXY, other conditions associated with tall stature, such as Marfan syndrome, homocystinuria, growth hormone excess, and hyperthyroidism, should also be considered.

Evaluation and Treatment

Treatment recommendations include evaluation and interventions for developmental and behavioral disorders that may be found in children and adolescents with XYY. Evaluations of speech-language, motor, cognitive, and social development are important during early childhood so that a treatment plan can be developed and early intervention therapies can be initiated if necessary. Psychological evaluation should be performed in children with any academic, social, or behavioral difficulties, with an emphasis on evaluation for specific learning disabilities, executive function impairments, and socioemotional disorders. Children with social deficits should be assessed for autism spectrum disorders. ADHD and executive functioning difficulties, as well as other behavioral and emotional regulation problems, should be treated with a combination of psychological interventions and psychopharmacology. Standard psychological treatment strategies may need to be adjusted to accommodate a child's cognitive and language abilities.

Physicians should be aware of and screen for medical features that can be associated with XYY, such as tics, tremors, scoliosis, seizures, sleep apnea, flat feet, clinodactyly, and radioulnar synostosis. Because XYY is sometimes confused with XXY, physicians should be aware that in most cases of XYY, puberty, testosterone levels, and fertility are normal, and this distinction is important for patients and their families.

Families should be provided with resources for support, including links to advocacy organizations such as KS&A (www.genetic.org) and Unique (www.rarechromo.org). Families should also be referred to local support organizations serving individuals with general developmental disabilities or mental health problems for help identifying local resources and community services.

45,X/Turner Syndrome

Epidemiology

Turner syndrome occurs in approximately 1 in 2,000 female live births, according to studies in which karyotypes were performed on thousands of consecutively live-born infants (Stochholm et al. 2006). Findings from these studies indicate that the majority of cases have mosaicism, and the prevalence of 45,X in females with TS is estimated to be less than 10%. In contrast, approximately 50% of females ascertained postnatally have a 45,X karyotype, with fewer cases of mosaicism. This finding suggests that the majority of females with TS remain undiagnosed because they may have normal or mild phenotype, and existing knowledge of TS may be skewed toward the 45,X karyotype and more severe characteristics.

Etiology

TS is caused by a complete (monosomy) or partial loss of one copy of the X chromosome, a structural defect in one of the X chromosomes, or mosaicism of a 45,X cell line with another cell line. In the approximately 50% of identified cases of TS with monosomy X (45,X), one of the X chromosomes is inherited as a result of a nondisjunction error during formation of the egg or the sperm. In this subgroup with 45,X, the single X chromosome is of maternal origin in 60%–80% of cases and of paternal origin in the remainder of cases. Notably, no factors (e.g., maternal or paternal age) are known to cause this skew (Frias and Davenport 2003).

Approximately 20%–35% of patients with TS have the mosaic form, typically with 45,X/46,XX or 45,X/46,X,iso(Xq), in which they have one 45,X cell line and one or more additional cell lines. The second cell line may contain one normal X chromosome and one structurally abnormal X or Y chromosome, such as an isochromosome X [46,X,i(Xq)], ring X [(46,X,r(X)], or isochromosome Y [46,X,i(Y)], or a normal 46,XX or 46,XY cell line. Mosaic karyotypes likely result from postfertilization mitotic errors in a normal zygote. A cell line with a Y chromosome is found in about 5% of cases with TS by routine karyotype alone and in about 10% in FISH studies for Y chromosome material.

The majority (99%) of 45,X fetuses are aborted spontaneously in the first trimester. Therefore, it has been speculated that at least part of the second chromosome is necessary for fetal survival (Frias and Davenport 2003).

Most of the clinical manifestations of TS are hypothesized to be caused by a loss of gene expression from the second X chromosome. However, only one such gene, *SHOX*, has been identified to date (Marchini et al. 2007). *SHOX* belongs to a family of homeobox genes, transcriptional regulators that are major controllers of developmental processes. Its expression during embryogenesis correlates with many of the phenotypic abnormalities present in TS. For instance, *SHOX* expression localized at the elbow, knee, and wrist in developing limbs results in skeletal abnormalities seen in TS, including cubitus valgus (wide carrying angle at the elbow) and genu valgum (knock knees). Decreased *SHOX* expression is a primary cause of the short stature associated with TS.

Haploinsufficiency of other genes that escape X-inactivation may cause maldevelopment of the lymphatic vessels, which contributes to many other medical features associated with TS. Absence or atypical development of peripheral lymphatics correlates with generalized lymphedema and cystic hygroma (collection of lymph fluid in the posterior neck). Severe lymphatic obstruction results in hydrops fetalis, which is a major factor in spontaneously aborted fetuses with 45,X (Kajii et al. 1980). In 45,X fetuses that survive, some of the dysmorphic features in TS, including webbed neck, low and upward-sweeping hairline, and low-set, prominent ears, result from a resolving cystic hygroma. Additionally, structural abnormalities of the heart and vascular system are more common in females with cystic hygroma and lymphedema, indicating that the abnormal lymphatic vessels may be responsible for the development of these abnormalities (Loscalzo et al. 2005).

Gonadal dysgenesis is a common feature in females with TS and is caused by increased atresia of germ cells. The ovaries in most cases are replaced by fibrous streaks. The oocyte loss is associated with meiotic pairing errors, the lack of both X chromosomes that normally remain active in ooctyes, and decreased expression of other genes that are important for ovarian function (Zinn 2001).

The X chromosome carries a high number of genes that influence cognition, and the deletion of one or more genes that escape X-inactivation has been hypothesized to cause the neurocognitive deficits in TS. Two such X chromosome regions, a small 10-megabase (Mb) interval of the distal Xp (Xp22.33) and a 4.96-Mb locus at Xp11.3, have been associated with the TS neurocognitive phenotype (Good et al. 2003; Ross et al. 2000).

Signs and Symptoms

Facial and Skeletal Features

As a result of fetal lymphatic obstruction, facial features of TS usually consist of low posterior hairline and neck webbing, downward slanting of the eyes, epicanthal folds, small or protruding jaw, and posterior rotation of the ears. Skeletal features associated with TS can include cubitus valgus, short metacarpals and metatarsals, scoliosis, kyphosis, and lordosis.

Short Stature

Short stature and growth failure are universal features of TS, resulting from *SHOX* haploinsufficiency, skeletal dysplasia, growth hormone secretion dysfunction, and estrogen deficiency. The growth failure starts in utero and progresses throughout childhood and adolescence. In a longitudinal study of girls with TS, height was in the 25th percentile at birth, the 5th percentile at 1 year, and the 3rd percentile at 2 years (Savendahl and Davenport 2000). Females untreated with growth hormone therapy achieve an average adult height 8 inches (or 3 standard deviations below the mean) shorter than their peers. Untreated adults with TS in the United States are on average 4 feet 8 inches (148 cm) (Ranke et al. 1983).

Sexual Development

Females with TS commonly have gonadal dysgenesis and pubertal delay. At birth, the ovaries are typically fibrotic, which results in streak ovaries, and there may be a hypoplastic uterus due to lack of estrogen (Modi et al. 2003).

The majority of girls with TS will not achieve a normal menstrual cycle; however, spontaneous pubertal development with menarche can occur (9% in girls with 45,X vs. 41% in girls mosaic for a 46,XX cell line) (Pasquino et al. 1997). Testosterone production from the adrenal glands may allow for pubic or axillary hair, but there is typically minimal or no breast development. Unassisted pregnancies are very uncommon. Infertile females with TS seeking reproductive options may seek use of assisted reproductive technologies involving oocyte donation and in vitro fertilization and embryo transfer.

Cardiovascular and Renal Abnormalities

Approximately 40% of individuals with TS have a structural abnormality of the cardiovascular system. Aortic coarctation with or without a bicuspid valve is present in 14%, a bicuspid valve alone in 10%, and aortic stenosis with or without regurgitation in 5%. The remaining cases involve other significant structural defects that require medical follow-up and often surgical intervention (e.g., hypoplastic left heart, atrial septal defects) (Sybert 1998). Hypertension, cardiac conduction defects, and mitral valve prolapse are also more common in individuals with TS than in the general population. Aortic dissection can occur at any age, typically at a median age of 35 years. Renal structural abnormalities are present in 30%–40% of females with TS, with increased likelihood for collection system malformations, horseshoe kidneys, malrotation, or multicystic/dysplastic kidneys (Bilge et al. 2000).

Ophthalmological and Otological Complications

Strabismus, usually an accommodative esotropia for farsightedness, occurs in one-third of girls with TS. Hearing loss is also common in TS, with a higher risk for conductive hearing loss secondary to chronic otitis media during childhood and for sensorineural hearing loss in adults.

Other Medical Problems

Infants with TS may have difficulties with early feeding (e.g., refusal to transition to solid food, gastroesophageal reflux), often attributed to oral-motor dysfunction. Gastrointestinal issues in TS can include celiac disease, an immune-mediated disease of the small intestines triggered by ingestion of gluten-containing grains (wheat, barley, and rye), which can lead to further growth failure and abdominal pain. Inflammatory bowel disease (Crohn disease and ulcerative colitis) is seen in about 3% of females with TS, and the diagnosis is often delayed because the presentation of growth retardation may be assumed to be part of the TS characteristics (Keating et al. 1978). Other gastrointestinal complications may include elevated liver enzymes and gastrointestinal bleeding as a result of vascular lesions in the intestines. There are additional increased risks for autoimmune hypothyroidism and both type 1 and type 2 diabetes.

Developmental, Cognitive, and Behavioral Issues

Although their overall level of intellectual function is within the average range in most cases, girls with TS may have developmental delays in infancy and may have a pattern of visuospatial perceptual problems resulting in a performance or nonverbal IQ that is lower than the verbal IQ by approximately 10–15 points (Rovet et al. 1995). Girls with TS who have a small ring X chromosome have an increased risk of intellectual disability. Differences in brain structure, including smaller parietal, parietal-occipital, and prefrontal volumes, have been associated with visuospatial processing difficulties in TS. As a result, girls with TS generally show weaknesses on such cognitive and achievement subtests as arithmetic, digit span, picture completion, coding, object assembly, and block design. Their general pattern of cognitive, behavioral, and psychosocial functioning may be similar to that of individuals with nonverbal learning disability, although this classification can be controversial and does not capture the full pattern of deficits in some individuals with TS. Internalizing problems (anxiety, depression, social withdrawal), and attention-deficit disorder with or without hyperactivity may occur (Mazzocco et al. 1998). Girls with TS may also have challenges in interpreting social cues and adapting to new situations.

Difficulties with adjustment and self-esteem may occur in late childhood or early adolescence as girls with TS begin to recognize differences in their stature, secondary sex characteristics, and learning. Studies of TS have revealed problems such as social immaturity, inattention, poor self-esteem, poor social competence, and decreased school performance, when compared with peers (Christopoulos et al. 2008). Interestingly, physical characteristics in TS did not correlate with psychosocial functioning, which suggests that these psychosocial issues may not be caused solely by short stature and may not improve entirely after treatment for short stature with growth hormone (van Pareren et al. 2005).

Diagnostic Evaluation and Differential Diagnosis

The characteristics of females with TS differ depending on whether diagnosis occurs during the prenatal period, infancy, childhood, adolescence, or adulthood. Cases are often diagnosed "incidentally" when routine prenatal monitoring is done or when cytogenetic studies are performed upon noting congenital abnormalities on ultrasound or an abnormal biochemical screening result. Suspicion of TS may occur because of the presence of increased nuchal thickness, cystic hygroma, generalized edema, hydrops fetalis, short femurs, or cardiac defects on routine prenatal ultrasounds.

Approximately half of females with TS are diagnosed at birth or during infancy or early childhood; the average age at diagnosis is 6.6 years (Sybert and McCauley 2004). Girls who are diagnosed at birth are likely to manifest the classic TS features of lymphedema, with puffy hands and feet, webbed neck, and the distinct dysmorphic features of prominent and low-set ears, epicanthal folds, short neck, high arched palate, low hairline, broad chest, and peripheral edema. Females with subtle physical features may be diagnosed in late childhood or early adolescence when they present with short stature, delayed puberty, and/or amenorrhea. Finally, females diagnosed in adulthood may present with premature menopause or infertility. Because the features of TS may be mild or subtle, a diagnosis of TS should be considered for any girls presenting with unexplained short stature.

In general, because their physical characteristics are more distinct, females with the 45,X karyotype are typically diagnosed earlier than those with mosaicism. Females suspected of having TS should have a chromosome analysis performed to confirm the diagnosis. If a peripheral blood karyotype is normal despite a clinical suspicion of TS, a tissue (e.g., skin) biopsy may be examined. If virilization is evident, FISH with Y probes should be performed to rule out 45,X/46,XY mosaicism, because females with Y chromosome material are at an increased risk of gonadoblastoma.

The differential diagnosis of TS includes conditions associated with lymphedema and short stature. Noonan syndrome, an autosomal dominant disorder with a prevalence of 1 in 1,000 to 1 in 2,500 live births, shares many features with TS, including lymphedema, webbed neck, short stature, and skeletal anomalies (e.g., broad thorax, scoliosis, cubitus valgus). However, most females with Noonan syndrome enter puberty spontaneously, and the congenital heart defects differ from those of TS. Other conditions that may present with lymphedema are trisomies 13, 18, and 21 and Proteus syndrome. The differential diagnosis for short stature is extensive, including medical issues such as growth hormone deficiency, hypothyroidism, celiac disease, renal disease, and inflammatory bowel syndrome, as well as many other genetic disorders and skeletal dysplasias.

Evaluation and Treatment

Females with TS should receive the same preventive medical care as the general population, in addition to having routine screening and evaluation for medical concerns related to TS. Comprehensive published guidelines for care providers include evidence-based recommendations for health supervision in TS (Bondy 2007; Frias and Davenport 2003).

Growth hormone replacement therapy is the standard of care for individuals with TS, and its efficacy depends on age at initiation, length of therapy before initiation of estrogen therapy, growth hormone dosage, and use of anabolic steroids. Age at growth hormone initiation appears to be the most important efficacy factor, and therapy should begin in infancy, or as soon as growth failure is noted, and continued until satisfactory adult height is achieved or until growth hormone is no longer beneficial (when growth rate is below 2–2.5 cm/year). Normalization of height has the potential to decrease physical challenges of short stature and to improve self-esteem and social interactions. However, parents and girls with TS should have realistic expectations of the height to be gained, because these girls will likely remain below average in height. Their growth should also be plotted on a TS growth chart. Adverse effects of growth hormone are rare but may include risk for intracranial hypertension, slipped capital femoral epiphysis, scoliosis, and diabetes.

Sex steroid replacement is needed for girls with TS who do not enter puberty spontaneously or who fail to complete the pubertal developmental process. With early growth hormone therapy, estrogen replacement therapy may be initiated at approximately age 12–13 years in the presence of elevated gonadotropin levels and lack of pubertal development, thereby allowing girls with TS to achieve sexual development and function.

All individuals with TS should have an echocardiogram or magnetic resonance imaging of the heart at the time of diagnosis, with blood pressure monitoring at every clinic visit. Hypertension should be treated immediately due to the risk for aortic dissection. Women considering pregnancy should consult with a cardiologist, because risk of dissection is increased during pregnancy overall. Also, all females with TS should have a renal ultrasound at the time of diagnosis to evaluate for kidney malformations.

Gastrointestinal diseases such as celiac or inflammatory bowel disease should be considered in girls with TS who present with poorer growth than expected or nonspecific complaints such as fatigue, abdominal pain, or lack of appetite. The incidence of autoimmune hypothyroidism in TS increases with age; therefore, thyroid function (thyroid stimulating hormone and thyroxine [T_4]) should be monitored yearly beginning in early childhood. Additionally, it is important to check fasting blood glucose and lipid profile annually in adolescents and adults with TS, and to encourage an active lifestyle and healthy diet. Routine vision evaluation and close surveillance for middle ear effusion should be considered for all girls with TS. Referral to an otolaryngologist may be necessary for girls with frequent otitis media episodes to assess their need for tympanostomy tubes and hearing evaluation, and adolescents and adults should have a hearing evaluation every 2–3 years due to an increased risk for sensorineural hearing loss.

Additionally, girls with TS require individualized assessment for developmental and socioemotional problems that can be associated with TS. Overall, infants and toddlers with TS should have developmental assessments to determine if early intervention therapies may be necessary. During the school-age years, comprehensive psychoeducational evaluations are recommended to identify any existing learning disabilities and/or attentional deficits and to develop a plan for school-based supports for learning problems if needed. Physical accommodations for short stature are also important to include in school educational plans. Additional psychological assessments and interventions for socioemotional problems, anxiety, adjustment, and social skills should also be undertaken and therapies initiated in these areas if needed.

Family support resources that are helpful for families include the Turner Syndrome Society of the United States (www.turnersyndrome.org) and the Turner Syndrome Support Society in the United Kingdom (www.tss.org.uk), as well as local support organizations serving individuals with general developmental or learning disabilities.

XXX/Trisomy X Syndrome

Epidemiology

Trisomy X (also known as 47,XXX, triple X, or triplo-X) occurs in approximately 1 in 1,000 female births; however, estimates are that only about 10% of cases are diagnosed (Nielsen and Wohlert 1990). Although nonmosaic 47,XXX karyotypes are the most frequent, mosaicism occurs in approximately 10% of cases and can occur in many combinations, such as 46,XX/47,XXX or 47,XXX/48,XXXX, or combinations including TS cell lines, such as 45,X/47,XXX or 45,X/46,XX/47,XXX (Nielsen and Wohlert 1990).

Etiology

Trisomy X occurs due to nondisjunction in which the X chromosomes fail to properly separate during cell division either during formation of the egg or after conception (known as postzygotic nondisjunction). Studies of the parental origin of the additional X chromosome in XXX have shown that approximately 60% of cases occur due to maternal meiosis I errors, 20% due to maternal meiosis II errors, and 20% due to postzygotic nondisjunction (Hassold et al. 2007). XXX has been shown to have a statistically significant correlation with advancing maternal age because of an increased likelihood of nondisjunction events during meiosis with increasing maternal age.

In typical 46,XX females, only one X chromosome in each cell is genetically active, and the other is inactivated through DNA methylation. However, particular segments of the X chromosome, known as the pseudoautosomal regions (PAR1 and PAR2), are not inactivated and remain genetically active (Cooke and Smith 1986). Approximately 5%–10% of genes on the X chromosome outside the PARs also escape X inactivation. In XXX, two of the three X chromosomes are inactivated; however, genes in the PARs and other genes that escape X inactivation are expressed from the three X chromosomes. It is hypothesized that the phenotypic abnormalities associated with XXX result from overexpression of the genes on the X chromosome that escape X inactivation (Rappold 1993). As with the other SCA variations, the specific genes involved in the phenotype of trisomy have not been identified. One exception is *SHOX*, which escapes X inactivation and is associated with the short stature seen in TS and the tall stature seen in supernumerary SCA conditions (Rao et al. 1997).

Signs and Symptoms

Physical Characteristics

Significant facial dysmorphology or striking physical features are not commonly associated with XXX; however, minor physical findings can be present, including epicanthal folds, hypertelorism (wide-spaced eyes), upslanting palpebral fissures, clinodactyly, overlapping digits, and flat feet. Hypotonia and joint hyperextensibility may also be present (Linden et al. 1988). See Figure 9–1 for photographs of common physical features in XXX and other SCA conditions. Length and weight at birth are usually normal for gestational age; however, stature typically increases in early childhood, and by adolescence most girls with XXX are at or above the 75th percentile for height (Linden et al. 1988). Body segment proportions typically show long legs, with a short sitting height (Ratcliffe et al. 1994). The average head circumference is below the 50th percentile, although a lot of variation occurs across individuals.

Medical Problems

Major medical problems are not present in most cases, although medical problems that may be associated with XXX include genitourinary abnormalities (ranging from unilateral kidney and renal dysplasia to ovarian malformations) and congenital heart defects (atrial and ventricular septal defects, pulmonic stenosis, and aortic coarctation) (Chudley et al. 1990;

Lin et al. 1993). Seizure disorders are present in approximately 15% of cases (Grosso et al. 2004; Olanders and Sellden 1975). Gastrointestinal problems, including constipation and abdominal pain, are also common concerns (Linden et al. 1988).

Pubertal onset and sexual development are usually normal in individuals with XXX; however, cases of ovarian or uterine dysgenesis have been described in children and young adults with XXX. Premature ovarian failure (POF) has been associated with XXX, but studies on the prevalence of POF in individuals with XXX have not been performed (Villanueva and Rebar 1983). In individuals with XXX, a large percentage of the reported cases of POF were also associated with other autoimmune diseases, including autoimmune thyroid disorder (Goswami et al. 2003). Although no direct studies have been reported of fertility in XXX, many reports of successful pregnancies have been described, and fertility is likely normal in most cases unless complicated by a genitourinary malformation or POF (Linden et al. 1988).

Developmental and Psychological Characteristics

Like individuals with the other SCA conditions, individuals with XXX have significant variability in neurodevelopmental and psychological features. Some have minimal involvement, whereas others have clinically significant problems requiring comprehensive intervention services and supports. Infants and toddlers are at increased risk for early delays in speech-language and motor development. Average age for walking is 16 months (range 11–22 months) and for first words is 18 months (range 12–40 months) (Linden et al. 1988). Expressive language may be more impaired than receptive language, with a pattern described as developmental dyspraxia in some patients. Speech and language deficits in older children and adults may include higher-level language difficulties, such as problems with language processing, verbal fluency, language comprehension, and pragmatic language (Bender et al. 1983; Linden et al. 1988; Pennington et al. 1980). Motor skill deficits may also be present. A study on motor skills in children with XXX showed delayed age for walking, motor planning difficulties, and weaknesses in fine motor skills and motor coordination (Salbenblatt et al. 1989).

Individuals with XXX have a wide range of cognitive skills, with full scale IQs ranging from 55 to 115 across various studies and mean full scale IQs typically between 85 and 90 (Bender et al. 1983; Pennington et al. 1980, 1982). Cognitive deficits and learning disabilities are more common than in the general population or in sibling controls. Intellectual disability occurs in approximately 5%–10% of individuals with XXX (Bender et al. 1986). IQ subscales most commonly reveal deficits in verbal IQ compared to nonverbal/performance IQ; however, cognitive deficits may be found in both verbal and non-verbal domains (Pennington et al. 1980; Ratcliffe 1999). Other findings may include attentional problems, executive function impairments, and decreased adaptive functioning skills. ADHD is present in 25%–35% of cases, with symptoms of inattention typically more significant than those of hyperactivity (Bender et al. 1993; Pennington et al. 1980).

Individuals with XXX also have increased risks for emotional problems, including anxiety, depression/dysthymia, and adjustment disorders (Bender et al. 1995; Linden et al. 1988). Anxiety symptoms may manifest as social avoidance or withdrawal, selective mutism, generalized anxiety, and/or separation anxiety, and can present at any age. Language deficits and social immaturity relative to peers may also contribute to some social difficulties. Other mental health disorders (e.g., adjustment disorders, mood disorders, psychotic disorders) have been associated with XXX, but more comprehensive studies are needed (Otter et al. 2009). Again, the variability in the phenotype needs to be emphasized because many females with XXX have minimal cognitive, social, or emotional difficulties.

Diagnostic Evaluation and Differential Diagnosis

Diagnosis of XXX occurs through prenatal amniocentesis or chorionic villi sampling, or in the postnatal period by a karyotype test or chromosome analysis performed for various presenting clinical features, including hypotonia, developmental delays, physical features, and cognitive-behavioral difficulties. Once a diagnosis is established, further evaluations are important to identify whether medical, developmental, or psychological conditions associated with XXX are present (see the following subsection, "Evaluation and Treatment"). A chromosome analysis should be considered for girls who present with motor or speech delays, learning or intellectual disabilities, and behavioral or psychological issues such as ADHD or anxiety. The evaluation of tall stature in females should also include karyotype analysis to evaluate for XXX.

The differential diagnosis for XXX should include other genetic conditions associated with developmental delays, cognitive impairments, or anxiety symptoms, including fragile X syndrome, Down syndrome mosaicism, and the other SCA variations in females (tetrasomy X and pentasomy X). Females with fragile X syndrome and those with trisomy X can present with similar early developmental delays and low muscle tone, as well as learning disabilities with symptoms of social anxiety in childhood and adulthood. A specific DNA test is needed to evaluate for fragile X. The differential diagnosis should also include other conditions associated with tall stature, including Marfan syndrome, homocystinuria, growth hormone excess, and hyperthyroidism.

Neuroimaging studies in individuals with XXX have shown that whole brain volumes are reduced compared to those of controls, with a slight reduction in amygdala size (Patwardhan et al. 2002; Warwick et al. 1999). One study also reported findings of white matter "high-intensity foci" in 27% of females with XXX, similar to those seen in other SCA groups (Hoffman et al. 2008; Tartaglia et al. 2008). The significance of neuropathological findings of these white matter abnormalities is not yet known; however, the findings suggest that gene dosage effects from sex chromosome genes may affect white matter development or function.

Evaluation and Treatment

Interventions for XXX vary throughout the life span and depend on the presence and severity of associated problems. For individuals of all ages, medical history and physical examination with an emphasis on clinical features are important at the time of diagnosis and yearly thereafter. Infants and children with XXX should undergo evaluation for congenital malformations, including renal abnormalities and congenital heart malformations. Medical evaluations for constipation, flat feet, thyroid problems, seizures, and tremor are important. Seizure subtypes including absence, partial, and generalized seizures are possible and have good responses to standard anticonvulsant treatments. Adolescents and adults presenting with late puberty, menstrual irregularities, or problems with fertility should be evaluated for hormonal abnormalities due to the increased risk for ovarian insufficiency associated with XXX.

Newly diagnosed infants and young children with XXX should have a developmental assessment that includes comprehensive evaluation of language, motor, and social development. Infants with a prenatal diagnosis should have close follow-up of their early developmental milestones and socioemotional development, with neurodevelopmental evaluations recommended at least yearly until age 5–6 years. Early intervention therapies are commonly needed, including speech therapy, occupational therapy, and/or physical therapy. For school-age children and adolescents, psychology, speech-language therapy, and occupational or physical therapy evaluations are important. Evaluation should focus on common problems in XXX, including learning or intellectual disabilities, speech and language disorders (including apraxia of speech), ADHD (most often with predominantly inattentive symptoms), executive dysfunction, anxiety disorders, social difficulties, other mental health problems, and motor skills deficits. Because the behavioral symptoms associated with learning disabilities,

ADHD, language comprehension deficits, and anxiety may have significant overlap, these comorbidities should be considered when developing a treatment plan. Individuals with XXX frequently need school-based services with Individualized Education Programs (IEPs), although the intensity of supports can range from minimal assistance to more intensive supports. For females with XXX who have associated ADHD, anxiety, or other mental health diagnoses, psychopharmacological medication treatments can be helpful. Medication choices are the same as in the general population; however, low starting dosages are recommended. Psychological therapy and counseling strategies may need to be modified based on receptive-expressive language and cognitive abilities. Assessment of adaptive functioning is important to identify strengths and weaknesses and to support any need for community services or disability supports.

Resources for family support should be provided to families. Support and advocacy organizations include, in the United States, KS&A (www.genetic.org); in Europe, Unique (www.rarechromo.org); and an international triplo-X Internet-based group (www.triplo-x.org). Families should also be referred to local support groups and organizations serving individuals with general developmental disabilities, learning disabilities, or mental health problems to help identify local resources and community services.

Other Variations of Sex Chromosome Aneuploidy

Other variations of SCA exist in which individuals have more than one extra X and/or Y chromosome. The conditions include 48,XXYY, 48,XXXY, 49,XXXXY, and 49,XXXYY in males and 48,XXXX and 49,XXXXX in females. In general, the overexpression of genes from the additional sex chromosomes leads to more significant involvement compared to the trisomy conditions, and these variations are typically associated with higher rates of dysmorphic features and associated medical problems. Similarly, early developmental delays are almost universal, and these individuals have higher rates of intellectual disability, autism spectrum disorders, and behavioral difficulties. Further discussion of these conditions is beyond the scope of this chapter; however, resources are available for additional information about these conditions (Linden et al. 1995; Tartaglia et al. 2008, 2011).

Outcomes

Individuals with SCA experience a wide range of outcomes. Many individuals have minimal manifestations or have overcome childhood learning disorders, allowing for occupational success in a wide range of careers. Others have more significant cognitive and psychological involvement and may require a variety of supports and services. In general, the outcomes of those diagnosed in the prenatal period have been found to be generally improved compared to the outcomes of individuals identified after birth, although individuals with a prenatal diagnosis can still have learning or emotional problems (Robinson et al. 1992). In general, individuals with mosaicism also have improved outcomes compared to those with nonmosaic SCA (Bender et al. 1986). Other genetic factors explaining the variability in severity of the phenotype have not yet been identified.

New Research Directions

Although SCA variations are the most common chromosomal abnormalities in humans, professional and public awareness is lacking, misperceptions about these conditions are widespread, and additional research into all the SCA variations is needed. Due to ascertainment bias, the current knowledge of SCA continues to be skewed toward a more severe phenotype, and an accurate understanding will be possible only if all individuals are diagnosed, such as through population-based screening. Consequently, controversies exist as to how, when, and whom to screen, and how parents should give consent prior to screening. Guidelines need to be developed regarding treatments and interventions following identification of new cases, and determination is needed regarding where and how these services will be delivered, because the volume of individuals identified would be significant based on the high prevalence of these conditions.

Research on medical problems associated with most SCA conditions and their treatments needs to be expanded. Evidence-based recommendations for evaluation and treatment of the multiple medical problems associated with TS are regularly reviewed and revised by a national working group (Bondy 2007); however, these recommendations are generally lacking for the other SCA subgroups, for which national consortiums have not yet been established. The endocrine problems associated with XXY and TS have been well described, but associated medical problems such as autoimmune disease, seizures, tremor, thyroid dysfunction, or other associated congenital malformations have not been well studied in all the SCA conditions.

The neurodevelopmental and psychological features of SCAs can cause significant difficulties academically, emotionally, and psychosocially in some individuals, although very few studies have been done on treatments and interventions to help patients with these problems. Longitudinal studies are also important to improve understanding of how these behavioral features change with advancing age. Further research is needed to better understand and contrast the neuropsychological profiles across SCA groups and to understand the differences in neurobiological functioning and development that occur due to the differences in sex chromosome gene dosage. The specific genes on the sex chromosomes and the genetic mechanisms responsible for the clinical phenotypes and variability in severity of symptoms need to be identified. Additional animal models need to be developed, and animal-based research on the neurobiological and behavioral effects of differences in sex chromosome gene dosage needs to be expanded. In addition, research into the effects of estrogen and androgen action on neurocognitive and behavioral functioning is important, especially in the XXY and TS groups.

Key Points

- Sex chromosome aneuploidy (SCA) conditions are estimated to occur in 1 in 400 births, making them the most common chromosomal abnormalities in humans. Despite the high incidence, the majority of individuals with SCA conditions are not diagnosed in a timely manner because there is significant variability in the clinical and neurodevelopmental phenotype.

- XXY is the most common SCA, with a prevalence between 1 in 581 and 1 in 917 male births based on newborn screening studies. Males with this condition are at an increased risk for developmental delays, speech-language disorders, learning disabilities, attention-deficit/hyperactivity disorder (ADHD), and other psychological issues. Medically, XXY is associated with hypergonadotropic hypogonadism, which usually becomes clinically significant by midpuberty, leading to the need for testosterone replacement therapy.

- Compared to individuals with XXY, males with XYY typically have normal pubertal development, testicular size, and testosterone levels. Similar to individuals with XXY, they are at an increased risk for developmental delays, learning disabilities, and ADHD symptoms.

- The characteristics of females with Turner syndrome (TS) differ depending on whether diagnosis occurs during the prenatal period, infancy, childhood, adolescence, or adulthood. Girls who are diagnosed at birth are likely to manifest the classic TS features of lymphedema with puffy hands and feet, webbed neck, and distinct dysmorphic features. Females with subtle physical features may be diagnosed in late childhood or early adolescence when they present with short stature, delayed puberty, and/or amenorrhea. Finally, females diagnosed in adulthood may present with premature menopause or infertility.

Recommended Readings

Cordeiro L, Tartaglia N, Roeltgen D, et al: Social deficits in male children and adolescents with sex chromosome aneuploidy: a comparison of XXY, XYY, and XXYY syndromes. Res Dev Disabil 33:1254–1263, 2012

Ross JL, Roeltgen DP, Kushner H, et al: Behavioral and social phenotypes in boys with 47,XYY syndrome or 47,XXY Klinefelter syndrome. Pediatrics 129:769–778, 2012

Tartaglia N, Cordeiro L, Howell S, et al: The spectrum of the behavioral phenotype in boys and adolescents 47,XXY (Klinefelter syndrome). Pediatr Endocrinol Rev 8 (suppl 1):151–159, 2010

Tartaglia N, Ayari N, Howell S, et al: 48,XXYY, 48,XXXY and 49,XXXXY syndromes: not just variants of Klinefelter syndrome. Acta Paediatr 100:851–860, 2011

van Rijn S, Swaab H, Aleman A, et al: Social behavior and autism traits in a sex chromosomal disorder: Klinefelter (47XXY) syndrome. J Autism Dev Disord 38:1634–1641, 2008

Visootsak J, Graham JM Jr: Social function in multiple X and Y chromosome disorders: XXY, XYY, XXXY, XXXY. Dev Disabil Res Rev 15:328–332, 2009

References

Abramsky L, Chapple J: 47,XXY (Klinefelter syndrome) and 47,XYY: estimated rates of and indication for postnatal diagnosis with implications for prenatal counselling. Prenat Diagn 17:363–368, 1997

Becker KL: Clinical and therapeutic experiences with Klinefelter's syndrome. Fertil Steril 23:568–578, 1972

Bender B, Fry E, Pennington B, et al: Speech and language development in 41 children with sex chromosome anomalies. Pediatrics 71:262–267, 1983

Bender B, Puck M, Salbenblatt J, et al: Cognitive development of children with sex chromosome abnormalities, in Genetics and Learning Disabilities. Edited by Smith SD. San Diego, CA, College Hill Press, 1986, pp 175–201

Bender BG, Linden MG, Robinson A: Neuropsychological impairment in 42 adolescents with sex chromosome abnormalities. Am J Med Genet 48:169–173, 1993

Bender B, Harmon RJ, Linden MG, et al: Psychosocial adaptation in 39 adolescents with sex chromosome abnormalities. Pediatrics 96:302–308, 1995

Bilge I, Kayserili H, Emre S, et al: Frequency of renal malformations in Turner syndrome: analysis of 82 Turkish children. Pediatr Nephrol 14:1111–1114, 2000

Boisen E, Rasmussen L: Tremor in XYY and XXY men. Acta Neurol Scand 58:66–73, 1978

Bondy CA: Care of girls and women with Turner syndrome: a guideline of the Turner Syndrome Study Group. J Clin Endocrinol Metab 92:10–25, 2007

Bruining H, Swaab H, Kas M, et al: Psychiatric characteristics in a self-selected sample of boys with Klinefelter syndrome. Pediatrics 123:e865–e870, 2009

Carothers AD, Filippi G: Klinefelter's syndrome in Sardinia and Scotland: comparative studies of parental age and other aetiological factors in 47,XXY. Hum Genet 81:71–75, 1988

Christopoulos P, Deligeoroglou E, Laggari V, et al: Psychological and behavioural aspects of patients with Turner syndrome from childhood to adulthood: a review of the clinical literature. J Psychosom Obstet Gynaecol 29:45–51, 2008

Chudley AE, Stoeber GP, Greenberg CR: Intrauterine growth retardation and minor anomalies in 47,XXX children. Birth Defects Orig Artic Ser 26:267–272, 1990

Coffee B, Keith K, Albizua I, et al: Incidence of fragile X syndrome by newborn screening for methylated FMR1 DNA. Am J Hum Genet 85:503–514, 2009

Cooke HJ, Smith BA: Variability at the telomeres of the human X/Y pseudoautosomal region. Cold Spring Harb Symp Quant Biol 51:213–219, 1986

Fonseka KG, Griffin DK: Is there a paternal age effect for aneuploidy? Cytogenet Genome Res 133:280–291, 2011

Frias JL, Davenport ML: Health supervision for children with Turner syndrome. Pediatrics 111:692–702, 2003

Geerts M, Steyaert J, Fryns JP: The XYY syndrome: a follow-up study on 38 boys. Genet Couns 14:267–279, 2003

Good CD, Lawrence K, Thomas NS, et al: Dosage-sensitive X-linked locus influences the development of amygdala and orbitofrontal cortex, and fear recognition in humans. Brain 126:2431–2446, 2003

Goswami R, Goswami D, Kabra M, et al: Prevalence of the triple X syndrome in phenotypically normal women with premature ovarian failure and its association with autoimmune thyroid disorders. Fertil Steril 80:1052–1054, 2003

Graham JM Jr, Bashir AS, Stark RE, et al: Oral and written language abilities of XXY boys: implications for anticipatory guidance. Pediatrics 81:795–806, 1988

Grosso S, Farnetani MA, Di Bartolo RM, et al: Electroencephalographic and epileptic patterns in X chromosome anomalies. J Clin Neurophysiol 21:249–253, 2004

Hagerman RJ: Neurodevelopmental Disorders: Diagnosis and Treatment. New York, Oxford University Press, 1999

Harvey J, Jacobs PA, Hassold T, et al: The parental origin of 47,XXY males. Birth Defects Orig Artic Ser 26:289–296, 1990

Hassold TJ, Hall H, Hunt P: The origin of human aneuploidy: where we have been, where we are going. Hum Mol Genet 16:R203–R208, 2007

Hoffman TL, Vossough A, Ficicioglu C, et al: Brain magnetic resonance imaging findings in 49,XXXXY syndrome. Pediatr Neurol 38:450–453, 2008

Iitsuka Y, Bock A, Nguyen DD, et al: Evidence of skewed X-chromosome inactivation in 47,XXY and 48,XXYY Klinefelter patients. Am J Med Genet 98:25–31, 2001

Kajii T, Ferrier A, Niikawa N, et al: Anatomic and chromosomal anomalies in 639 spontaneous abortuses. Hum Genet 55:87–98, 1980

Keating JP, Ternberg JL, Packman R: Association of Crohn disease and Turner syndrome. J Pediatr 92:160–161, 1978

Laron Z, Hochman IH: Small testes in prepubertal boys with Klinefelter's syndrome. J Clin Endocrinol Metab 32:671–672, 1971

Leggett V, Jacobs P, Nation K, et al: Neurocognitive outcomes of individuals with a sex chromosome trisomy: XXX, XYY, or XXY: a systematic review. Dev Med Child Neurol 52:119–129, 2010

Lin HJ, Ndiforchu F, Patell S: Exstrophy of the cloaca in a 47,XXX child: review of genitourinary malformations in triple-X patients. Am J Med Genet 45:761–763, 1993

Linden MG, Bender BG, Harmon RJ, et al: 47,XXX: what is the prognosis? Pediatrics 82:619–630, 1988

Linden MG, Bender BG, Robinson A: Sex chromosome tetrasomy and pentasomy. Pediatrics 96:672–682, 1995

Lorda-Sanchez I, Binkert F, Maechler M, et al: Reduced recombination and paternal age effect in Klinefelter syndrome. Hum Genet 89:524–530, 1992

Loscalzo ML, Van PL, Ho VB, et al: Association between fetal lymphedema and congenital cardiovascular defects in Turner syndrome. Pediatrics 115:732–735, 2005

Marchini A, Rappold G, Schneider KU: SHOX at a glance: from gene to protein. Arch Physiol Biochem 113:116–123, 2007

Mazzocco MM, Baumgardner T, Freund LS, et al: Social functioning among girls with fragile X or Turner syndrome and their sisters. J Autism Dev Disord 28:509–517, 1998

Modi DN, Sane S, Bhartiya D: Accelerated germ cell apoptosis in sex chromosome aneuploid fetal human gonads. Mol Hum Reprod 9:219–225, 2003

Morris JK, Alberman E, Scott C, et al: Is the prevalence of Klinefelter syndrome increasing? Eur J Hum Genet 16:163–170, 2008

Nielsen J, Wohlert M: Sex chromosome abnormalities found among 34,910 newborn children: results from a 13-year incidence study in Arhus, Denmark. Birth Defects Orig Artic Ser 26:209–223, 1990

Olanders S, Sellden U: Electroencephalographic investigation, in Females With Supernumerary X Chromosomes: A Study of 39 Psychiatric Cases. Edited by Olanders S. Göteborg, Sweden, University of Göteborg, 1975, pp 77–85

Otter M, Schrander-Stumpel CT, Curfs LM: Triple X syndrome: a review of the literature. Eur J Hum Genet 18:265–271, 2009

Ottesen AM, Aksglaede L, Garn I, et al: Increased number of sex chromosomes affects height in a nonlinear fashion: a study of 305 patients with sex chromosome aneuploidy. Am J Med Genet A 152A:1206–1212, 2010

Pasquino AM, Passeri F, Pucarelli I, et al: Spontaneous pubertal development in Turner's syndrome. Italian Study Group for Turner's Syndrome. J Clin Endocrinol Metab 82:1810–1813, 1997

Patwardhan AJ, Brown WE, Bender BG, et al: Reduced size of the amygdala in individuals with 47,XXY and 47,XXX karyotypes. Am J Med Genet 114:93–98, 2002

Pennington B, Puck M, Robinson A: Language and cognitive development in 47,XXX females followed since birth. Behav Genet 10:31–41, 1980

Pennington BF, Bender B, Puck M, et al: Learning disabilities in children with sex chromosome anomalies. Child Dev 53:1182–1192, 1982

Ranke MB, Pfluger H, Rosendahl W, et al: Turner syndrome: spontaneous growth in 150 cases and review of the literature. Eur J Pediatr 141:81–88, 1983

Rao E, Weiss B, Fukami M, et al: Pseudoautosomal deletions encompassing a novel homeobox gene cause growth failure in idiopathic short stature and Turner syndrome. Nat Genet 16:54–63, 1997

Rappold GA: The pseudoautosomal regions of the human sex chromosomes. Hum Genet 92:315–324, 1993

Ratcliffe S: Long-term outcome in children of sex chromosome abnormalities. Arch Dis Child 80:192–195, 1999

Ratcliffe S, Butler G, Jones M: Edinburgh study of growth and development of children with sex chromosome abnormalities, IV. Birth Defects Orig Artic Ser 26:1–44, 1990

Ratcliffe SG, Pan H, Mckie M: The growth of XXX females: population-based studies. Ann Hum Biol 21:57–66, 1994

Robinson A, Bender B, Borelli J, et al: Sex chromosomal abnormalities (SCA): a prospective and longitudinal study of newborns identified in an unbiased manner. Birth Defects Orig Artic Ser 18:7–39, 1982

Robinson A, Bender BG, Linden MG: Prognosis of prenatally diagnosed children with sex chromosome aneuploidy. Am J Med Genet 44:365–368, 1992

Ross JL, Roeltgen D, Kushner H, et al: The Turner syndrome–associated neurocognitive phenotype maps to distal Xp. Am J Hum Genet 67:672–681, 2000

Ross JL, Samango-Sprouse C, Lahlou N, et al: Early androgen deficiency in infants and young boys with 47,XXY Klinefelter syndrome. Horm Res 64:39–45, 2005

Ross JL, Roeltgen DP, Stefanatos G, et al: Cognitive and motor development during childhood in boys with Klinefelter syndrome. Am J Med Genet A 146A:708–719, 2008

Rovet J, Netley C, Bailey J, et al: Intelligence and achievement in children with extra X aneuploidy: a longitudinal perspective. Am J Med Genet 60:356–363, 1995

Salbenblatt J, Meyers DC, Bender BG, et al: Gross and fine motor development in 47,XXY and 47,XYY males. Pediatrics 80:240–244, 1987

Salbenblatt JA, Meyers DC, Bender BG, et al: Gross and fine motor development in 45,X and 47,XXX girls. Pediatrics 84:678–682, 1989

Samango-Sprouse C: Mental development in polysomy X Klinefelter syndrome (47,XXY; 48,XXXY): effects of incomplete X inactivation. Semin Reprod Med 19:193–202, 2001

Savendahl L, Davenport ML: Delayed diagnoses of Turner's syndrome: proposed guidelines for change. J Pediatr 137:455–459, 2000

Schwartz ID, Root AW: The Klinefelter syndrome of testicular dysgenesis. Endocrinol Metab Clin North Am 20:153–163, 1991

Simpson JL, de la Cruz F, Swerdloff RS, et al: Klinefelter syndrome: expanding the phenotype and identifying new research directions. Genet Med 5:460–468, 2003

Stewart DA, Bailey JD, Netley CT, et al: Growth, development, and behavioral outcome from mid-adolescence to adulthood in subjects with chromosome aneuploidy: the Toronto study, in Children and Young Adults With Sex Chromosome Aneuploidy. Edited by Evans HJ, Hamerton JL, Robinson A. New York, Wiley-Liss for the March of Dimes Birth Defect Foundation, 1991, pp 131–188

Stochholm K, Juul S, Juel K, et al: Prevalence, incidence, diagnostic delay, and mortality in Turner syndrome. J Clin Endocrinol Metab 91:3897–3902, 2006

Swerdloff RS, Lue Y, Liu PY, et al: Mouse model for men with Klinefelter syndrome: a multifaceted fit for a complex disorder. Acta Paediatr 100:892–899, 2011

Sybert VP: Cardiovascular malformations and complications in Turner syndrome. Pediatrics 101:E11, 1998

Sybert VP, McCauley E: Turner's syndrome. N Engl J Med 351:1227–1238, 2004

Tartaglia N, Davis S, Hench A, et al: A new look at XXYY syndrome: medical and psychological features. Am J Med Genet A 146A:1509–1522, 2008

Tartaglia N, Cordeiro L, Howell S, et al: The spectrum of the behavioral phenotype in boys and adolescents 47,XXY (Klinefelter syndrome). Pediatr Endocrinol Rev 8 (suppl 1):151–159, 2010

Tartaglia N, Ayari N, Howell S, et al: 48,XXYY, 48,XXXY and 49,XXXXY syndromes: not just variants of Klinefelter syndrome. Acta Paediatr 100:851–860, 2011

van Pareren YK, Duivenvoorden HJ, Slijper FM, et al: Psychosocial functioning after discontinuation of long-term growth hormone treatment in girls with Turner syndrome. Horm Res 63:238–244, 2005

van Rijn S, Swaab H, Aleman A, et al: X chromosomal effects on social cognitive processing and emotion regulation: a study with Klinefelter men (47,XXY). Schizophr Res 84:194–203, 2006

van Rijn S, Swaab H, Aleman A, et al: Social behavior and autism traits in a sex chromosomal disorder: Klinefelter (47XXY) syndrome. J Autism Dev Disord 38:1634–1641, 2008

Villanueva AL, Rebar RW: Triple-X syndrome and premature ovarian failure. Obstet Gynecol 62(Suppl):70S–73S, 1983

Visootsak J, Graham JM Jr: Social function in multiple X and Y chromosome disorders: XXY, XYY, XXYY, XXXY. Dev Disabil Res Rev 15:328–332, 2009

Walzer S, Bashir A, Silbert A: Cognitive and behavioral factors in the learning disabilities of XXY and XYY boys. Birth Defects Orig Artic Ser 26:45–58, 1990

Warwick MM, Doody GA, Lawrie SM, et al: Volumetric magnetic resonance imaging study of the brain in subjects with sex chromosome aneuploidies. J Neurol Neurosurg Psychiatry 66:628–632, 1999

Wikstrom AM, Painter JN, Raivio T, et al: Genetic features of the X chromosome affect pubertal development and testicular degeneration in adolescent boys with Klinefelter syndrome. Clin Endocrinol (Oxf) 65:92–97, 2006

Zinn AR: The X chromosome and the ovary. J Soc Gynecol Investig 8 (suppl 1):S34–S36, 2001

Zinn AR, Ramos P, Elder FF, et al: Androgen receptor CAGn repeat length influences phenotype of 47,XXY (Klinefelter) syndrome. J Clin Endocrinol Metab 90:5041–5046, 2005

C H A P T E R   1 0

DISORDERS OF LEARNING

Dyslexia, Dysgraphia, Dyscalculia, and Other Symbolic Dysfunctions

Ingrid N. Leckliter, Ph.D.
Janice L. Enriquez, Ph.D.

Learning disabilities and disorders (LDs) are common in the general population. Prevalence estimates range broadly from 1% to 30% (Goldstein and Schwebach 2009). The variability among the different systems that operationally define LDs confounds precise estimates. Yet primary and specialty care providers can expect to have patients with LD in their practices (Bravender 2008). Rather than seeking help with concerns about LD or about school or vocational performance per se, the patient is likely to have main presenting concerns about comorbid conditions such as attention-deficit/hyperactivity disorder (ADHD) and/or related factors such as anxiety. In working with patient populations with known medical conditions such as epilepsy, chromosomal syndromes, teratogenic exposures, and preterm birth, health care professionals may find that once an individual is medically stable, concerns about LDs are primary.

LDs are chronic neurodevelopmental conditions that affect long-term adjustment and educational, vocational, and economic attainment; however, they respond to intervention, particularly targeted intervention. Functioning is improved by early identification and interventions that address the core, aberrant neurocognitive processes that underpin LDs. Early response can reduce the risk for secondary socioemotional sequelae and potentially improve long-term outcomes. Consequently, our primary goals in this chapter are to help clinicians to 1) identify risk, 2) refer patients suspected of having LDs for appropriate assessment and obtain evidence-based recommendations for individualized intervention, and 3) promote patient self-advocacy.

Nomenclature and Operational Definitions

Conceptually, most authorities agree that LDs are a heterogeneous group of conditions that cause individuals to have unexpected challenges acquiring and developing specific academic skills even though they possess normal intelligence and properly functioning senses and despite receiving appropriate instruction. However, the use of biomarkers such as genetic tests or neuroimaging to identify LDs in the *individual* has yet to emerge. Consequently, to arrive at a diagnosis in the absence of such physiological tests, physicians must depend on results from psychological, neuropsychological, and educational tests administered and interpreted by colleagues in allied health care and educational fields.

Since the term *learning disabilities* was first introduced by Samuel A. Kirk in 1962, the definition and associated labels have been modified frequently. Different labels, definitions, and classification practices are associated with the various systems and parties involved in the care and education of and advocacy for individuals with LDs. In the United States, at least three sets of systems are used, and the nomenclature varies according to the system. For example, the public education system uses the term *specific learning disabilities* (SLD). Behavioral and mental health providers use the DSM-IV-TR term *learning disorder*. Medical doctors, such as neurologists, and allied health care professionals who practice in medical settings, such as clinical neuropsychologists, may use the ICD-10 diagnosis *symbolic dysfunction* or more specific diagnoses such as *dyslexia* or *dyscalculia*. Complexity also accrues because some systems are in the process of revision. For example, the DSM diagnostic system is pending revision in DSM-5, scheduled to replace the current DSM-IV-TR (American Psychiatric Association 2000) in May 2013. A similar update will occur for the World Health Organization's (2001) *International Statistical Classification of Diseases and Related Health Problems, 10th Revision*, ICD-10, which will be replaced by ICD-11 around 2014 or 2015.

These differences in nomenclature may hinder efforts to properly identify or diagnose individuals with LDs and hamper their access to appropriate services. Such differences also drain limited public and private resources. For example, an individual diagnosed via private neuropsychological assessment with a learning disorder, such as dyscalculia, may not be able to access publicly funded special education services if his or her school's specialists determine he or she does not have an SLD. An example of this is *Forest Grove School District v. T.A.* (2009). Despite two school district evaluations and one private neuropsychological assessment, Forest Grove School District in Oregon determined that T.A., a high school freshman at the time of his first evaluation, did not qualify for special education services under the Individuals With Disabilities Education Act. The district also deemed him ineligible for accommodations under Section 504 of the Rehabilitation Act. T.A.'s parents originally asked the district to evaluate him for SLDs, but the district determined that he did not have SLDs. After T.A. underwent a private neuropsychological assessment in his junior year, the district's multidisciplinary team reexamined him. The district still concluded that his disorders did not have a "severe adverse effect" on his academic performance and that his "problems did not have a 'severe, significant' impact on his education" (Dixon et al. 2010, p. 3). The multidisciplinary team arrived at this decision despite agreeing with the multiple clinical diagnoses that the private neuropsychological assessment identified, including ADHD, dyscalculia, various neurocognitive deficits, marijuana addiction, and depression. The district declined to provide T.A. with an Individualized Education Program (IEP). Consequently, his parents kept him in a private therapeutic boarding school to which they had transferred him during his junior year. After this case proceeded through due process, district court judicial review, and reversal by the Ninth Circuit Court of Appeals, the U.S. Supreme Court agreed to hear it. In 2009, the justices voted 6 to 3 that Forest Grove School District did not comprehensively assess all areas of suspected disability, failed to propose an IEP of any kind for T.A., and thereby failed to provide him a free appropriate public education (FAPE). The Supreme Court remanded the case to the district court with instructions to reconsider its decision. The newspaper *The Oregonian* (Portland, Oregon) estimated that the school district's potential legal fees could reach approximately 1% of its general fund plus approximately $500,000 in attorney fees and $65,000 in tuition reimbursement to T.A.'s parents if the court favored his parents (Owen 2009).

After the Supreme Court remanded the case, both lower courts decided the family was not entitled to reimbursement because T.A.'s parents had enrolled him in the therapeutic school "solely because of his drug abuse and behavioral problems" and *not* because he had special learning needs. The parents' response to a single question on the therapeutic school's 18-page admissions application formed the basis of the courts' determinations. At the time of this writing, it is uncertain whether any further actions will occur. Later in this chapter, we review how health care professionals may help their patients obtain comprehensive assessments, and we suggest areas of suspected disability that school districts might examine (see "Systems Anchor Identification of LDs").

Because of the possible ramifications associated with different classification systems, we use the term *learning disorders* (LDs) or more specific diagnoses such as dyslexia, dysgraphia, and dyscalculia unless specifically referring to the educational disability category *specific learning disability* (SLD). As the aforementioned case illustrates, this distinction in nomenclature is significant and not merely a matter of semantics. Furthermore, this usage reflects our training and practice. In this chapter, as noted earlier, we define LDs as unexpected challenges in acquiring and developing specific academic skills even though the individual possesses normal intelligence and properly functioning senses and has received appropriate instruction. LDs are due to limitations in core neurocognitive processes that underpin the efficient acquisition of target skills the individual attempts to acquire. Hence, individuals with LDs learn less efficiently than their typically developing peers. Furthermore, genetic constitution and/or developmental, medical, or acquired factors (e.g., preterm birth, metabolic disorder, toxic exposures, traumatic brain injuries) may be the etiological factor(s) that limit these core neurocognitive processes. Most professionals agree that LDs are not the result of limited exposure to appropriate instructional opportunities and practices.

Signs and Symptoms: Onset and Developmental Course

In this chapter, we focus on four LD phenotypes commonly identified across literatures: dyslexia, dysgraphia, dyscalculia, and nonverbal learning disorder (NLD). Adhering to common medical neurological conventions for nomenclature, terms that begin with the *a-* prefix, such as *alexia, agraphia*, and *acalculia*, refer to the loss of skills and abilities that were formerly evident, due perhaps to a stroke, traumatic brain injury, or other adverse brain events. In our view and that of the DSM-5 working committees, these are acquired *neurocognitive* disorders (Cluster 1), and they are distinct from LDs, which are *neurodevelopmental* disorders (Cluster 2). In both clusters, cognitive processes such as attentional control, memory, learning, and comprehension are disturbed and abnormalities, alteration, or dysfunction in the neural substrate is present. Among neurodevelopmental disorders, however, "the brain's 'normal' potential is never reached" (Sachdev et al. 2009, p. 2003). By contrast, the cognitive deficits found among neurocognitive disorders represent a *decline* from previous cognitive functioning levels (Jeste et al. 2010).

We do not address in this chapter other neurodevelopmental dysfunctions or disorders that may adversely affect an individual's achievement, such as specific language impairment, dyspraxia, syndrome of sensory processing/integration disorder, central auditory processing disorder, or autism spectrum disorders. Some of these conditions are less well defined (e.g., central auditory processing disorder, sensory processing/integration disorder, dyspraxia), and the scientific evidence for their management and treatment is limited. Also, they, as well as other conditions, are classified elsewhere. For example, DSM-5 will classify specific language impairment under communication disorders. In contrast, reflecting the different views and nomenclatures in the field, Virginia Berninger, an educational psychologist and a distinguished researcher, neuroscientist, and interventionist in the field of language-based learning disabilities, prefers the term *oral and written language learning disability*, noting that the condition is the same as specific language impairment (Berninger and Richards 2010).

Presenting Concerns

Surveillance for developmental irregularities can alert health care providers that the patient is at risk for LDs, even before the individual has experienced years of academic failure. When developmental surveillance has been inconsistent, providers are often alerted to the possible risk of LDs through any of the following common general factors: concerns about inattention, lack of follow-through or impersistence on effortful mental tasks (i.e., "laziness"), excessive time spent on homework or job-related activities, inability to meet new performance expectations on the job, notable disparity in the individual's pattern of academic performance (e.g., arithmetic is much better than reading), failure to recall previously learned information from one day to the next, fatigue, task avoidance, distractibility, anxiety, somatic complaints (e.g., headaches, stomachaches), dysphoric mood, low self-esteem, oppositional behaviors, conduct problems, and substance use or abuse.

Fortunately, emerging longitudinal studies are mapping the identifiable, albeit at times overlapping, trajectories of LDs. Knowledge of these trajectories will enhance developmental surveillance. For example, some research studies have detected signs as early as infancy that an individual, as he or she matures, will develop dyslexia and poor reading (e.g., Molfese 2000). Others have reported that infants understand basic numerical concepts. With knowledge such as this about early development, even before formal education begins, we can predict risk and offer early intervention to mitigate the chances of adverse outcome.

In the following subsections, we present an overview of the emerging definitions of each LD phenotype and tables that list the most common features of the developmental trajectories. A health care professional who encounters these or similar concerns should request assessment for the suspected LD or LDs, because many may co-occur.

Dyslexia

The overarching feature of dyslexia, as with all LDs, is the individual's unexpected difficulty in acquiring an academic skill, in this case reading. Intense debate about how to operationalize "unexpected" is ongoing, however. For example, some have argued for a "discrepancy model," wherein the individual's reading skills are significantly below his or her intellectual ability. This definition, however, frequently fails to identify those individuals with high-average or better cognitive ability who struggle to learn to read. Others have argued for a model in which reading achievement falls below a certain criterion (e.g., <25th percentile for age or grade), and a subset of this group has suggested that specific patterns of academic strengths and weaknesses also may be important. Yet others have argued for a definition of dyslexia, as well as other LDs, that includes the presence of specific patterns of neurocognitive processing strengths and deficiencies in addition to unexpected difficulties learning the target academic skills. Although deficiencies in language-based phonological processing are the most common, deficiencies in one or more of the following core neurocognitive processes are present in individuals with dyslexia: phonemic awareness; phonological coding and memory; efficient application of the sound-symbol (phoneme-grapheme) code to accurately read novel words; storage of written words; rapid automatic naming; executive functions such as response inhibition; and the ease or efficiency with which the individual switches mental sets (Berninger 2006; Shaywitz et al. 2008). These deficiencies are functionally manifest across the life span, as described in Table 10–1. Their presence should trigger referral for assessment of suspected dyslexia.

Dysgraphia

Unexpected difficulties in producing written script (i.e., problems with handwriting and spelling) define dysgraphia. Deficiencies in one or more of the following core neurocognitive processes are present: fine motor coordination and sequencing such as coordinating and rapidly tapping the index finger to the thumb; rapidly and accurately tapping each of the four fingers in succession on the thumb; storage and retrieval of written letters and words; verbal working memory; rapid automatic naming and rapid set-shifting; and language skills such as syntax and morphology. As an individual matures, when these skills are deficient, they interfere with the automaticity with which the individual writes, possibly compromising higher-level functions required for composition, such as forming ideas or planning and holding an organizational strategy in mind (Berninger and May 2011; Hamstra-Bletz and Blöte 1993). Table 10–2 shows the developmental trajectory of functional symptoms associated with dysgraphia. Their presence should trigger referral for assessment.

TABLE 10–1. Developmental trajectory of dyslexia

Toddler, preschool, kindergarten	Elementary, middle school	High school, postsecondary, vocation, career
Has biological parents and/or siblings with history of speech-language disorder and/or dyslexia	Has trouble distinguishing and/or manipulating speech sounds	Has difficulty remembering names of people and places
Has articulation delay	Has difficulty recalling the sounds associated with letters	Reads slowly (particularly material outside of personal areas of interest)
Mis-sequences syllables when speaking	Cannot recall basic personal information such as date of birth or telephone number	Does not finish assignments or tests on time
Has trouble saying and generating rhymes	"Forgets" the same word from one sentence to the next	Has difficulty learning foreign language
Has trouble learning color names	Misreads function words such as *an*, *from*, and *too*	Does not read for pleasure
Has difficulty learning letter and/or number names	Has dysfluent oral reading	Avoids reading in public (e.g., restaurant menus)
	Takes too long to do homework	May inordinately sacrifice recreational time for study time
	Seems unable to focus or sustain attention during language arts	May earn unexpectedly poor scores on high-stakes tests such as the Graduate Record Examination (GRE) or Medical College Admission Test (MCAT)
	"Hates" reading	
	Is poor at spelling	
	Overuses general terms such as *stuff* and *things* instead of specific vocabulary	

Dyscalculia

Someone with dyscalculia has unexpected difficulties acquiring numerical computation and mathematics reasoning skills, including deficits in the acquisition of basic computational skills such as addition, subtraction, multiplication, and division. Procedural and working memory deficits are related to dyscalculia and are evidenced by inaccurate retrieval of math facts and

TABLE 10–2.   Developmental trajectory of dysgraphia

Toddler, preschool, kindergarten	Elementary, middle school	High school, postsecondary, vocation, career
Has delayed motor milestones	Has difficulty rapidly tapping index finger to thumb	Demonstrates more knowledge through speech than writing
May have participated in early intervention occupational therapy	Has difficulty rapidly sequencing the four fingers to touch the thumb in succession	Uses poor syntax, grammar, and organization
Is uninterested in or rushes through fine motor activities such as coloring, drawing, and cutting and pasting	Writes letters or words that are unrecognizable, reversed (*b/d*), inverted (*u/n*), or transposed (*who/how*)	Has lack of writing automaticity, which interferes with composition content and length
Has a tight, awkward, immature pencil grasp	Writes with many erasures and overwriting	Does not complete written assignments or tests within time limits
	Spells poorly	
	Demonstrates more labored writing and spelling during spontaneous retrieval than during copying	
	Writes letters and words with irregular sizes and spacing	
	Uses excessive pressure against writing surface, which may dimple the back of the page	
	Complains of hand fatigue or cramps	
	Is distressed when writing is required	
	Avoids writing	
	Demonstrates less of a preference for the style of script (in middle school and particularly among girls)	

increased response time. A fundamental lack of the ability to represent numerical magnitudes on a spatially oriented number line, or *number sense*, may be directly related to dyscalculia (von Aster and Shalev 2007).

Table 10–3 shows the developmental trajectory of functional symptoms associated with dyscalculia.

TABLE 10–3. Developmental trajectory of dyscalculia

Toddler, preschool, kindergarten	Elementary, middle school	High school, postsecondary, vocation, career
Has delayed knowledge of basic concepts (e.g., *bigger, shorter, largest, same*) Is delayed in acquisition of rote counting Does not display 1:1 correspondence in counting by end of kindergarten	Is overreliant on finger and verbal counting strategies (that may be erroneous) rather than shifting to retrieval of math facts from long-term memory Has slow and effortful retrieval of math facts, with high error rate Has problems with spatial organization and alignment when writing numerals Has difficulties applying sequenced procedures to compute solutions Has difficulties detecting and self-correcting errors Has difficulties attending to and discerning relevant from irrelevant information	Has difficulty abstracting principles and transferring procedural knowledge across tasks and contexts Has difficulty with geometry and calculus Has lower levels of income and employment relative to expectations based on intellect and reading skills

Studies have suggested that infants possess a biologically based preverbal number system that allows them to understand simple quantities as early as age 6 months. Preschoolers have a verbal understanding of numbers as well as simple addition and subtraction. The detection of dyscalculia increases during kindergarten and beyond in parallel with cognitive maturation and educational opportunities (Geary 2000). More diagnoses occur during elementary school years than in early years. Up to 65% of children diagnosed with dyscalculia by the third grade showed early signs of dyscalculia in kindergarten within a longitudinal study (Mazzocco 2007).

Nonverbal Learning Disorder

NLD is a syndrome (Rourke 1987) that is more variably defined and operationalized than the LDs discussed in the three preceding subsections. NLD consists primarily of unexpected difficulties in acquiring several skill sets that benefit the development of age-appropriate, independent adaptive functioning. Visual, spatial, executive, and organizational skills, such as the ability to find the way in new locales, plan and organize workspace and/or products, and accurately discern facial affective expressions, are among the most relevant and adversely affected skills. Psychomotor speed and dexterity, bilateral tactile-perceptual skills, abstract problem solving, arithmetic and mathematics, reading comprehension, and social and emotional skills also are affected, although these vary throughout the course of the life span (Tsatsanis and Rourke 2008).

Because deficiencies in nonverbal cognitive processes are characteristic of NLD, verbal composite scores usually exceed nonverbal composites (Verbal Comprehension Index >Perceptual Reasoning Index) on traditional tests of intelligence (e.g., the Wechsler scales). These areas of strength, such as in rote verbal skills, may be so well developed that LD is not suspected during the first 5–10 years of life. This is because many basic academic skills are acquired via rote verbal repetition. However, as individuals mature beyond early elementary school, rote learning is deemphasized and planning, organizing, abstraction, synthesizing, and responding to more complex, novel social contexts come to the fore. Hence, risk for NLDs may more likely be detected after the early elementary years. Whether the NLD phenotype should be used in clinical practice is controversial given the overlap in symptoms with autism spectrum disorders, particularly Asperger disorder, and with other childhood disorders that "vary in genetic, brain pattern, timing of brain insult, as well as other factors" (Spreen 2011, p. 5). Table 10–4 shows the developmental trajectory of functional symptoms associated with NLD.

Assessment Purposes and Goals

Assessment for LDs has multiple purposes and goals. The primary ones are 1) to establish entitlement eligibilities, such as for special education services, vocational accommodations under the Americans With Disabilities Act of 1990 (P.L. 101-336), or Social Security and Supplemental Security Income disability programs; 2) to identify the core neurocognitive deficits that underpin the LDs and render differential mental health or medical diagnoses; and 3) to recommend targeted treatments and appropriate accommodations based on the documented neurocognitive deficits. Accordingly, when a health care professional makes a referral, he or she should clarify the main questions for which the evaluation is being requested. Referral questions drive the assessment process and help define the individual tests to be administered and interpreted. A different, emerging identification process, which relies less on standardized assessment, is known as response to intervention (RTI). It has the dual purpose of diminishing risk of LD (by providing early intervention) and identifying individuals with LD (i.e., those who do not respond to intervention). RTI has its own set

TABLE 10–4. Developmental trajectory of nonverbal learning disorder

Toddler, preschool, kindergarten	Elementary, middle school	High school, postsecondary, vocation, career
May have a medical condition (e.g., uncomplicated calossal agenesis, chromosome 22q11.2 deletion syndrome, early shunted hydrocephalus, cranial irradiation of childhood brain cancers) that confers an element of risk	Demonstrates right-left and spatial confusion	Has difficulty with route learning and reading maps
Demonstrates low levels of exploratory play	Has difficulty interpreting facial expressions and gestures	Experiences disorientation and confusion while changing classrooms
Appears relatively uninterested in tactile exploration, fine motor, or construction play	Has difficulty with 1:1 correspondence in counting	May have notably improved and neat handwriting after much overpractice
Has poor coordination that may interfere with gusto at play and feeding times	Has difficulty recognizing and copying letters and numbers	Rarely achieves >6th-grade equivalent in mathematics
Has delayed acquisition of gross and fine motor milestones	Resists writing and drawing	Has problems with scheduling and managing time
Is verbally chatty and accurately parrots words but with limited comprehension	Talks rather than does	Has difficulties budgeting and managing a checkbook
Is distractible and off-task, and may be diagnosed with attention-deficit/ hyperactivity disorder	May participate in occupational therapy	Has difficulties performing tasks that require measurement skills and dealing with ratios and fractions (e.g., carpentry, following recipes)
	Is stronger at word recognition/decoding and spelling than at math	Has difficulty listening to lectures while simultaneously taking notes
	Performs spatial misalignments when writing numerals and math problems	Experiences challenges in social relationships, ranging from withdrawal and social neglect to teasing, bullying, and victimization
	Does not understand place values in math (e.g., tens, hundreds)	May experience anxiety and/or depression
	Has difficulty with time (e.g., reading analog clock, reading calendar, predicting how long a project will take)	
	Has difficulty discerning and following patterns	

of controversies (see "Is Diagnostic Assessment Necessary Before Intervening?" below). At this time, despite some of RTI's philosophical strengths, expert consensus endorses comprehensive individually administered evaluations that identify a pattern of neurocognitive strengths and weaknesses as well as achievement deficits consistent with the pattern of neurocognitive weaknesses (Hale et al. 2010).

Epidemiology

Within the United States, the lifetime prevalence rate of LDs is estimated overall at 9.7% (Altarac and Saroha 2007). Severe disabilities occur at a rate of 1.5%, mild disabilities at a rate of 4%–5% (Goldstein and Schwebach 2009). The remaining disabilities are of moderate severity. LDs occur more in boys than in girls, although in the past decade boys and girls had similar rates of dyscalculia (Stock et al. 2006). In addition, prevalence is higher in individuals in low-income communities (Altarac and Saroha 2007). Variable estimates are attributed to differing operational definitions of LDs between and within disciplines, the range of tests used to examine LDs, and limitations in study methodologies, such as sample size. Also, cross-cultural differences in educational practices, such as nomenclature, contribute to variable estimates. For example, in the United Kingdom, learning disabilities equate with what are referred to as intellectual disabilities in the United States (Lin 2003).

In the general population, rates of dyslexia range from 5% to 17% (Semrud-Clikeman et al. 2005), with 27% of high school seniors and 36% of fourth graders falling below basic reading comprehension standards in the United States. Dysgraphia varies between 5% and 33% (Overvelde and Hulstijn 2011). Dyscalculia occurs in approximately 5%–13% of school-age children, although the rate is typically about 6%, with variability across countries (Barbaresi et al. 2005; Mazzocco and Myers 2003). In one of the most comprehensive longitudinal studies estimating dyscalculia in children from kindergarten age to age 19 years, cumulative incidence estimates varied between 5.9% (Minnesota regression formula), 9.8% (discrepancy model), and 13.8% (low achievement). NLDs occur infrequently, being present in only 10%–29% of individuals affected with LDs.

Etiologies
Family Medical History, Heritability, and Genetic Transmission

Multiple interacting variables contribute to LDs. Genetic factors explain about 50% of the variation in reading development (Goldstein and Schwebach 2009), and they explain 40%–67% of the variation in mathematics development (Shalev et al. 2001). However, heritability estimates for LDs may vary based on intelligence, socioeconomic status, or both. For example, the heritability of dyslexia for individuals with average IQs is 0.72, but it is 0.43 for those with IQs less than average. There is a high familial incidence of LDs, particularly dyslexia and dyscalculia (Raskind 2001; Shalev et al. 2001). For example, children of a parent who has dyslexia are eight times more likely to have it than those whose parents developed appropriate reading skills. Chromosomes 6p and 15p are commonly identified with dyslexia, and other candidate genes are also being explored (Mattson et al. 2011).

Medically Related Risks

Childhood medical conditions and some genetic syndromes are associated with LDs. For example, relative to the general population, individuals with Klinefelter syndrome or Noonan syndrome are at increased risk for dyslexia. About 3% of individuals with spina bifida myelomeningocele (SBM) have dyslexia (Pierpont et al. 2010). Dyscalculia and NLD are common phenotypes of Turner syndrome, fragile X, chromosome 22q11.2 deletion syndrome, and SBM (Mazzocco and McCloskey 2005). Compared to the general population, children with seizure disorder or epilepsy are at much greater risk for LDs (Fastenau et al. 2008).

Early Birth and Developmental History

Early birth risk factors for developing LDs include prematurity, very low birth weight, low 5-minute Apgar score, low maternal education, late or no prenatal care, and maternal prenatal use or abuse of tobacco, alcohol, or other substances (Stanton-Chapman et al. 2001). For example, prenatal cocaine exposure increases the risk for LDs by 2.8 times (Morrow et al. 2006). Preterm birth is often associated with developmental delay, including delays in language, phonological processing, and cognitive and motor functioning. Furthermore, preterm children are at increased risk for language disorders and neurocognitive as well as academic deficits during preschool years and beyond (Baron and Rey-Casserly 2010; Johnson et al. 2011).

Environmental Risks

Several environmental risk factors, such as single-parent homes, early lack of environmental stimulation, and exposure to high-density urban environments, with concomitant high risk for accidents and violence, are associated with later development of LDs (Pastor and Reuben 2008). Children of families with more resources and opportunities to stimulate basic literacy and numeracy are more likely than those without such means to enter school better equipped with fundamental academic skills. For example, children from backgrounds with low income, low parent education, and a single parent often enter kindergarten without fundamental math skills. This gap widens with maturity. Early exposure to domestic or community violence may predispose children to socioemotional dysfunction and cognitive limitations that may compromise their potential for learning in school.

Traumatic brain injury or other central nervous system insults, such as neurotoxic exposures (e.g., inhalant use, lead poisoning), may cause LDs. Early occurrence of LDs disrupts normal neurocognitive development that is crucial for later academic skills. These deficiencies may not be evident in younger children because some neurocognitive processes, such as certain executive functions, do not come online until later years.

Differential Diagnosis and Determining Intervention Needs

Systems Anchor Identification of LDs

As we stated above in "Nomenclature and Operational Definitions," the operational definitions and identification or diagnosis of LDs are anchored in the systems the individual encounters. School districts often complete psychoeducational or other multidisciplinary assessments (e.g., speech and language, occupational therapy) to determine whether a student has an SLD and is eligible for special education services. Federal law, state regulations, district guidelines, and the operating procedures of multidisciplinary teams all influence this process. The results are useful in preparing the eligible student's IEP. They establish the student's present levels of performance and guide decisions about goals and benchmarks the student will work toward in special education. Goals and benchmarks provide data to help determine whether the student is making adequate educational progress. Assessments through the school district also may help identify special strategies and accommodations (e.g., graphic organizers, electronic texts, extra time) or related services (e.g., speech-language therapy, adaptive physical education) that could benefit the student.

Parents can refer their child to the school district and request an initial assessment (at public expense) to determine whether the student has an SLD or another disability (e.g., other health impairment, autism, serious emotional disability) that might entitle the child to special education services. Health care professionals should urge, and perhaps even help, parents put this request in writing to the attention of the school's principal. Templates and sample letters can be obtained from advocacy organizations and Web sites (e.g., Cortiella 2009; National Dissemination Center for Children With Disabilities 2002). Relying solely on oral communication with the student's teacher may not be sufficient to trigger this process, particularly in a timely manner. Also, as illustrated in the *Forest Grove School District v. T.A.* (2009) Supreme Court decision, the health care professional can be very helpful to parents by assisting them in considering and identifying all areas of suspected disability so that school personnel can perform adequate, comprehensive assessments to establish a FAPE. One advocacy organization uses the acronym CHAMPS as a mnemonic aid to an overview of areas in which disabilities may be suspected: **c**ommunication, **h**ealth and living skills, **a**cademics, **m**otor, **p**erceptual, and **s**ocial/emotional (Matrix Parent Network+Resource Center 2012).

If school personnel do not suspect that the student has a disability, they can refuse the parents' request for initial assessment, but they must provide the parents with a written explanation for the refusal and the basis for their decision. The parents have a right to due process and can appeal this decision. However, many parents find it less stressful to pursue a private assessment with a specialist such as a clinical psychologist or neuropsychologist. Often, this action moves them into the medical system of care for a diagnosis. When parents ask a primary care or specialty physician to make a referral for an independent assessment, the physician needs to thoughtfully formulate the referral question. Many third-party insurers do not reimburse for educational assessments of SLDs because the insurers consider these assessments within the province of the school district. In particular, they rarely cover testing to establish the individual's levels of academic achievement and to determine whether the levels differ from expectations (e.g., based on age, grade, or cognitive ability).

Hence, the referral questions posed to the clinical psychologist or neuropsychologist should emphasize concerns about the student's patterns of neurocognitive strengths and the potential weaknesses that underpin the suspected LDs. For example, the referring professional might ask whether the individual demonstrates neurocognitive processing weaknesses that potentially lead to dyslexia. He or she may simultaneously note the individual's strengths, such as achievement at expected levels in mathematics. This information can be identified from the psychoeducational testing results the school may have already completed, a report card review, or parent report. Due to the many comorbidities that accompany LDs, the referral questions also should describe concerns related to the potentially adverse functional impact on the student's daily activities or emotional state (e.g., difficulty following written instructions, inability to take notes or complete required projects within deadlines, inability to participate in small-group learning teams, task avoidance, excessive fatigue, anxiety, somatic complaints, dysphoria). Psychological assessments, particularly neuropsychological assessments, are designed to identify the core neurocognitive deficits that underpin learning disorders. Adequate, comprehensive neuropsychological assessments lead to the formulation of individualized, often evidence-based recommendations for interventions and accommodations.

Is Diagnostic Assessment Necessary Before Intervening?

Historically, as a consequence of how LDs have been operationalized, many students had to experience several years of failure before their LDs were identified and they were provided with appropriate interventions (often referred to as the wait-to-fail model of identification). Response to Intervention (RTI) is an educational model that germinated from efforts to replace the wait-to-fail model with a more supportive approach to identification and intervention. The foundational stages of RTI are to 1) intervene early among students who function at or below a cutoff criterion for low achievement and prevent the occurrence of learning disabilities, particularly among individuals for whom environmental factors might be important moderators; 2) closely monitor progress and intensify intervention when students continue to lag; and 3) identify individuals who do not respond to intervention as expected. At stage 3, RTI may lead to a comprehensive assessment to determine whether an underlying SLD accounts for the student's learning difficulties. Despite the idealism behind RTI, one of its primary shortcomings is the absence of initial comprehensive assessments. Without such an assessment, deficient neurocognitive processes unique to the individual cannot be identified, so targeted and individualized interventions cannot be offered. Increased intensity of educational intervention alone may not be a sufficient intervention for students with LDs, and critics of RTI have described it as an undesirable transition from the wait-to-fail to a "watch them fail" approach (Reynolds and Shaywitz 2009).

General Medical Examination

For all individuals suspected of having LDs, a general medical examination is an important first step because it can rule out potential sensory causes of academic underachievement (e.g., poor vision, poor hearing) and other physical factors that may interfere with optimal neurocognitive processes (e.g., exposures to neurotoxins such as lead, metabolic disorders, sleep disorders, thyroid disorders). Also, the physician can consider referrals for genetic and metabolic testing to determine whether chromosomal anomalies or inborn errors of metabolism may be present.

Comorbidities and Differential Diagnosis

Primary care physicians have a unique opportunity to ensure that LDs are not missed in their patients who present with concerns about attention, overactivity, poor response control, oppositional behavior, somatic complaints, anxiety, or dysphoric mood. Comorbid conditions are as high as 40% between the different LDs and other behavioral or psychiatric disorders (Mayes and Calhoun 2006). Children diagnosed with dyslexia are often at risk for other conditions such as externalizing behaviors, delinquency, and later antisocial personality disorders. Dysgraphia co-occurs with language disorder, dyslexia, working memory deficits, and ADHD (Sundheim and Voeller 2004). Individuals with NLDs are at risk for social difficulties, internalizing symptoms, and in some cases suicide. In addition, LDs sometimes co-occur; dyscalculia and dyslexia co-occur in up to 43% of cases, and dyscalculia and dysgraphia co-occur in up to 50% of cases.

In tandem with referral to a neuropsychologist or clinical psychologist, appropriate referrals are often made to other health care specialists to consider whether comorbidities exist. Clinical speech-language pathologists are helpful in identifying the presence of phonological, speech, and language disorders; verbal dyspraxia; dysnomia; or semantic-pragmatic language disorder. Clinical occupational therapists provide comprehensive assessments for fine motor concerns and motor planning deficits, such as dyspraxia or sensory processing differences, and they are able to provide appropriate recommendations to develop adaptive and functional skills. In addition, given the incidence of comorbidity between LDs and behavioral and socioemotional dysfunction, a referral to a mental health specialist is also typically appropriate.

Neuroimaging: Identified Abnormalities

Neuroanatomical regions are of interest when considering LDs. Nonimpaired readers demonstrate differences in neural activation patterns when compared to individuals with dyslexia. The neural system for reading includes an anterior system, a region surrounding the inferior frontal gyrus, thought to be related to articulation and word analysis; and two posterior systems, including the parietotemporal region, which is related to word analysis, and the occipitotemporal region, which serves as the *visual word-form area* and allows for reading fluency by integrating phonology (sounds) with orthography (print) through some yet unknown mechanism. Shaywitz and Shaywitz (2008) identified several studies that suggest that the parieto-temporal system is "pivotal in mapping the visual percept of print into the phonological structures of language" (p. 1334). Nonimpaired children demonstrate significant activation in the inferior frontal gyrus and the parietotemporal and occipitotemporal regions of the left hemisphere. However, children with dyslexia display increased bilateral activation in the inferior frontal gyri when compared to nonimpaired readers, with activation in the right occipitotemporal area and decreased activation within the left parietotemporal and occipitotemporal regions. Children with dyslexia appear to compensate when reading by relying on the posterior medial occipitotemporal region, which is a memory-based system (Shaywitz and Shaywitz 2008).

Neuroanatomical abnormalities related to dyscalculia vary with development, although specific areas are notably associated with this disability. A developmental shift appears to occur from childhood to adulthood with regard to mathematical processing. Children demonstrate more neural activation of frontal regions (e.g., anterior cingulate gyri), whereas adults display more activation in the intraparietal sulci, with a corresponding decrease in prefrontal activation over time (von Aster and Shalev 2007). The horizontal and anterior sections of the intraparietal sulcus are also associated with either numerical processing or spatial as well as object processing in adults (Simon and Rivera 2007). Posterior parietal areas are strongly associated with numerical competence, and the frontal lobes, subcortical structures, and cerebellum are also implicated in mathematical processing. These findings are consistent in studies examining Turner syndrome. Specifically, within this population, abnormal activations in the intraparietal sulci and parietal lobes occur with numerical tasks (Mazzocco and McCloskey 2005).

Disruptions in white matter and anomalous right hemisphere function are implicated in the NLD phenotype. Fibers connecting the subcortical and limbic systems with cortical areas and fibers connecting to the frontal region also are of interest within NLD (Rourke 1987).

Interventions

Pharmacological Interventions

Although pharmaceutical products are routinely used to manage LD comorbidities such as ADHD and anxiety, they are not routinely used to directly treat LDs or their underlying neurocognitive deficits or to improve academic performance. Very few drugs have been used specifically to treat LDs. In the mid-1980s and early 1990s, piracetam was studied in children with LDs because of its benefits in helping individuals with stroke recover language functions such as comprehension and writing. Tallal et al. (1986) reported on a double-blind, placebo-controlled study of children with dyslexia and found that a daily piracetam dose of 3,300 mg over a 12-week trial significantly improved rate and accuracy (i.e., fluency) of reading and writing. Other studies did not find a significant main effect, however (e.g., Ackerman et al. 1991), and our physician colleagues do not prescribe piracetam for LDs. However, because fluency is one of the most difficult aspects of LD to improve and piracetam does not adversely affect neuron growth or function (Britz et al. 2006), perhaps further investigation is merited, particularly as it may potentiate the benefit of educational intervention among individuals who have certain patterns of neurocognitive deficits associated with dyslexia (Ackerman et al. 1991).

Nonpharmacological Interventions

Free Appropriate Public Education

Although egalitarianism is the core of America's founding principles, in our clinical experience, access to effective interventions often hinges on families' private resources. The ability of public schools to offer the intensity and quality of evidence-based interventions that have been shown by science to work is restricted by their limited resources, including insufficient finances and lack of adequately trained educators. Compared to general education, publicly funded special education programs prevent worsening of academic failure among students with LD, but they rarely accelerate academic progress (e.g., Hanushek et al. 2002; Torgesen et al. 2001). Targeted, evidence-based interventions do accelerate academic progress, however. Scammacca et al. (2007) concluded that some of these interventions could be offered at relatively low cost; the average was about $2,400 per student, but one program cost as little as $150 per student. The use of trained paraprofessionals, small groups (rather than one-to-one instruction), and shorter instructional periods (e.g., 10- to 15-minute sessions rather than 50-minute sessions) lowered costs.

Intervening Early

In addition to concluding that evidence-based intervention in the public schools need not be cost prohibitive, Scammacca et al. (2007) also concluded that intervening early (before grade 3), while the brain has greater plasticity, is crucial and has the potential to reduce the incidence of LDs. Indeed, some scientists have suggested that an optimal window of opportunity may exist during the first few years of school, when the student will require less effort to develop skills than in later elementary school years or beyond (Shaywitz et al. 2008). Efficacy studies of a number of targeted, evidence-based interventions revealed associated changes in brain activation, metabolism, organization, and the expression of genetic vulnerability (Berninger and May 2011; Berninger and Richards 2010; Klingberg 2010; Shaywitz and Shaywitz 2008). Furthermore, functional activation and emerging tractography studies of white matter networks suggest that specific, individualized intervention changes the underlying neural connectivity and brain functioning; these patterns differ relative to the individual's responsiveness to intervention (Davis et al. 2010, 2011). Beginning early in the school years to remediate difficulties benefits children because of both the greater plasticity of younger brains and the prevention of multiple failure experiences that reduce motivation. Early intervention forestalls the development of feelings of hopelessness and helplessness and the resulting social concomitants that come from students' repeated failures. Substantially more research is needed to develop interventions for individuals who do not respond and for individuals at later stages of development (Scammacca et al. 2007).

Formal Curricula and Evidence-Based Interventions That "Work"

Part of the U.S. Department of Education, the Institute of Education Sciences has developed the What Works Clearinghouse (http://ies.ed.gov/ncee/wwc/reports), whose reports provide rigorous reviews and rate the quality and efficacy studies of curricula, products, intervention programs, and educational practices. For example, the reports extracted in July 2011 for LDs reflected two of 15 interventions—the Lindamood Phoneme Sequencing (LiPS) program and Read Naturally—with research studies meeting evidence standards (e.g., use of a comparison group, efficacy attributed solely to the intervention) that demonstrated positive or potentially positive effects on at least one student outcome. Important caveats regarding the utility of these reports should be noted, however. The prescribed nature of the interventions and their materials fail to adequately address the idiosyncratic differences of nonresponders and their need for individually attuned instruction (Berninger and May 2011). No algorithms exist to guide educators or interventionists in their selection of effective interventions. Hence, there is a need for comprehensive clinical assessments; they provide diagnoses, identify neurocognitive patterns, and drive recommendations for individualized intervention.

Consultations With Other Specialists and Private Tutoring

In light of the developmental trajectory and relatively higher frequency of language-based LDs such as dyslexia and dysgraphia, consulting with other health care specialists is often useful. Some speech-language pathologists develop specialized expertise in interventions to enhance the acquisition of reading and writing skills in LD populations (Goldsworthy and Lambert 2010). Families with private resources also often seek tutoring or enroll their students in franchised learning centers. The Association of Educational Therapists (www.aetonline.org) is a good resource for families to identify professional and board-certified educational therapists. The International Dyslexia Association also lists nationwide resources, such as tutors, educational therapists, private schools, and educational advocates (www.interdys.org). Some franchised learning centers offer evidence-based interventions (e.g., the Lindamood-Bell Learning Processes offers LiPS; www.lindamood-bell.com), but others offer services that do not have a scientific base that supports their efficacy. Some families ask whether to seek consultation with optometric specialists, but "scientific evidence does not support the claims that visual training, muscle exercises, ocular pursuit-and-tracking exercises, behavioral/perceptual vision therapy, 'training' glasses, prisms, and colored lenses and filters are effective direct or indirect treatments for learning disabilities" (American Academy of Pediatrics et al. 2009, p. 818).

Parent-Supported In-Home Programs and Strategies

Families often ask what they can do at home to supplement education intervention and services that might be provided as part of their child's FAPE. Some evidence-based programs that improve core neurocognitive skills such as working memory are available through interactive software and are guided by weekly phone consultations with a trained coach (Holmes et al. 2009). Other interactive programs and software, although not yet evaluated in and of themselves, are based on sound scientific evidence that memory strategies, such as humorous, memorable visual images, lyrics, or scenarios, improve the encoding and retrieval of facts (e.g., addition and multiplication tables; Mastropieri and Scruggs 1998).

In our experience, family harmony can often be quite disrupted when parents attempt to tutor their child with LD themselves. Both parties often end up frustrated with each other, and this may set the stage for development of secondary behavioral or mental health problems. The family is an important resource and refuge for the individual with LD after long school days of academic struggle. Families often benefit from professional guidance to enhance children's experience of competence and success at home and in community settings (e.g., through experience with athletic teams, art, or music) so each child's strengths are recognized and developed as his or her academic weaknesses are also being addressed. Long-term outcome studies show that these avocations often can turn into vocations or help to establish supportive social networks (Spreen 1988).

Mental and Behavioral Health Interventions for Parent Guidance, Family Support, Coping Skills, and Life Enrichment

A child or adult with LD may experience the subtleties of life as far more complex than do individuals without LDs. In addition to academic deficits, other areas of functioning may be compromised. For a parent, advocating on behalf of a child with LD may be marked by many moments of frustration and challenge. Therefore, it is important for individuals with LD, as well as their families, to be adequately informed and supported as they face the socioemotional and behavioral challenges that may arise. Resources that are easy to access, such as films (see, e.g., Redford 2012), and online and in-person support groups, such as the International Dyslexia Association (www.interdys.org), are helpful.

Resilience factors are important to consider given the potential for negative outcomes such as undereducation and school dropout, underemployment, criminal activity, and substance use, as well as persistent, untreated mental health conditions and suicide. However, within a study conducted over a 20-year span, predictors of success among individuals diagnosed with LD included self-awareness of limitations and strengths; active engagement in different aspects of life (e.g., community, social, work); and the ability to seek advice and accept responsibility when needed, to create and follow through on goals, to offer support to others in social relationships, and, importantly, to develop strong and intimate peer and family relationships to help cope with stress and combat emotional instability (Goldberg et al. 2003). Similarly, the National Longitudinal Study of Adolescent Health found that an individual's degree of connection with parents and school was strongly associated with reduced risk for emotional and behavioral problems (Svetaz et al. 2000).

Several areas of support may be offered to individuals with LD and their families. Given the incidence of mental health issues, referral to an individual and/or a family therapist is appropriate. Evidence-based treatments, such as cognitive-behavioral therapy (CBT), have gained significant support through multimodal studies of anxiety. One such CBT-based program, which also has several variants depending on the developmental level of the child, is the Coping Cat curriculum for children ages 6–13 years. Participants in this program are taught the cognitive, emotional, and behavioral aspects of anxiety; triggers to anxiety; coping techniques; and practice skills gained within the environment. Group and parent CBT may also assist in supporting the child or adolescent. CBT is effective in treating depression in children and adolescents, with the latter group benefiting also from interpersonal therapy, a time-limited treatment to decrease depressive symptoms and improve social functioning within significant relationships. Evidence-based treatments for disruptive behaviors include behavior and skills therapy, and parent management training, such as Parent-Child Interaction Therapy or the Positive Parenting Program (Triple P), along with anger management coping skills. Information on all of these programs is available at the Association for Behavioral and Cognitive Therapies Web site (www.abct.org). In addition to these treatments, children and adolescents may benefit from social skills training due to the high prevalence of peer rejection and bullying, which, in turn, limit opportunities to gain social skills. Involvement in extracurricular activities is often recommended to strengthen self-esteem and expand social networks. Equally important, assistance with developing functional living skills may be required. Parents may gain support through meeting with other families of children diagnosed with LD or by pursuing family counseling or individual treatment.

New Research Directions

Etiology

Studies involving neuroimaging and identification of candidate genes and loci related to LDs are currently under way, with most research in these areas involving dyslexia (Berninger and Richards 2010). Quantitative genetic studies could elucidate to what degree math skills, and which ones in particular (e.g., computational vs. problem solving), are independent. Longitudinal quantitative genetic studies would be beneficial to identify genetic and environmental influences on response to treatment. In addition, molecular genetic studies may in the future identify linkage of DNA markers for dyscalculia (Petrill and Plomin 2007). Possible epigenetic processes are hypothesized and will likely continue to evolve with future findings, the advent of more advanced quantitative techniques, and the development of more precise and unitary definitions of LDs.

Intervention

Recent imaging studies suggest individual differences in response to intervention. Specifically, different activation levels are found between children who respond and those who do not respond to reading intervention in areas involving the left hemisphere posterior superior temporal and middle temporal gyri (Davis et al. 2011). Targeted drug treatments may be developed to synergistically enhance the efficacy of current nonpharmacological interventions.

Early intervention, prior to the beginning of formal education, also is an important area of study. One promising program, Tools of the Mind, effectively develops the executive function skills of preschoolers by using play, visual aids, and peer interaction embedded in all activities, including lessons of reading and math. Cognitive control strongly predicts academic functioning. Tools of the Mind has produced promising results among preschoolers from disadvantaged backgrounds (Diamond et al. 2007).

Prevention

Although the neural signature can be identified in groups of individuals with certain LDs, the brain imaging and other methods used to do so must be refined before they can provide biomarkers in the individual. Once biomarkers can identify LDs in the individual, professionals will be able to identify early risk and provide intervention earlier, perhaps preventing the full expression of the neurobiological vulnerabilities that underpin LDs.

Key Points

- Learning disorders (LDs) are operationally defined by the system the individual encounters and are a heterogeneous group of neurodevelopmental conditions.

- Although neural networks are aberrant and learning disorders are chronic, LDs do respond to intervention with varying degrees of benefit.

- Primary care physicians, psychiatrists, and other medical specialists can optimize the developmental trajectory and prognosis for individuals with LD by making appropriate referrals for comprehensive assessments and intervention, making diagnoses, carefully assessing and diagnosing any comorbid conditions, providing treatment when appropriate, and promoting the individual's unique strengths beyond academics.

- Practitioners need to know the resources in their communities and inform and empower families to advocate effectively within and across all levels of systems serving individuals with learning disorders. Parents need information in order to be advocates. Practitioners should be able to provide parents with Web sites and addresses for further information; many are provided in the chapter's text.

- Learning disorders often co-occur with other medical and behavioral or mental health conditions. Some of these conditions may be prevented by early detection of the LD; others need to be identified, managed, and treated concurrently with the LD.

Recommended Readings

Berninger VW, Wolf BJ: Teaching students with dyslexia and dysgraphia: lessons from teaching and science. Baltimore, MD, Paul H. Brookes Publishing, 2009

Shaywitz SE: Overcoming dyslexia: a new and complete science-based program for reading problems at any level. New York, Knopf, 2003

Thompson S: The source for nonverbal learning disorders. East Moline, IL, LinguiSystems, 1997

Timmons J, Wills J, Kemp J, et al: Charting the course: supporting the career development of youth with learning disabilities. Washington, DC, Institute for Educational Leadership, National Collaborative on Workforce and Disability for Youth, 2010

Willis J: Learning to Love Math: Teaching Strategies That Change Student Attitudes and Get Results. Alexandria, VA, Association for Supervision and Curriculum Development, 2010

Wright PWD, Wright PD: Wright's Law: Special Education Law, Second Edition. Hartfield, VA, Harbor House Law Press, 2007

References

Ackerman PT, Dykman RA, Holloway C, et al: A trial of piracetam in two subgroups of students with dyslexia enrolled in summer tutoring. J Learn Disabil 24:542–549, 1991

Altarac M, Saroha E: Lifetime prevalence of learning disability among US children. Pediatrics 119(suppl):S77–S84, 2007

American Academy of Pediatrics, Section on Ophthalmology, Council on Children with Disabilities; American Academy of Ophthalmology, American Association for Pediatric Ophthalmology and Strabismus; et al: Joint statement—learning disabilities, dyslexia and vision. Pediatrics 124:837–844, 2009

American Psychiatric Association: Diagnostic and Statistical Manual of Mental Disorders, 4th Edition, Text Revision. Washington, DC, American Psychiatric Association, 2000

Americans With Disabilities Act of 1990, Pub. L. No. 101-336, sec. 2, 104 Stat. 328

Barbaresi WJ, Katusic SK, Colligan RC, et al: Math learning disorder: incidence in a population-based cohort, 1976–82. Ambul Pediatr 5:281–289, 2005

Baron I, Rey-Casserly C: Extremely preterm birth outcome: a review of four decades of cognitive research. Neuropsychol Rev 20:430–452, 2010

Berninger VW: A developmental approach to learning disabilities, in Handbook of Child Psychology, 6th Edition, Vol 4. Edited by Renninger KA, Sigel IE, Damon W, et al. Hoboken, NJ, Wiley, 2006, pp 420–452

Berninger VW, May MO: Evidence-based diagnosis and treatment for specific learning disabilities involving impairments in written and/or oral language. J Learn Disabil 44:167–183, 2011

Berninger VW, Richards T: Inter-relationships among behavioral markers, genes, brain and treatment in dyslexia and dysgraphia. Future Neurol 5:597–617, 2010

Bravender T: School performance: the pediatrician's role. Clin Pediatr (Phila) 47:535–545, 2008

Britz R, Bester MJ, da Silva A, et al: Piracetam: its possible mode of action in children with learning disabilities and its effect on in vitro cell growth. Early Child Dev Care 176:285–298, 2006

Cortiella C: Sample letter: requesting evaluation. July 22, 2009. Available at: http://www.ncld.org/checklists-a-more/checklists-worksheets-a-forms/sample-letter-requesting-evaluation. Accessed April 19, 2012.

Davis N, Fan Q, Compton DL, et al: Influences of neural pathway integrity on children's response to reading instruction. Front Syst Neurosci 4:150, 2010

Davis N, Barquero L, Compton DL, et al: Functional correlates of children's responsiveness to intervention. Dev Neuropsychol 36:288–301, 2011

Diamond A, Barnett S, Munro S: Preschool program improves cognitive control. Science 317:1387–1388, 2007

Dixon SG, Eusebio EC, Turton WJ, et al: Forest Grove School District v. T.A. Supreme Court case: implications for school psychology practice. J Psychoeduc Assess 29:103–113, 2010

Fastenau P, Shen J, Dunn D, et al: Academic underachievement among children with epilepsy. J Learn Disabil 41:195–207, 2008

Forest Grove School District v T.A., 129 S Ct 2484 (2009)

Geary DC: From infancy to adulthood: the development of numerical abilities. Eur Child Adolesc Psychiatry 9 (supp 2):S11–S15, 2000

Goldberg R, Higgins E, Raskind M, et al: Predictors of success in individuals with learning disabilities: a qualitative analysis of a 20-year longitudinal study. Learn Disabil Res Pract 18:222–236, 2003

Goldstein S, Schwebach AJ: Neuropsychological basis of learning disabilities, in Handbook of Clinical Child Neuropsychology. Edited by Reynolds CR, Fletcher-Janzen E. New York, Springer Science+Business Media, 2009, pp 187–202

Goldsworthy C, Lambert K: Linking the Strands of Language and Literacy: A Resource Manual. San Diego, CA, Plural Publishing, 2010

Hale J, Alfonso V, Berninger V, et al: Critical issues in response-to-intervention, comprehensive evaluation, and specific learning disabilities identification and intervention: an expert white paper consensus. Learn Disabil Q 33:223–236, 2010

Hamstra-Bletz L, Blöte A: A longitudinal study on dysgraphic writing in primary school. J Learn Disabil 26:689–699, 1993

Hanushek EA, Kain JF, Rivkin SG: Inferring program effects for specialized populations: does special education raise achievement for students with disabilities? Rev Econ Stat 84:584–599, 2002

Holmes J, Gathercole SE, Dunning DL: Adaptive training leads to sustained enhancement of poor working memory in children. Dev Sci 12:F9–F15, 2009

Jeste D, Blacker D, Blazer D, et al: Neurocognitive disorders: a proposal from the DSM-5 Neurocognitive Disorders Work Group. American Psychiatric Association. 2010. Available at: http://www.dsm5.org/Proposed%20Revision%20Attachments/APA%20Neurocognitive%20Disorders%20Proposal%20for%20DSM-5.pdf. Accessed April 19, 2012.

Johnson S, Wolke D, Hennessy E, et al: Educational outcomes in extremely preterm children: neuropsychological correlates and predictors of attainment. Dev Neuropsychol 36:74–95, 2011

Kirk SA: Educating Exceptional Children. Boston, MA, Houghton Mifflin, 1962

Klingberg T: Training and plasticity of working memory. Trends Cogn Sci 14:317–324, 2010

Lin J-D: Intellectual disability: definition, diagnosis and classification. J Med Sci 23:83–90, 2003

Mastropieri MA, Scruggs TE: Constructing more meaningful relationships in the classroom: mnemonic research into practice. Learn Disabil Res Pract 13:138–145, 1998

Matrix Parent Network+Resource Center: Assessments. 2012. Available at: http://www.matrixparents.org/pdf/packetsArticles/AssessmentPacket.pdf. Accessed April 20, 2012.

Mattson T, Zuchelli A, Onkamo N, et al: SNP variations in the 7q33 region containing DGKI are associated with dyslexia in the Finnish and German populations. Behav Genet 41:134–140, 2011

Mayes S, Calhoun S: Frequency of reading, math, and writing disabilities in children with clinical disorders. Learn Individ Differ 16:145–157, 2006

Mazzocco MM: Defining and differentiating mathematical learning disabilities and difficulties, in Why Is Math So Hard for Some Children? The Nature and Origins of Mathematical Learning Difficulties and Disabilities. Edited by Berch DB, Mazzocco MM. Baltimore, MD, Paul H Brookes Publishing, 2007, pp 29–48

Mazzocco MM, McCloskey MM: Math performance in girls with Turner or fragile X syndrome, in Handbook of Mathematical Cognition. Edited by Campbell JI. New York, Psychology Press, 2005, pp 269–297

Mazzocco M, Myers G: Complexities in identifying and defining mathematics learning disability in the primary school-age years. Ann Dyslexia 53:218–253, 2003

Molfese DL: Predicting dyslexia at 8 years of age using neonatal brain response. Brain Lang 72:238–245, 2000

Morrow C, Culbertson J, Accornero V, et al: Learning disabilities and intellectual functioning in school-aged children with prenatal cocaine exposure. Dev Neuropsychol 30:905–931, 2006

National Dissemination Center for Children With Disabilities: Sample letters: requesting an initial evaluation for special education services. 2002. Available at: http://www.ldonline.org/article/14620. Accessed April 19, 2012.

Overvelde A, Hulstijn W: Handwriting development in grade 2 and grade 3 primary school children with normal, at risk, or dysgraphic characteristics. Res Dev Disabil 32:540–548, 2011

Owen W: U.S. Supreme Court rules against Forest Grove School District in case involving ex-student with special needs. OregonLive.com, September 20, 2009. Available at: http://www.oregonlive.com/news/index.ssf/2009/06/us_supreme_court_rules_against_1.html. Accessed April 20, 2012.

Pastor PN, Reuben CA: Diagnosed attention deficit hyperactivity disorder and learning disability: United States, 2004–2006. Vital Health Stat 10 (237):1–14, 2008

Petrill S, Plomin R: Quantitative genetics and mathematical abilities/disabilities, in Why Is Math So Hard for Some Children? The Nature and Origins of Mathematical Learning Difficulties and Disabilities. Edited by Berch DB, Mazzocco MM. Baltimore, MD, Paul H Brookes Publishing, 2007, pp 307–324

Pierpont W, Weismer S, Roberts A, et al: The language phenotype of children and adolescents with Noonan syndrome. J Speech Lang Hear Res 53:917–932, 2010

Raskind W: Current understanding of the genetic basis of reading and spelling disability. Learn Disabil Q 24:143–157, 2001

Redford J: The D Word: Understanding Dyslexia. HBO Documentary Films, 2012

Reynolds CR, Shaywitz SE: Response to intervention: ready or not? Or, from wait-to-fail to watch-them-fail. Sch Psychol Q 24:130–145, 2009

Rourke B: Syndrome of nonverbal learning disabilities: the final common pathway of white-matter disease/dysfunction? Clin Neuropsychol 1:209–234, 1987

Sachdev P, Andrews G, Hobbs MJ, et al: Neurocognitive disorders: cluster 1 of the proposed meta-structure for DSM-V and ICD-11. Psychol Med 39:2001–2012, 2009

Scammacca N, Vaughn S, Roberts G, et al: Extensive Reading Interventions in Grades K–3: From Research to Practice. Portsmouth, NH, RMC Research Corporation, Center on Instruction, 2007

Semrud-Clikeman M, Fine JG, Harder L: Providing neuropsychological services to students with learning disabilities, in Handbook of School Neuropsychology. Edited by D'Amato RC, Fletcher-Janzen ER, Reynolds C. Hoboken, NJ, Wiley, 2005, pp 403–424

Shalev RS, Manor O, Kerem B, et al: Developmental dyscalculia is a familial learning disability. J Learn Disabil 34:59–65, 2001

Shaywitz SE, Shaywitz BA: Paying attention to reading: the neurobiology of reading and dyslexia. Dev Psychopathol 20:1329–1349, 2008

Shaywitz SE, Morris R, Shaywitz BA: The education of dyslexic children from childhood to young adulthood. Annu Rev Psychol 59:451–475, 2008

Simon R, Rivera S: Neuroanatomical approaches to the study of mathematical ability and disability, in Why Is Math So Hard for Some Children? The Nature and Origins of Mathematical Learning Difficulties and Disabilities. Edited by Berch DB, Mazzocco MM. Baltimore, MD, Paul H. Brookes Publishing, 2007, pp 283–306

Spreen O: Learning Disabled Children Growing Up: A Follow-Up Into Adulthood. New York, Oxford University Press, 1988

Spreen O: Nonverbal learning disabilities: a critical review. Child Neuropsychol 30:1–26, 2011

Stanton-Chapman T, Chapman D, Scott K: Identification of early risk factors for learning disabilities. J Early Interv 24:193–206, 2001

Stock P, Desoete A, Roeyers H: Focusing on mathematical disabilities: a search for definition, classification and assessment, in Learning Disabilities: New Research. Edited by Randall S. New York, Nova Science Publishers, 2006, pp 29–62

Sundheim ST, Voeller KK: Psychiatric implications of language disorders and learning disabilities: risks and management. J Child Neurol 19:814–826, 2004

Svetaz MV, Ireland M, Blum R: Adolescents with learning disabilities: risk and protective factors associated with emotional well-being: findings from the National Longitudinal Study of Adolescent Health. J Adolesc Health 27:340–348, 2000

Tallal P, Chase C, Russell G, et al: Evaluation of the efficacy of piracetam in treating information processing, reading and writing disorders in dyslexic children. Int J Psychophysiol 4:41–52, 1986

Torgesen JK, Alexander AW, Wagner RK, et al: Intensive remedial instruction for children with severe reading disabilities: immediate and long-term outcomes from two instructional approaches. J Learn Disabil 34:33–58, 2001

Tsatsanis KD, Rourke BP: Syndrome of nonverbal learning disabilities in adults, in Adult Learning Disorders. Edited by Wolf LE, Schreiber HE, Wasserstein J. New York, Psychology Press, 2008, pp 159–190

von Aster MG, Shalev RS: Number development and developmental dyscalculia. Dev Med Child Neurol 49:868–873, 2007

World Health Organization: International Statistical Classification of Diseases and Related Health Problems, 10th Revision. Geneva, World Health Organization, 2001

CHAPTER 11

SPEECH AND LANGUAGE DISORDERS IN CHILDHOOD

A Neurodevelopmental Perspective

Ann M. Mastergeorge, Ph.D.

Signs, Symptoms, and Developmental Course

In DSM-5, which is expected to replace DSM-IV-TR (American Psychiatric Association 2000) in 2013, speech and language disorders will fall under the heading of neurodevelopmental disorders, and the term *language disorders* will be used to describe language behaviors that are different from those expected for a child's chronological age. The definition of language disorders by the American Speech-Language-Hearing Association is influenced primarily by Bloom and Lahey's (1978) conceptual model of the structure of language and the domains that are affected if this structure is disrupted. A language disorder may involve one or more of the following: 1) the form of language (phonology, morphology, syntax), 2) the content of language (semantics), 3) the function or use of language in social communication (pragmatics). The various patterns emphasize that language disorders encompass many different kinds of disruption in the integration of content, form, and use. The term describes the conditions of children who have difficulty learning the form of language (a disruption of form), children who can talk easily and readily but who have little meaning in their communication (a disruption of content), and children who use forms to communicate ideas but not in the conventional manner (a distortion of the interactions among content, form, and use). In sum, a language disorder is an impairment in the ability to 1) receive and/or process a symbol system, 2) represent concepts or symbol systems, and/or 3) transmit or use symbol systems.

Language disorders are heterogeneous, vary in levels of severity, and are generally categorized by the type of exhibited symptoms. Children with language disorders typically share four common symptoms. First, children with language delays almost always show a *deficiency in the quantity of language learned*, comprehended, and produced. Generally, these children have a sparse verbal repertoire. Limited early vocalizations, limited vocabulary, and slow learning of new words are often the first signs of a problem with learning language. These symptoms initially might be considered to be a delay in language or late emergence of language (characteristics of "late talkers") but may later be characterized as a language disorder if the symptoms persist.

A second common symptom of children with language disorders is a *deficiency in grammar.* Children with this deficiency generally have difficulty learning, comprehending, and producing language with adequate grammatical elements. Due to limited syntax, their sentences may be shorter, simpler, and often devoid of variety in language content. Their language often lacks various grammatical morphemes, such as the plural *s*, the present progressive *ing*, and articles, pronouns, and prepositions, to name a few. The syntactic or morphological deficiencies may range from subtle to very pronounced, depending on the severity of the disorder.

Third, children with language disorders may have *inadequate social communication skills.* These children may have difficulty initiating a conversation or maintaining a topic, may fail to share interest or request objects or actions, and may have difficulty understanding the rules of turn-taking in conversations.

A fourth symptom involves *deficient nonverbal communication skills.* Children with this deficiency may be delayed or impaired in their use of gestures and body language, facial expressions, and intonation and phrasing patterns, as well as their understanding of gestures to convey communicative intentions.

The developmental course of language disorders is variable. Symptomatology may range from the late emergence of language—a language delay—to more complicated diagnoses of disorders of language that may include one or more domains of language. Importantly, one must comprehend the continuum of typical development, recognize late onset of development, and be aware of the risks for delays and speech and language disorders. Pediatric surveillance and parental concerns (e.g., Bishop and McDonald 2009) may provide important diagnostic information regarding indicators of a language delay or disorder that suggest the necessity of a speech and language evaluation. Overall, those physicians caring for young children (pediatricians, family practice physicians, and child psychiatrists) are in a position to iden-tify delays early using recommended guidelines for consistent surveillance and screening of speech and language skills from infancy and throughout the school-age years. The American Academy of Pediatrics recommends that surveillance—the ongoing process of assessing the child's development and behavior—be performed at all health supervision visits. In addition, a formal screening instrument should be administered at the 9-, 18-, and 30-month visits—or at 24 months if the child is unlikely to be seen at a 30-month time point (McQuiston and Kloczko 2011).

Determining whether a developmental difference is significant and warrants further evaluation requires an understanding of the parameters of typical developmental language milestones. In terms of the acquisition of these milestones, it has been widely argued that the acquisition of language is a robust phenomenon given that the development of language occurs for children in a universal fashion (Rice et al. 2005). For instance, typically de-veloping infants are intrinsically wired with many of the foundational skills necessary for learning language, and these skills (e.g., speech discrimina-tion, production of early speech sounds) become more specialized over the first year. In general, a complex interaction between biological and envi-ronmental experiences is necessary to develop communicative competence. *Communicative competence* is the knowledge and implicit awareness that speakers of a language possess and use in order to communicate effectively (Hymes 2001), and this pivotal skill is honed over the course of develop-ment, beginning in infancy. Language development is an early pivotal skill with roots in early infancy, and thus physicians need to understand the con-tinuum of typical developmental language milestones, because as the pro-fessionals interfacing with families and their infants and children on a regular basis, they are in a position to assess whether a child is at risk for or has a delay in communicative development.

The typical acquisition and the variability of language milestones are indicated by many studies of language development (e.g., Bates et al. 1992; Bishop et al. 2003; Fenson et al. 1994; Joseph et al. 2002; Vicari et al. 2000). For example, in a seminal study conducted by Fenson et al. (1994), the av-erage word production of children age 2 years was 312 words, with a range from 7 to 668 words. One factor that accounts for this variability is the amount of language that children are exposed to in the early language-learning years. In addition, language skills have been associated with early literacy skills and the emergence of reading and written language; there-fore, a disruption in typical development may be associated with long-term negative outcomes for academic language-related skills such as reading, written language, and verbal problem-solving skills (Bishop et al. 2003). The developmental course of language disorders is highly variable and linked to a variety of issues, including early symptoms of language disorders, the type and severity of the disorder, and individual language profiles. Current screening measures do not reliably predict persistent language delay versus maturational lag followed by recovery. Factors that have been associated with early delays in expressive language include family history of language delay, low socioeconomic status, and the richness of the language environment (Bailey et al. 2004; Horowitz et al. 2003). Those children who continue to manifest speech and language delays typically require targeted and specific assessment and intervention. Early intervention programs often set a percentage delay standard to determine eligibility, which typically is 20%–30% below chronological age in one or more domains of development. Many speech-language pathologists use a criterion of 1.25 standard deviations below the mean on standardized measures or below the 10th percentile as a clinical cutoff for identifying a child in need of therapeutic services. In sum, given the heterogeneity of language disorders, as well as the comorbidity of language disorders with other neurodevelopmental phenotypes, it is necessary to understand the genetic and environmental influences that may mitigate or exacerbate the course of symptomatology.

Epidemiology

Communication disorders are among the most prevalent disabilities in early childhood. Prevalence studies suggest that 13%–18% of children ages 18–36 months present with late talking or expressive language delays, and at age 4 years, approximately 50% of the late talkers still present with language difficulties. The majority of preschool children with identified disabilities have speech, language, and communication impairments. In fact, approximately 5%–8% of children experience speech and language delays or disorders sometime during the preschool years, between ages 36 and 60 months (Bishop 2006; McQuiston and Kloczko 2011). Language disorders in preschool children are strongly associated with later-appearing academic problems, as well as emotional and behavioral disorders. About 10%–15% of school-age children have speech, language, or hearing disorders. Tomblin et al. (1997) conducted a case-control epidemiological review study of prenatal and perinatal risk factors in 177 children with specific language impairment (SLI), compared to 925 children without sensory, developmental, or language impairments, and did not find correlates for these risk factors. They did, however, postulate that environmental differences (e.g., elevated rates of learning problems in fathers, poorer educational attainment by both parents) may indicate the influence of the environment on gene expression (epigenetic influences), with environmental differences compounding genetic liabilities or buffering children from a speech and language impairment.

Genetic Risk Factors

There is a growing literature examining the genetic and environmental etiology of variance in language skills and disorders (e.g., Stromswold 2008). The field has revealed a number of interesting candidate regions for disorders of speech and language, but no specific candidate genes have been identified and sufficiently interrogated to be referred to as a candidate gene for speech and language disorders. Overall, rather than being affected by a "gene for language," SLI appears to be more affected by patterns of inheritance that do not correspond to any known dominant or recessive pattern. A case study of a three-generational family in which SLI affected 50% of children of an affected parent demonstrated a causal mutation on chromosome 7 (the forkhead box P2 gene, or *FOXP2*); however, this gene does not regulate language but rather regulates activity and appears to have an effect on the regulatory functions of speech and language (Bishop 2006; Fisher 2005). Genomewide scans have identified at least four chromosomal regions, on chromosomes 2, 13, 16, and 19, that may influence language impairments (Fisher 2005). Deciphering the genetic basis of speech and language disorders is under way, and this molecular genetic approach has potential for aiding in understanding and extrapolating the neurological pathways underlying speech and language disorders.

Developmental and Environmental Risk Factors

The environmental context in which a child is raised has long been recognized as crucial to determining developmental, including language, outcomes. Risk for language delays and disorders has long been associated with socioeconomic factors and economic deprivation. Maternal and family variables—in particular, socioeconomic indicators—have been implicated in the development of language in young children. The mother's education level and the family's socioeconomic status are considered to be proxy measures of environmental support for language learning and predictors of language impairment (Dollaghan et al. 1999; Tomblin et al. 1997). Other studies (e.g., Pan et al. 2005; Zubrick et al. 2007) have yielded mixed evidence but found maternal language and literacy to be a significant predictor of language growth in children, and lower vocabulary and reading levels in mothers were found to be directly related to lower levels of vocabulary in their children. Furthermore, maternal depression may be a mediating factor.

Overall, the environmental variables that appear to be more predictive than others for development of future language disorders are 1) high birth order (Hoff-Ginsberg 1998; Pine 1995; Tallal et al. 1989), 2) low maternal education (Paul 1991; Rice et al. 1999), and 3) single-parent home (Andrews et al. 1995; Miller and Moore 1990). A population-based investigation of birth risk factors for school-identified SLI (Stanton-Chapman et al. 2002) suggested that very low birth weight, low 5-minute Apgar scores, later or no prenatal care, high birth order, and low maternal education are associated with the highest individual population-level risk for language impairment. In addition, SLI was indicated to be more prevalent in males than females.

Animal Models

Studies have been conducted to identify genetic factors that increase susceptibility to developmental disorders of speech and language. For example, *FOXP2* has been implicated in a severe monogenic speech and language disorder (Fisher 2006). Gross chromosomal arrangements disrupting *FOXP2* have been identified in isolated cases of speech and language delay (Lai et al. 2001; Scharff and White 2004) and have provided avenues for exploration of neurogenetic mechanisms that contribute to the capacity for speech and language (Fisher et al. 2003). The identification of these genetic variances facilitates the use of animal models to explore whether an earlier version of this gene could be present in animals such as rodents and birds and provides an opportunity to understand the neuromolecular environment necessary for the evolution of vocal learning in nonlinguistic species.

Studies of expression patterns in nonspeaking species have provided insights into the potential role of the gene FoxP2 (Jarvis et al. 2000; Scharff and White 2004). Neuroanatomical and genetic investigations of bird species have indicated the presence of structures in the forebrain that are involved in vocal control for both production and learning of songs and that appear to be common for all vocal learners. For instance, two studies to address FoxP2 in songbirds (Brainard and Doupe 2002; Jarvis et al. 2000) found a notable concordance in the spatiotemporal central nervous system (CNS) expression patterns in birds and mammals; these levels of patterns and expression are comparable in relation to vocal control structures and may show some species-specific differences related to variability in vocal plasticity. Other studies have examined the spatiotemporal patterning of FoxP2 in nonhuman primates during brain development (e.g., Haesler et al. 2004; Jarvis et al. 2000), with the goal of understanding differences and similarities in primate evolution that will enhance the understanding of speech mechanisms.

In sum, studies of the FoxP2 gene in animals may provide evidence regarding the neural environments necessary for vocal learning to occur and also may help in determining more precisely the influences *FOXP2* has on the development of neural circuitry in humans. Additionally, key aspects of human vocal communication patterns involve neurogenetic mechanism modifications evident in nonspeaking animals that may provide an understanding of region-specific language roles in CNS structures. Future studies suggested by Fisher (2006) include targeted knockouts of FoxP2 in mice, with the goal of gaining developmental, anatomical, and behavioral insights into the gene function that implicates speech and language functions in humans.

Language Phenotypes in Neurodevelopmental Disorders

Language disorders are widely recognized as hallmark symptoms in other developmental disabilities, often presenting as a comorbidity component in disabilities such as autism spectrum disorder, attention-deficit/hyperactivity disorder, intellectual disabilities (e.g., Down syndrome), and learning disabilities, to name a few (Geurts and Embrechts 2008; Yoder and Warren 2004). Rice and Warren (as discussed in Rice 2004) argue that there is a need for consideration of the ways in which language disorders appear across clinical conditions, given the genetic and biobehavioral investigations within other neurodevelopmental disorders and the significance of shared symptoms of language disorders (Rice et al. 2005).

Early work in the area of SLI and behavioral, emotional, and social difficulties focused on the prevalence of psychiatric disorders, particularly behavioral difficulties, in children with SLI (e.g., Baker and Cantwell 1982; Beitchman et al. 1989). Research studies have suggested that the presence of social difficulties in children with SLI leads to social withdrawal, shyness, difficulties in peer relationships, and conduct and emotional difficulties (Durkin and Condi-Ramsden 2007; Lindsay et al. 2007). In addition, children with SLI show a delayed pattern of linguistic growth, accompanied by some aspects of deviant growth, and have developmental and language timing mechanism deviance when compared to children with language disorders (Rice 2004; Smith and Morris 2005).

Although communication deficits are part of the diagnostic criteria for autism spectrum disorder, children with this disorder vary widely in their communication skills, with some remaining nonverbal throughout their lives and others displaying adequate skills to participate in conversation. In a study by Lord et al. (2004), a subset of children with autism who were nonverbal appeared to have a deviant language system when compared to a subset of children with autism who had verbal communication skills and a diagnosis of language delay.

More is understood about the early lexical development of children with autism than of those with SLI. For children with autism, the symptom of delayed language is usually the primary referral concern. Furthermore, in autism, in contrast to SLI, pragmatic language impairments are not secondary but rather are a hallmark and primary feature.

As discussed in Chapter 3, fragile X syndrome (FXS) is the most common form of inherited mental retardation and is often comorbid with autism (Bailey et al. 1998). Although the language development of FXS is not as well understood as that of other disorders, the individuals' delays in language development appear to be congruent with their nonverbal language delays (Abbeduto and Murphy 2004). Boys with FXS acquire expressive language skills more slowly than girls with FXS; however, similar to children with Williams syndrome, children with FXS have a relative strength in verbal abilities when compared to their visual and spatial skills across cognitive tasks (Bailey et al. 2004).

In contrast to children with some of the other language phenotypes, children with Williams syndrome have a delay in language development and make developmental errors that are consistent with those of typically developing children at younger ages. Children with Williams syndrome have a pattern of language skills being greater than nonverbal skills, whereas children with SLI have the opposite pattern, with nonverbal skills being greater than language skills (Mervis 2004).

Children with Down syndrome present with a disordered language system, with vocabulary skills less impaired than grammatical abilities (Yoder and Warren 2004), and have an overall slower acquisition of language. Unlike children with the other language phenotypes described, children with Down syndrome have significant problems in speech production (Abbeduto and Murphy 2004).

Thus, each of these neurodevelopmental disorders has a signature pattern of language development and impairment that defines the norm for that disorder, although individual differences are marked in all of the disorders and range from near-normal language functioning to severe language impairments and lack of verbal language.

Diagnostic Evaluation of Speech and Language Disorders

Because of the variety of communication disorders, many different assessment and intervention tools are used by professionals. The purpose of assessment is not only to determine a child's skills in a particular area, but also to use the information obtained during the assessment to determine a diagnosis and to target specific areas for intervention. In general, communication assessment has four purposes: 1) to identify skills that a person does and does not possess in a particular area of communication; 2) to guide the design of intervention for enhancing a person's skills in a particular area of communication; 3) to monitor a person's communicative performance and progress over time; and 4) to determine whether a person meets eligibility requirements for educational and therapeutic services (Friberg 2010; Justice 2010).

In general, speech-language professionals use their clinical skills and knowledge of current research to design a highly individualized, sensitive, comprehensive, nonbiased, and family-centered assessment for each person. While performing the clinical activities necessary to assess a child's language skills, clinicians gather quantitative data by measuring the communicative behaviors they observe. They make efforts to describe communicative behaviors in ways that are observable and measurable—for example, by stating that they are measuring "the number of times a child correctly responds to two-part verbal directions" rather than "language competence." Overall, measurement is an integral part of clinical assessment. Thus, a clinician's diagnostic judgment should be based on both qualitative and quantitative data generated by repeated measurements of specific language behaviors in different response modes and under varied stimulus conditions (Friberg 2010; Hegde 1996). Most important is that diagnostic decisions should never be based solely on the analysis of a single diagnostic test.

Psychometric tests play an important role in the identification of children with language impairments. These tests provide important diagnostic information about language functions and are used to compare a child's performance to normative data. Many diagnostic tests and empirical research guidelines exist for assessing communicative disorder risk, delay, and disability in infants and toddlers, as well as in preschoolers and school-age children. Early language precursors, such as gestures, reciprocal interactions, and imitation in play and in speech, can be assessed very early in development. A variety of diagnostic tests are used during the assessment process, and intervention criteria should be based on standardized measures of both receptive language and expressive language. The assessment process is generally systematic and comprehensive in scope and usually involves the following sequence: completing developmental screening (and making a referral if specified), administering the assessment protocol, interpreting the assessment findings, identifying a disorder, determining a diagnosis, and developing an intervention plan.

The diagnostic tools used in a speech and language evaluation allow the clinician to determine the diagnosis. In general, a language disorder diagnosis is based on the language assessment criteria from a variety of standardized and nonstandardized tools used to determine whether the individual's communication skills 1) are markedly discrepant from what is considered typical development and 2) interfere to a significant degree with the individual's performance in major life settings such as home and school. Information is generally included from the following assessment procedures: case history (includes prenatal and birth history, medical history, developmental history, general behavior, and educational history), parent interview, standardized measures, parent report measures, language sampling, orofacial examination (to check speech structures of the face and mouth, as well as gross anatomical and physiological deviations that may be associated with the speech and language disorder), and hearing screening. Overall, assessments are conducted to assess language understanding, speech production, nonverbal communicative behaviors (e.g., gestures, pointing), and the function and use of language. These assessment areas are directly related to types of language disorders and provide evidence for diagnostic criteria for communication disorders.

Types of Language Disorders and Diagnostic Criteria

Childhood speech and language disorders have traditionally been classified into mutually exclusive categories using a medical model of diagnosis based on etiological or contributory factors. Currently, the most widely used diagnostic classification system for determining a speech and language disorder is DSM-IV-TR. In the forthcoming DSM-5, a major revision for categorizing communication disorders is proposed, and diagnostic categories have been added and changed, with specific rationales based on current research and empirical studies. The proposed communication disorders will be included under the diagnostic category of neurodevelopmental disorders and comprise the following: language impairment, late language emergence (LLE), specific language impairment (SLI), social communication disorder (SCD), speech sound disorder (SSD), childhood onset fluency disorder, and voice disorder. Although the DSM-5 criteria are not yet finalized, information in this chapter is based on the most current information available from the DSM-5 committee; however, further changes may appear in the final publication, due in 2013.

Language Impairment

Under the proposed DSM-5 criteria, children with language impairment have language abilities that are below age expectations in one or more of the following: comprehension, production, pragmatics, and written language. Generally, diagnosis with language impairment indicates that children have lower abilities in language than chronological-age peers throughout their developmental trajectory (e.g., Bishop et al. 2003; Catts et al. 2002; Tomblin and Zhang 2006). Symptoms must be present in early childhood; however, the severity and impact of this impairment may not be fully manifested until later, when more specific cognitive demands are placed on the individual in the language and learning environment of the classroom; then, the impairment may be seen to coexist with other disorders such as learning disabilities.

Late Language Emergence

The LLE category is defined as delayed language onset with developmental language trajectories below expectations for children ages 8–36 months, based on age-referenced developmental criteria. LLE may be observed in children up to age 4–5 years. During clinical visits, physicians can inquire about language abilities, especially if the parent raises concerns that a child is not talking or has very limited interest in repeating words, or both. Some of the indicators include having a limited vocabulary, few word combinations, limited use of gestures, and difficulty following verbal commands—all of which affect functional and social use of language in a variety of contexts—without evidence of any other diagnosed disabilities or significant delays in other domains. Well child developmental surveillance will often flag such cases as needing further follow-up. Identifying toddlers with LLE provides an opportunity to refer these children to early intervention and may mitigate the development of a language impairment (Tager-Flusberg and Cooper 1999; Watt et al. 2006; Wetherby et al. 2003).

Specific Language Impairment

SLI is diagnosed when a child's language development is deficient with no obvious explanation, including no intellectual impairment or hearing loss, and the child has typical nonverbal cognitive performance. The prevalence of SLI has been estimated to be around 7%, although this may vary depending on the diagnostic criteria used and the child's age (Tomblin et al. 1997). Children with SLI have significant difficulty learning to talk, despite showing typical development in all other areas. In general, language development is delayed, with delayed development of grammatical forms and the presence of a limited vocabulary (Bishop 2006). Parents may become concerned about the immaturity of their child's speech and mention this during a visit to the pediatrician. The physician should be concerned if the child presents with typical development in other areas but appears to have significant difficulty with grammatical aspects of speech. For example, a 7-year-old child may use simplified speech more indicative of a preschool-age child and produce sentences such as "me go there" instead of "I went there." In sum, the inclusionary criteria state that language skills are below age-level expectations and nonverbal cognitive skills are at age-level expectations (and may exceed expectations). Unlike some of the other diagnostic categories of language impairment, SLI is suggestive of a genetic influence and is considered to resemble complex genetic disorders in which there are known patterns of inheritance in families that do not correspond to a specific known dominant or recessive pattern of occurrence (Bishop 2002; Fisher 2005; Vargha-Khadem et al. 2005). A candidate gene on chromosome 6 has been identified as significant in that it provides contributions of a shared type for SLI and reading disability (e.g., Rice et al. 2009), and other studies have identified trait loci on chromosomes 16 and 19 for SLI (e.g., Falcaro et al. 2008). Overall, multiple genetic and environmental risk factors appear to be implicated in SLI, and SLI appears to be a disorder with dimensions of impairment.

Social Communication Disorder

SCD is described as a disorder of pragmatic skills and is diagnosed when the social aspects of children's communication skills are limited, with difficulty using language appropriately in social contexts. Children with SCD have intact vocabulary and sentence structure abilities, but they do not use language in typical ways in social communication contexts to engage in typical childhood banter, discourse, and conversation that is appropriate and meaningful to the context. These children may sound like "little professors," as many have an unusually sophisticated vocabulary; however, they often use odd words and phrases, have difficulty initiating and sustaining conversation, and are challenged by understanding social cues. These difficulties particularly affect their social interactions and relationships with peers.

Speech Sound Disorder

SSD is defined as a disorder in which the speech output (production) does not include speech sounds that are appropriate for development. Parents may mention that they are concerned that others do not seem to understand their child's speech or that the preschool teacher requested that a parent see the pediatrician about the issue. These production difficulties, often referred to as phonological disorders or articulation problems, include deviant phonological processes such as final consonant deletion (e.g., "boa" for "boat"), substitutions (e.g., "tup" for "cup"), and vowel distortions, to name a few. This disorder may coexist with other disorders, including cleft palate, apraxia, and cerebral palsy, any of which may further affect the severity of the SSD. The impact on severity is most significant in the area of childhood apraxia of speech (Lewis et al. 2006; Smith and Morris 2005). In this disorder, children have a limited repertoire of sounds, a significant rate of sound omissions and distortions, and an inconsistent pattern of errors, which all affect the severity level of the intelligibility rating. Notably, articulation disorders generally respond to intervention strategies that focus on specific deviant phonological processes that are evident in the child's speech production. Apraxia, on the other hand, is a *severe* phonological disorder and requires protracted, intensive intervention with specific skills targeted to enhance articulatory motor movements and sequences, since these are also severely affected in this disorder.

Childhood Onset Fluency Disorder

Childhood onset fluency disorder is called "stuttering" in DSM-IV, but a change in the diagnostic label has been recommended to be consistent with the World Health Organization's (2001) *International Statistical Classification of Diseases and Related Health Problems,* Tenth Revision (ICD-10). The essential feature of this disorder is a disturbance in the normal fluency and time patterning of speech that is inappropriate for the individual's age, with the onset usually occurring between ages 2 and 7 years. This disorder is characterized by frequent occurrences of the following fluency disruptions: sound and syllable repetitions (e.g., "Wh-wh-wh-why is he going?"), sound prolongations (e.g., "Eeeeeat the cereal"), whole-word repetitions (e.g., "He-He-He is a boy"), and circumlocutions (word substitutions to avoid problematic words). The extent of the stuttering behaviors varies depending on the situation, and the stuttering is often more severe when the individual is under special pressure to communicate. Stress and anxiety may exacerbate the dysfluency, and as the child becomes aware of the difficulty in speaking, he or she may develop mechanisms for avoiding the dysfluencies. Stuttering suggests that neurological pathways are implicated. This disorder has similarities with other tic disorders that wax and wane and are linked to abnormalities in basal ganglia function.

Voice Disorder

A voice disorder involves abnormalities in the area of vocal quality, pitch, loudness, and duration that persist over a period of time. Because the voice is affected, this disorder may also diminish effectiveness of communicative interactions and social participation. Symptoms of a voice disorder may include hoarse or harsh-sounding speech, and parents may report that their children talk loudly and seem to be straining their voice when speaking. A pediatrician should decide whether voice problems indicate a need for follow-up with an ear, nose, and throat specialist. Sometimes voice disorders require medical intervention for possible vocal nodules, and subsequent language intervention may be necessary to help children use a modal pitch that does not strain their vocal cords. Voice atypicalities often go unnoticed by parents, and thus clinicians should interview parents of children with voice disorders to determine the history of unusual voice patterns and possible need for follow-up care. When voice problems in children go undetected and untreated, they can lead to damage to the vocal cords and vocal tract.

Language Intervention in Speech and Language Disorders

In recent years, emphasis on the use of evidence-based practice in speech-language pathology has been growing (e.g., Dollaghan 2004; Goldstein 2002; Justice and Fey 2004; Meline and Paradiso 2003). Evidence-based practice stresses that clinical decision making should entail consideration of evidence from multiple sources: systematic research, the clinician's own clinical experience, and the values and preferences of the person(s) being served. Apel and Scudder (2005) suggested that additional advantages of evidence-based practice include better accountability to clients and their families. As characterized by the American Speech-Language-Hearing Association (2006), the process entails four steps: framing the clinical question, finding the evidence, assessing the evidence, and making the clinical decision. The use of this four-step process in the field of speech and language pathology can both improve and validate clinical services, and it promotes increased interactions between clinicians and researchers.

Overall, treatment in communication disorders is designed to change the way children interact with their verbal community, as well as the way the verbal community interacts with children (e.g., Hegde and Maul 2006). Clinicians promote naturalistic maintenance of newly taught language skills by changing the communicative behaviors of people who typically interact with the children in treatment. Given the range of communication disorders, a specific treatment plan should be individualized; however, all treatment plans should be designed in partnership with caregivers, teachers, and others who are consistent communication partners for the child receiving services. In treating language disorders, clinicians generally use the following guidelines for treatment:

1. Select target behaviors based on the principles of a targeted behavior selection framework. (Parents and caregivers along with teachers should be partners in selecting the skills to be taught.)

2. Establish baselines to understand the pretreatment levels of the selected target behaviors and to compare progress the child makes (or does not make) during treatment.
3. Choose intervention procedures and approaches based on evidence-based practices when possible.
4. Begin treatment based on the target behaviors selected.
5. Select probes for initial treatment response or behavior change.
6. Promote maintenance by training parents and others to support and help generalize the behaviors in the home and other contexts.
7. Provide postdismissal follow-up assessment to ascertain skill maintenance and generalization, and provide booster treatment sessions if skills are not maintained.

In summary, the basic treatment plan, probe, and maintenance procedures should be clear from the treatment onset, and these all need to be supported by parents and teachers. All of the elements of the basic sequence of treatment should be described in a written plan and then discussed with caregivers and teachers, with the goal of providing relevant activities, contexts, and opportunities for skills to be acquired naturalistically across clinical, home, and classroom environments. In addition, important intervention principles should be considered, including the following: early intervention, parental involvement, naturalistic environments, social interactions, functional outcomes, least restrictive environment, discourse-level skills, and speech and language skills in the academic environment.

Early Intervention

Early therapeutic intervention is a primary prevention strategy aimed at keeping a disorder from developing (especially if a child is considered at risk for developing a language delay) or at least reducing the disorder's severity. Many young children with language delays may have a developmental disorder such as autism spectrum disorder, an intellectual or global developmental disorder, or an acquired disorder such as a brain injury, or they may be vulnerable to developing a disorder due to various risk factors. Empirical evidence demonstrates that early language intervention is an effective tactic for reducing the negative outcomes associated with early language difficulties (e.g., Reynolds et al. 2001; Ward 1999) and that interventions can be implemented early in development. Further, an abundance of empirical evidence supports positive developmental outcomes for early communication intervention with infants and toddlers (Mahoney et al. 1999; Mitchell et al. 2006; Olswang et al. 1998), as well as preschool-age children (e.g., Justice et al. 2008; La Paro et al. 2004).

Parental Involvement

Parents play a critical role in fostering language development (Tamis-LeMonda et al. 2001) and should be provided with specific information to help them enhance their children's language-learning environment early in developmental surveillance and in early intervention contexts. For instance, the number of words children experience in their interactions with family members contributes to the speed with which children learn new words and the types of words they learn (Hart and Risley 1995). The following basic principles of family-centered practice (Dunst 1993) are recommended for clinicians: making the family rather than the individual the unit of intervention; fostering the family's sense of competence and independence in the intervention; respecting the parents' rights and responsibility to determine what is best for their child (in terms of treatment); helping to mobilize resources for coordinated, normalized service delivery; and developing a collaborative relationship with the family.

The shift to family-centered practice is evident in health care as well as education. Although family involvement was mandated by the Education for All Handicapped Children Act of 1975 (EHA; P.L. 94-142) in the Individualized Education Program (IEP) process, the EHA amendments of 1986 (P.L. 99-457) and the Individuals with Disabilities Education Act Amendment enacted in 1990 (IDEA; P.L. 101-496) and reauthorized in 1997 and 2004 require movement toward family-centered practice. Family-centered practice is essential when working with infants and toddlers but also should be utilized with preschool children if possible. Many current studies use parent-mediated interventions to promote precursor language skills (e.g., gestures, turn-taking, joint attention) and to actively involve parents in language interventions by training them to use specific strategies and techniques to facilitate children's language skills, with parents thereby playing key roles and implementing effective practices in language intervention treatment (e.g., Coulter and Gallagher 2001; Girolametto et al. 2006; Law et al. 2004).

Naturalistic Environments

The provision of services in children's natural environments plays a critical part in language interventions for very young children. The EHA amendments of 1986 mandate that infants and toddlers (ages birth to 3 years) who are at risk for or who have disabilities should have Individualized Family Service Plans, case management, and a comprehensive plan of services, and that the intervention should be provided in naturalistic environments. Working in the child's natural environments promotes development of language opportunities in the context of familiar activities and routines. Working in the home environment also helps parents (guided by the therapist) to learn specific language stimulation strategies. For example, during snack time, the therapist might observe the parent preparing a snack and subsequently engaging with the child. The therapist can use the context of this activity to provide specific strategies to the parent and structure the snack routine to encourage the child's use of requesting behaviors. In these naturalistic environments, the parents are considered to be partners in the intervention, with the direction and guidance of the clinician.

Social Interactions

Rather than participating in rote drill and practice tasks, children with language disorders should be engaged in meaningful interactions with others to have opportunities to apply new language forms, content, and use (McQuiston and Kloczko 2011). When a child is engaged in meaningful social interactions, his or her use of emerging forms and functions is recognized as having communicative value. For example, instead of asking a child to look at pictures and repeat the name of pictured objects, a parent can engage the child in joint play with objects, which requires asking for an actual toy and requesting particular actions. This approach provides more meaningful, authentic opportunities for communicating and engaging children in intervention.

Functional Outcomes

Language interventions should target outcomes that are meaningful and that have value in home, school, and community contexts, and these interventions should be considered within a developmental framework (Tager-Flusberg et al. 2009). For instance, if a child is working on grammatical development, a language goal that targets repetition of 10 noun phrases (e.g., "the dog," "the plate," "the ball") in an intervention session has little developmental relevance or functional value. A more relevant developmental goal would be for the child to use noun phrases to specify requests, such as using phrases for commenting or requesting during mealtime routines (e.g., "I like butter," "want more milk," "no more peas").

Least Restrictive Environment

Providing language intervention to children in the least restrictive environment is mandated by federal law. IDEA stipulates that children with disabilities are to be educated with their peers to the greatest extent possible. Many children with language disorders receive their language intervention through "pull-out" therapies, usually provided in a resource room or language therapy room outside the classroom. This pull-out model has garnered criticism because children are removed from the context in which they need to learn to perform—inside the classroom (e.g., Bashir et al. 1998). The premise behind least restrictive environment, in contrast, is that children need to "learn, practice, and apply skills with their classmates in the communicative context of the classroom" (DiMeo et al. 1998, p. 39). This model promotes providing therapy to children directly in their classrooms and using a consultative or collaborative model in which speech-language pathologists and teachers work together to develop and monitor children's language goals.

Discourse-Level Skills

Language intervention for school-age children requires an intensive focus on discourse-level skills—that is, using language for narrative and conversational purposes. Instructional discourse can be very challenging for children with language disorders because it requires the integration of form, content, and use, all of which may be areas of challenge and weakness for these children. Because classroom discourse is not usually accompanied by visual cues to assist with the interpretation of the discourse, children have to rely on their linguistic skills for interpretation. Interventions should focus on providing ample opportunities for a child to participate in discourse at various levels of complexity—including conversation, narrative, and instructional discourse—with the clinician providing intervention strategies, including multisensory supports, to maximize participation and acquisition of discourse skills (e.g., Merritt et al. 1998).

Academic Speech and Language Skills

Children with language disorders often struggle with academic requirements, including reading, writing, and spelling; therefore, language intervention should focus on developing skills that are critically linked to success in these areas (Justice and Schuele 2004). One area of particular difficulty for children with language impairments is phonological awareness, which is the ability to attend to units of sound that make up continuous speech; low ability in this area is a key deficit in children with dyslexia (see Chapter 10, "Disorders of Learning"). During preschool years, children with such difficulties are slower than others in phonological awareness games such as making rhymes, and during early elementary grades, these children have difficulty identifying the number of syllables in words and the associations between letters and their phonetic sounds. Problems with phonological awareness contribute to the deficits in reading and spelling that are prevalent among children with language disorders (Catts et al. 2002). Integrating specific literacy goals in the language intervention is increasingly important for these children; children should be prompted to think about the phonological composition of words (e.g., the word *dog* has three sounds, whereas the word *dogs* has four sounds). Children with language impairments have difficulty with tasks that require a conscious reflection on language (e.g., "Circle all of the nouns in this passage," "Is the word *caterpillar* considered to be a long or short word?"); therefore, providing learning opportunities for them to be frequently engaged in these metalinguistic tasks is an important aspect of language intervention for school-age children.

Outcomes

Language disorders are heterogeneous, vary in severity, and often co-occur with other neurodevelopmental disorders. Differentiating language delay, language deviance, and late language emergence requires continued surveillance of emerging and deviant language skills. Children with persistent language disorders are at high risk for developing learning disabilities, including disabilities in reading and written language. Interventions for children with both language delays and language disorders have more positive predicted language outcomes when the interventions are early and targeted and when parents and teachers are involved with the goal of generalizing language behaviors across contexts. Studies of language acquisition have been sensitive to the need for age-referenced benchmarks, but little attention has been given to the goal of determining specificity of language treatment by investigating how these normative benchmarks are tied into children's biological mechanisms in interaction with environmental influences (Fisher et al. 2003).

New Research Directions

Across different dimensions of language disorders, individual profiles consist of relative areas of strength and weakness in each of the developmental language disorders, suggesting that the dimensions of speech, semantics, syntax, and pragmatics warrant differentiation in descriptions of symptoms of language disorders. Currently, research is needed to provide systematic comparisons of dimensions across disorders at greater levels of specificity. For instance, the contrast between delayed versus deviant aspects of language acquisition demonstrates considerable promise in providing an overarching perspective on the ways in which language impairments can be specifically manifested. Clearly, this contrast plays out differently across various dimensions of language and might be better clarified through additional studies of longitudinal growth data across clinical conditions (Hayiou-Thomas 2008). In addition, future studies need to examine issues related to the underlying timing mechanisms at work in various neurodevelopmental disorders, as well as the ways in which communication disorders are connected to underlying neurocognitive and genetic factors. Advances in genetics and neurocognitive measurement promise new avenues of inquiry (e.g., Bishop 2002; Fisher et al. 2003; Newbury and Monaco 2010)—and potentially for treatment.

At the same time, routine developmental surveillance must be conducted to determine language symptomatology that indicates children who are at risk for speech and language problems. In addition, early intervention for young children with language impairments should be monitored to track positive developmental outcomes. Individualized language intervention targets for these very young children should be chosen to ensure successful communicative attempts that continue to build on other specific communicative skills. The pediatric clinician is in a unique position to identify delays early, and the impact that this early identification may have on the road to positive language developmental outcomes is significant. Language development provides the best early correlate to cognitive development, and because communication delays can result in significant comorbid dysfunction, a child's speech and language functioning should be a major consideration in surveillance and screening, with the goal of significantly enhancing both prevention and early intervention approaches in the future.

Key Points

- A language disorder may involve a disruption in one or more of the following areas: 1) the form of language (phonology, morphology, syntax); 2) the content of language (semantics); and 3) the function or use of language in social communication (pragmatics).

- Language disorders are heterogeneous, vary in levels of severity, and are generally categorized by the types of exhibited symptoms.

- Children with language disorders typically share four common symptoms: 1) a deficiency in quantity of language learned, comprehended, and produced; 2) a deficiency in grammar; 3) inadequate social communication skills; and 4) deficient nonverbal communication skills.

- The developmental course of language disorders is variable, with symptomatology ranging from late emergence of language to more complicated diagnoses of language disorders.

- Communication disorders are among the most prevalent disabilities in early childhood. Language disorders in preschool are strongly associated with later-appearing academic problems as well as emotional and behavioral disorders.

- Language phenotypes in neurodevelopmental disorders are common and often present as a comorbidity component in disabilities such as autism spectrum disorder, attention-deficit/hyperactivity disorder, intellectual disabilities, and learning disabilities.

- Types of language disorders have been revised in the forthcoming DSM-5 to include the following under the diagnostic category of neurodevelopmental disorders: language impairment, late language emergence, specific language impairment, social communication disorder, speech sound disorder, childhood onset fluency disorder, and voice disorder.

- Early intervention is a primary prevention strategy aimed at keeping a disorder from developing or, at least, reducing the severity of the disorder.

- Language interventions should utilize evidence-based practices, include functional outcomes, involve parents, engage children in meaningful social interactions, and provide intervention in the least restrictive environment. Language interventions for school-age children should focus on discourse-level skills and academic-related speech and language skills, including reading, writing, and spelling, and should include intensive and comprehensive classroom interventions.

Recommended Readings

Joseph RM, Tager-Flusberg H, Lord C: Cognitive profiles and social-communicative functioning in children with autism spectrum disorder. J Child Psychol Psychiatry 43:807–821, 2002

Law J, Garrett Z Nye C: The efficacy of treatment for children with developmental speech and language delay/disorder. J Speech Lang Hear Res 47:924–943, 2004

Mervis CB: Cross-etiology comparisons of cognitive and language development, in Developmental Language Disorders: From Phenotypes to Etiologies. Edited by Rice ML, Warren SF. Mahwah, NJ, Erlbaum, 2004, pp 153–186

McQuiston S, Kloczko N: Speech and language development: monitoring processes and problems. Pediatr Rev 32:230–239, 2011

Tager-Flusberg H, Rogers S, Cooper J, et al: Defining spoken language benchmarks and selecting measures of expressive language development for young children with autism spectrum disorders. J Speech Lang Hear Res 52:643–652, 2009

References

Abbeduto L, Murphy MM: Language, social cognition, maladaptive behavior and communication in Down syndrome and fragile X syndrome, in Developmental Language Disorders: From Phenotypes to Etiologies. Edited by Rice ML, Warren SF. Mahwah, NJ, Erlbaum, 2004, pp 77–97

American Psychiatric Association: Diagnostic and Statistical Manual of Mental Disorders, 4th Edition, Text Revision. Washington, DC, American Psychiatric Association, 2000

American Speech-Language-Hearing Association: 2006 Schools Survey. Rockville, MD, American Speech-Language-Hearing Association, 2006

Andrews H, Goldberg D, Wellen N, et al: Prediction of special education placement from birth certificate data. Am J Prev Med 11:55–61, 1995

Apel K, Scudder RR: Integrating evidence-based practice instruction into the curriculum. Perspectives on Issues in Higher Education 8:10–14, 2005

Bailey DB, Mesibov GB, Hatton DD, et al: Autistic behavior in young boys with fragile X syndrome. J Autism Dev Disord 28:499–508, 1998

Bailey DB, Heebeler K, Scarborough A, et al: First experiences with early intervention: a national perspective. Pediatrics 113:887–896, 2004

Baker L, Cantwell DP: Language acquisition, cognitive development, and emotional disorder in children, in Children's Language, Vol 3. Edited by Nelson KE. Hillsdale, NJ, Erlbaum, 1982, pp 286–321

Bashir AS, Conte B, Heerde SM: Language and school success: collaborative challenges and choices, in Language Intervention in the Classroom. Edited by Merritt DD, Cullatta B. San Diego, CA, Singular Publishing, 1998, pp 1–36

Bates E, Thal D, Janowsky J: Early language development and its neural correlates, in Handbook of Neuropsychology, Vol 7: Child Neuropsychology. Edited by Rapin I, Segalowitz SJ. Amsterdam, The Netherlands, Elsevier, 1992, pp 69–110

Beitchman J, Hood J, Rochon J, et al: Empirical classification of speech/language impairment in children. J Am Acad Child Adolesc Psychiatry 28:118–123, 1989

Bishop DV: The role of genes in the etiology of specific language impairment. J Commun Disord 35:311–328, 2002

Bishop DV: What causes specific language impairment in children? Curr Dir Psychol Sci 15:217–221, 2006

Bishop DV, McDonald D: Identifying language impairment in children: combining language test scores with parental report. Int J Lang Commun Disord 44:600–615, 2009

Bishop DV, Price T, Dale P, et al: Outcomes of early language delay: etiology of transient and persistent language difficulties. J Speech Lang Hear Res 46:561–575, 2003

Bloom L, Lahey M: Language Development and Language Disorders. New York, Wiley, 1978

Brainard M, Doupe AJ: What songbirds teach us about learning. Nature 417:351–358, 2002

Catts H, Fey M, Tomblin J, et al: A longitudinal investigation of reading outcomes in children with language impairments. J Speech Lang Hear Res 45:1142–1157, 2002

Coulter L, Gallagher C: Evaluation of the Hanen Early Childhood Educators programme. Int J Lang Comm Disord 36:264–269, 2001

DiMeo JH, Merritt DD, Cullatta B: Collaborative partnerships and decision making, in Language Intervention in the Classroom. Edited by Merritt DD, Cullatta B. San Diego, CA, Singular, 1998, pp 37–98

Dollaghan CA: Evidence-based practice in communication disorders: what do we know, and when do we know it? J Commun Disord 37:391–400, 2004

Dollaghan CA, Campbell T, Paradise J, et al: Maternal education and measures of early speech and language. J Speech Lang Hear Res 42:1432–1443, 1999

Dunst C: Implications of risk and opportunity factors for assessment and intervention practices. Topics Early Child Spec Educ 13:143–153, 1993

Durkin K, Condi-Ramsden G: Language, social behavior, and the quality of friendships in adolescence with and without a history of specific language impairment. Child Dev 78:1441–1457, 2007

Education for All Handicapped Children Act of 1975, Pub. L. 94-142, sec. 1, 89 Stat. 773

Education of the Handicapped Act Amendments of 1986, Pub. L. 99-457, sec. 1(a), 100 Stat. 1145

Falcaro M, Pickles A, Newbury DF, et al: Genetics and phenotypic effects of phonological short-term memory and grammatical morphology in specific language impairment. Genes Brain Behav 7:393–402, 2008

Fenson L, Dale PS, Reznick JS, et al: Variability in early communicative development. Monogr Soc Res Child Dev 59:1–185, 1994

Fisher SE: Dissection of molecular mechanisms underlying speech and language disorders. Appl Psycholinguist 160:636–645, 2005

Fisher SE: How can animal studies help to uncover the roles of genes implicated in human speech and language disorders? in Transgenic and Knockout Models of Neuropsychiatric Disorders. Edited by Fisch GS, Flint J. Totowa, NJ, Humana Press, 2006, pp 127–149

Fisher SE, Lai C, Monaco A: Deciphering the genetic basis of speech and language disorders. Ann Rev Neurosci 26:57–80, 2003

Friberg J: Considerations for test selection: how do validity and reliability impact diagnostic decisions? Child Lang Teach Ther 26:77–92, 2010

Geurts H, Embrechts M: Language profiles in ASD, SLI, and ADHD. J Autism Dev Disord 38:1931–1943, 2008

Girolametto L, Greenberg J, Weitzman E: Facilitating language skills: inservice education for early childhood educators and preschool teachers. Infants & Young Children 19:36–46, 2006

Goldstein H: Communication intervention for children with autism: a review of treatment efficacy. J Autism Dev Disord 32:373–396, 2002

Haesler S, Wada K, Nshedjan A, et al: FoxP2 expression in avian vocal learners and non-learners J Neurosci 24:3164–3175, 2004

Hart B, Risley T: Meaningful Differences in the Everyday Experience of Young American Children. Baltimore, MD, Paul H. Brookes Publishing, 1995

Hayiou-Thomas M: Genetic and environmental influences on early speech, language and literacy development. J Commun Disord 41:397–408, 2008

Hegde MN: A Coursebook on Language Disorders in Children. San Diego, CA, Singular, 1996

Hegde MN, Maul C: Language Disorders in Children: An Evidence-Based Approach to Assessment and Treatment. Boston, MA, Pearson Education/Allyn & Bacon, 2006

Hoff-Ginsberg E: The relation of birth order and socioeconomic status to children's language experience and language development. Appl Psycholinguist 19:603–629, 1998

Horowitz SM, Irwin JR, Briggs-Gowan MJ et al: Language delay in a community cohort of young children. J Am Acad Child Adolesc Psychiatry 42:932–937, 2003

Hymes D: On communicative competence, in Linguistic Anthropology: A Reader. Edited by Duranti A. Malden, MA, Blackwell, 2001, pp 53–73

Individuals with Disabilities Education Act Amendments of 1990, Pub. L. 101-476, sec. 1(a), Oct. 30, 1990, 104 Stat. 1103[reauthorized 1997, 2004]

Jarvis E, Ribeiro S, da Silva ML, et al: Behaviourally driven gene expression reveals song nuclei in hummingbird brain. Nature 406:628–632, 2000

Joseph RM, Tager-Flusberg H, Lord C: Cognitive profiles and social-communicative functioning in children with autism spectrum disorder. J Child Psychol Psychiatry 43:807–821, 2002

Justice LM: When craft and science collide: Improving therapeutic practices through evidence-based innovations. Int J Speech Lang Pathol 12:79–86, 2010

Justice LM, Fey ME: Evidence-based practice in schools: integrating craft and theory with science and data. ASHA Lead, September 21, 2004, pp 4–5, 30–32

Justice LM, Schuele M: Phonological awareness: description, assessment, and intervention, in Articulation and Phonological Disorders, 5th Edition. Edited by Bernthal J, Bankson N. New York, Allyn & Bacon, 2004, pp 376–406

Justice LM, Pullen PC, Pence K: Influence of verbal and nonverbal references to print on preschoolers' visual attention to print during storybook reading. Dev Psychol 44:855–866, 2008

Lai C, Fisher S, Hurst J, et al: A novel forkhead-domain gene is mutated in a severe speech and language disorder. Nature 313:519–523, 2001

La Paro KM, Justice L, Skibbe LE, et al: Relations among maternal, child, and demographic factors and the persistence of preschool language impairment. Am J Speech Lang Pathol 13:291–303, 2004

Law J, Garrett Z, Nye C: The efficacy of treatment for children with developmental speech and language delay/disorder. J Speech Lang Hear Res 47:924–943, 2004

Lewis DA, Freebaim LA, Hansen AJ, et al: Dimensions of early speech sound disorders: a factor analytic study. J Commun Disord 39:139–157, 2006

Lindsay G, Dockrell JE, Strand S: Longitudinal patterns of behaviour problems in children with specific speech and language difficulties: child and contextual factors. Br J Educ Psychol 77:811–828, 2007

Lord C, Shulman, C, DiLavore P: Regression and word loss in autistic spectrum disorders. J Child Psychol Psychiatry 45:936–955, 2004

Mahoney G, Kaiser A, Girolametto L, et al: Parent education in early intervention: a call for a renewed focus. Topics Early Child Spec Educ 19:131–140, 1999

McQuiston S, Kloczko N: Speech and language development: monitoring processes and problems. Pediatr Rev 32:230–239, 2011

Meline T, Paradiso T: Evidence-based practice in schools. Lang Speech Hear Serv Sch 34:273–283, 2003

Merritt DD, Barton J, Cullatta B: Instructional discourse: a framework for learning, in Language Intervention in the Classroom. Edited by Merritt DD, Cullatta B. San Diego, CA, Singular, 1998, pp 143–174

Mervis CB: Cross-etiology comparisons of cognitive and language development, in Developmental Language Disorders: From Phenotypes to Etiologies. Edited by Rice ML, Warren SF. Mahwah, NJ, Erlbaum, 2004, pp 153–186

Miller BC, Moore KA: Adolescent sexual behavior, pregnancy, and parenting: research through the 1980s. J Marriage Fam 52:1025–1044, 1990

Mitchell S, Brian J, Zwaigenbaum L, et al: Early language and communication development of infants later diagnosed with autism spectrum disorder. J Dev Behav Pediatr 27:69–78, 2006

Newbury DF, Monaco AP: Genetic advances in the study of speech and language disorders. Neuron 68:309–320, 2010

Olswang L, Rodriguez B, Timler G: Recommending intervention for toddlers with specific language learning difficulties. Am J Speech Lang Pathol 7:23–32, 1998

Pan B, Rowe ML, Singer JD, et al: Maternal correlates of growth in toddler vocabulary production in low income families. Child Dev 76:763–782, 2005

Paul R: Profiles of toddlers with slow expressive language development. Top Lang Disord 11:1–13, 1991

Pine J: Variation in vocabulary development as a function of birth order. Child Dev 66:272–281, 1995

Reynolds A, Temple J, Robertson D, et al: Long-term effects of an early childhood intervention on educational achievement and juvenile arrest. JAMA 285:2239–2346, 2001

Rice ML: Growth models of developmental language disorders, in Developmental Language Disorders: From Phenotypes to Etiologies. Edited by Rice ML, Warren SF. Mahwah, NJ, Erlbaum, 2004, pp 207–240

Rice ML, Spitz RV, O'Brien M: Semantic and morphosyntactic language outcomes in biologically at-risk children. J Neurolinguistics 12:213–234, 1999

Rice ML, Warren SF, Betz SK: Language symptoms of developmental language disorders: an overview of autism, Down syndrome, fragile X, specific language impairment and Williams syndrome. Appl Psycholinguist 26:7–27, 2005

Rice ML, Smith SD, Gayán J: Convergent genetic linkage and associations to language, speech and reading measures in families of probands with specific language impairment. J Neurodev Disord 1:264–282, 2009

Scharff C, White SA: Genetic components of vocal learning. Ann NY Acad Sci 1016:325–347, 2004

Smith SD, Morris CA: Planning studies of etiology. Appl Psycholinguist 26:97–110, 2005

Stanton-Chapman T, Chapman D, Bainbridge N, et al: Identification of early risk factors for language impairment. Res Dev Disabil 23:390–405, 2002

Stromswold K: The genetics of speech and language impairments. N Engl J Med 359:2381–2383, 2008

Tager-Flusberg H, Cooper J: Present and future possibilities for defining a phenotype for specific language impairment. J Speech Lang Hear Res 42:1275–1278, 1999

Tager-Flusberg H, Rogers S, Cooper J, et al: Defining spoken language benchmarks and selecting measures of expressive language development for young children with autism spectrum disorders. J Speech Lang Hear Res 52:643–652, 2009

Tallal P, Ross R, Curtiss S: Familial aggregation in specific language impairment. J Speech Hear Disord 54:167–173, 1989

Tamis-LeMonda CS, Bornstein MH, Baumwell L: Maternal responsiveness and children's achievement of language milestones. Child Dev 72:748–767, 2001

Tomblin J, Smith E, Zhang X: Epidemiology of specific language impairment: prenatal and perinatal risk factors. J Commun Disord 30:325–344, 1997

Vargha-Khadem F, Gadian DG, Copp A, et al: FOXP2 and the neuroanatomy of speech and language. Nat Rev Neurosci 6:131–138, 2005

Vicari S, Caselli M, Tonucci F: Asynchrony of lexical and morphosyntactic development in children with Down syndrome. Neuropsychologia 38:634–644, 2000

Ward S: An investigation into the effectiveness of an early intervention method for delayed language development in young children. Int J Lang Comm Dis 34:243–264, 1999

Watt N, Wetherby A, Shumway S: Prelinguistic indicators of language outcome at three years of age. J Speech Lang Hear Res 49:1224–1237, 2006

Wetherby AM, Goldstein H, Cleary J, et al: Early identification of children with communication disorders: concurrent and predictive validity of the CSBS Developmental Profile. Infants Young Child 16:161–174, 2003

World Health Organization: International Statistical Classification of Diseases and Related Health Problems, 10th Revision. Geneva, World Health Organization, 2001

Yoder P, Warren S: Early predictors of language in children with and without Down syndrome. Am J Ment Retard 4:285–300, 2004

Zubrick S, Taylor C, Rice M, et al: Late language emergence at 24 months: an epidemiological study of prevalence, predictors, and covariates. J Speech Lang Hear Res 50:1562–1592, 2007

Index

Page numbers printed in **boldface** *type refer to tables or figures.*